THE JOURNEY HOME
Our Evolving Consciousness

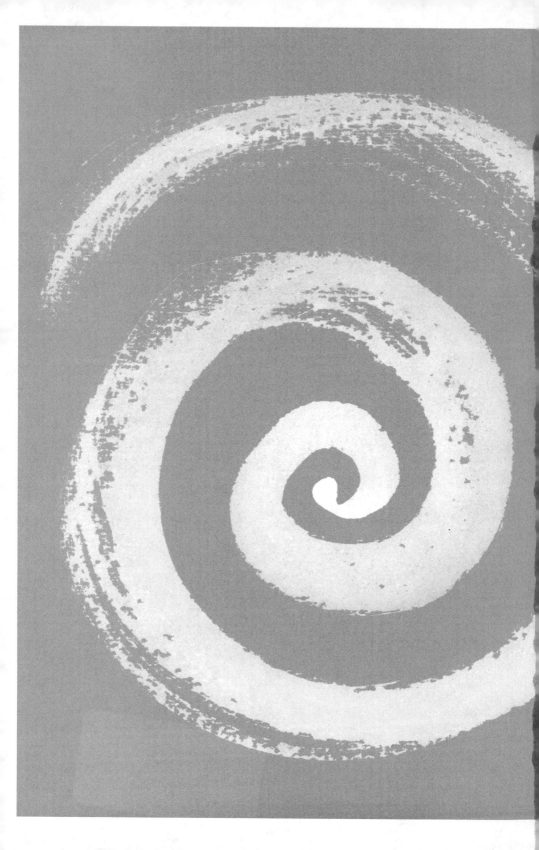

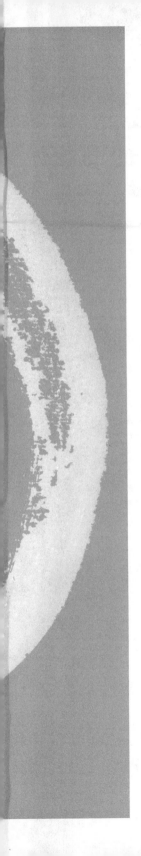

THE JOURNEY HOME
Our Evolving Consciousness

by Kathy Oddenino

JOY PUBLICATIONS

Requests for information or permission to make copies of any part of this work may be addressed to:
    Joy Publications
    133A Lee Drive, Annapolis, MD 21403-4043 USA

Printed in the United States of America
ISBN 0-923081-06-2

Current Printing 10 9 8 7 6 5 4 3 2 1

Cover painting by Branntler. Personal collection.

Edited by Margaret Martin
Text and cover design/production by Hannah Kleber

This book is dedicated to the millions of people who are searching for the wisdom to understand themselves.

The key to understanding ourself is to understand our dual soul and spirit as the integrated lifeforce energy of our physical body. We must have this wisdom before we can end the fear and confusion within our intellectual mind and live in the comfort and joy of who we are.

I have written this book for you as a beacon of light in the darkness to enhance your journey home as an evolving consciousness.

TABLE OF CONTENTS

INTRODUCTION

I have written this book as food for the soul of every person with an open mind who is willing and excited about thinking cyclically as an integrated trinity of minds, emotions, and feelings. As I complete this book, I am seeing the consciousness changes that are taking place within individuals and within our society as we continue the search for our internal self. Our search is changing our mental and emotional focus as we look internally to discover who we are instead of looking externally at others. Since I have always been interested in the journey home for our soul that we have lived as human beings, I can't help but remember that we have not always been so obsessively focused on the external reality of our lives.

I am a metaphysical philosopher who lives and breathes with an understanding of who we are, why we are here, and how everything in life relates to everything on earth and within the universe. A philosopher is literally a lover of wisdom. From a soul and spirit perspective, our purpose as humans is to seek the wisdom and love of our Divine Nature, which means that each of us is a natural philosopher. Metaphysics is the first division of philosophy because it was our first concept of philosophy as we devoted our search within the invisible world to help us remember the soul and spirit within ourselves. Our original search was to understand the invisible soul and spirit within us as the fractal pattern from which we created the design of our physical body. Internally we knew that we had created ourselves from an invisible trinity of consciousness energy. As we spent time on earth the consciousness of our soul and spirit began to fade, which inspired us to seek the knowledge to understand why.

For most of our historical past we have understood that we are more than our physical body. It wasn't until the seventeenth century that science and philosophy split and science began to focus more on "how" things work as a technology rather than "why" they work as a philosophy. The Industrial Revolution began the expansion of technology, and oddly enough, it followed a period in our history that was considered the "Age of Enlightenment." In our soul journey the Age of Enlightenment was the period when we seriously focused our mind on religion in a self-centered manner, and we forgot the foundation of ourselves as a dual soul and spirit.

My focus from birth has been to understand the consciousness of the dual soul and spirit. At the age of two I was in total communication with many of my parallel past soul lives that had lived with the identical focus that I now live in this lifetime. Being in touch with my dual soul lives and my universal mind gave me a head start because I could use the information that was learned in my past lives, my universal mind, and my present life to live the physical experiences and relate the information to my life and to other people with an active and passive consciousness.

Living with the focus of my mind working in a cyclic fashion, while I have been living in a physical world that thinks intellectually, has not always been comfortable for me. Now I am very comfortable with my trinity of consciousness because I have spent a lifetime being educated by my spirit consciousness to help me understand the precise relationship of our lives to who we are as human beings. During my childhood and until their deaths my mother and father were my ballast. Their role has now been taken over by my children and grandchildren. When a deep and unconditional love is present, it truly does not matter if the consciousness levels are identical, as long as the mind is open. This difference within families has more to do with the aware consciousness of everything in life having and being in relationship than it does with the developing soul's evolution, which will be revealed with age.

During my lifetime I have had multiple opportunities to make the choice to begin again. The difference between the societal consciousness and my consciousness level is extreme, and this difference has required a constant level of balance for me. I am aware of the importance of the collective consciousness becoming a consciousness of love and how very important love is to humanity and earth at this moment in time. The major denial of all of humanity to change is created by a fear of the unknown. It is my intention to help humanity to understand that the unknown is the emotion of love, and when we change our thinking, emotions, and feelings we will change the world and make it a better place for our families and ourselves.

Each of us is living and evolving with or without a consciousness of the journey home that our soul is living. As I have lived the physical experiences of being a student, a nurse, mother, teacher, and writer my canvas of life has expanded, and I have never been protected from life. That is not the role of our soul and spirit. The concept of "miracles" is part of our imagination. Life is our miracle. The concept of "mystery" only defines our ignorance. Life is designed by our soul and spirit as our moment-by-moment opportunity to expand our consciousness. Our soul and spirit is not above "shock therapy" to motivate us to change our thinking and emotions. The interpretation of our life experience always originates within our specific level of conscious awareness. When the multiple disciplines of science or technology function from an external level of consciousness that does not believe in the soul and spirit, the perception of life is distorted and limited by those individuals within the disciplines and those who accept the "facts" from these disciplines as truth. Our external viewpoint limits us to one-third of the "whole," and we physically create our world from that limited perception which is devoid of ethical values.

The purpose of our search is to understand ourselves as a trinity of consciousness that is living within a physical body. We are one being as a spirit consciousness, dual soul mind and emotions, and a living physical body. We have eternal life as a soul and spirit. We have a finite physical body that our soul and spirit re-creates from inherent memory.

Through the ages of our evolution we have separated ourself down to the finest of chemicals, which form our cells, without truly finding the relationship that we have as a soul and spirit to our physical matter. In this book we are going to look at each part of ourself, both visible and invisible, to understand the physical connection of our soul and spirit to our physical body and life experiences. If we can consciously understand that we have evolved as a consciousness while living our physical experiences of life, we can see the logic of changing our beliefs and behaviors. Understanding ourselves as an evolving consciousness allows us to accept change gracefully without judging or blaming ourselves for who we have been and what we have done.

My years of education, both formal and informal, have given me a wonderful exposure to life and the many disciplines of science. Because of the knowledge that I have I can clearly understand that we are at no time in the history of our consciousness evolution separate as matter, soul, and spirit. As my universal mind continues teaching me and I see the relationship of my formal knowledge to what I hear from my soul and spirit consciousness, I see the beauty and wisdom of who we are. Our invisible self is constantly interpenetrated into our visible self as our lifeforce energy that allows our physical matter to function in its "mysterious" or consciously unknown way. It is the miracle of our interpenetrated spirit that teaches us to consciously evolve as a soul in physical matter. As a trinity of consciousness, life is our miracle. Each of our physical lives is a cycle of expression for our living soul. Each life provides us with opportunities of growth and change as the evolution of our dual soul consciousness.

Our soul sees each life as we see each grain of sand on a beach. The only difference is the way our soul sees each life in all three dimensions. When we look at a grain of sand we see it only within the singular perception of our intellect. We fail to see the energy of the sand that is moving and changing right before our eyes. Each grain of sand is an atomic marvel of chemicals, movement, color, sound, tone, and vibration.

Can you imagine building a sand castle with one grain of sand? Our soul could not evolve if it had only one life to live. What would a beach look like with our limited perception if it had only one grain of sand? We would step on the grain of sand without recognizing it under our feet. One grain of sand would not feel like a beach to any of our senses or to our foot that would stand upon the sand.

Each life that we live is important but it is minuscule in relationship to the whole. Each life leaves a soul print within us in the same way that we leave our footprints in the sand of a beach. Our soul is our dual mind and emotions. The soul prints that are left within us are the levels of consciousness that our soul mind and emotions lived during a physical lifetime. Only our growth of mental and emotional consciousness is taken with our soul and spirit into a new lifetime.

When we use our consciousness as an integrated trinity of consciousness, we use it as a cyclic mind and loving emotions. All that we have ever learned is stored within our consciousness memory. My knowledge of metaphysical philosophy comes from my past lives when I lived as a philosopher. The equality, truth, harmony, love, and beauty of who we are and how we were created is as fresh in my mind today as it was then. The only difference is that during multiple lives I have expanded the knowledge and understand it even better than I did when I was first teaching it.

The identity of past lives is not important. The knowledge that we gain from our past lives must also evolve with other lives. Therefore, it is important to access the stored memory of our mind and emotions as a total consciousness not as a singular past life memory. In addition, we must continue to evolve in this lifetime so our information fits the times of society. Religion is a good example of how we obsessively attach ourselves to ancient information that no longer fits the times. The parable of Moses wandering in the wilderness with the children of Israel after their captivity is the story of the human species wandering in the wilderness of our transitional consciousness after coming out of the total captivity of our immature soul mind. When we lived totally in our immature soul we were children of our consciousness. Before we can reach the promised land of our mature loving soul as a transitional consciousness, we have wandered through the maze of our old primitive beliefs and behaviors, revisiting them before we can release them.

Moses lived about 1650 B.C. He was given this prophecy as a way of helping humanity that had already been in the wilderness of their ignorant minds for thousands of years, but it was interpreted as a physical reality from the fear within our mind. The parable that refers to the Israelites as "the chosen ones" does not mean what it has been interpreted to mean. The Israelites were being told that it would be they who wandered in the wilderness of ignorance for the longest period if they continued with their fighting. Nearly four thousand years later the information found in biblical literature continues to be the foundation of our various cultures. The interpretation of biblical information came from the minds and emotions of the people of the time, which was based upon superstition, symbols, and rituals of even earlier times. Religion is an external creation of ancient man and it has never discovered the soul and spirit information that is concealed in the words of Moses. Moses was a philosopher. Other great philosophers were Pythagoras, Hippocrates, Galen, Socrates, Aristotle, Plato, Jesus, Galileo, and Einstein. This list is incomplete, but it is important that we understand these people who integrated science and philosophy.

A philosopher seeks the wisdom to understand creation as one unit of consciousness that works together in harmony such as man, nature, earth, and the universe. The metaphysical philosopher seeks the wisdom of the "one" creation of the invisible soul and spirit integrated into the visible matter of our body, nature, earth, and the universe. When we study the different scientific disciplines with the perception of "one universal creation" versus "one physical life" our conclusions are different. We can see the duality of the opposites, the fractal pattern of life, evolution, harmony, beauty, truth, equality, and we can see the love, balance, and integrity with which we were created.

Although our aware consciousness is focused only upon the present life, our mature soul is in touch with the entire spectrum of our lives. When our dual soul consciousness begins to change its focus, medicine thinks we are mentally ill as we access other memory nodes that are soul memory nodes or prints within our subconscious soul mind. Therein we see the reflection of our limited intellectual consciousness with its singular and linear focus of judging our human experiences as right or wrong from our external perception. Our soul memory nodes are infinite and it is only our limited intellect and ego that keeps us from realizing our full potential of consciousness. Our intellect is limited by our ego beliefs, such as "We only live one life." Our ego beliefs act like a buried electronic fence to keep our intellect contained within certain boundaries of thought and emotions.

As our intellect has evolved, we have begun to unravel some of the mysteries of our invisible matter but we have failed thus far to connect this knowledge to our eternal soul and spirit consciousness. Perhaps this is because we have given the power of our soul and spirit over to religion and we no longer feel capable of being personally responsible for the health and wealth of our soul and spirit. We have also given the power of our mind and body over to medical science and we feel helpless to be who we want to be as healthy, clear-minded human beings. We are not willing to use the entire spectrum of our consciousness as male, female, and spirit because it is not understood. Our linear perception of the external world has distracted us from the beauty, equality, truth, and love of our internal world.

Each part of the trinity of consciousness that lives within us as our male, female, and spirit exists in *enfinite* levels of consciousness. The enfinite levels of consciousness within our trinity of consciousness are the many mansions of our mind that we can use to focus on the stored knowledge that we have accumulated. The many mansions of our mind function as libraries or computer chips that contain universal and soul memory nodes as the memory of each and every past life. In lives when our intellect has lived without awareness our subconscious intellect stored the fear from our sensory response to life around our intellect and captured it in the cosmic shell of our ego.

As we become aware of ourselves, other people, nature, earth, and the universe, we expand our conscious awareness of the relationship that exists between all of us as living beings that are evolving. We release our subconscious fears and begin to love our life and ourselves as we expand our consciousness of our internal wisdom, truth, love, and equality.

In traditional medicine, technology now allows physicians to "photograph" radiologically the body and the brain into extremely thin slices to detect disease as well as the function of the human body. Our consciousness also exists in extremely thin levels of electromagnetic energy that are just beginning to be detected but are not yet understood by science. Science can now find people who use their left brain and others who use both the left and right brain to a degree. For many years we have been living the transition from our left brain to our right brain, and as the technology of science expands, our understanding will expand and we will soon be able to validate the transition that we are experiencing. We could be understood now if the perception of the scientific mind understood the invisible soul and spirit consciousness.

The lack of scientific understanding does not mean that our dual soul as a male and female consciousness and our spirit consciousness do not exist. It simply means that we have not yet accepted that they exist because we have no physical "proof." Proof can never be found if the metaphysical philosophy that stimulates our mind to seek the knowledge of the relationship does not exist.

The best way to define the multiple levels of consciousness is to explore the different relationships and behaviors that we live from generation to generation within families and within cultures. As knowledge affects each individual and erases ignorance, we will find the consciousness that we live becoming more equally balanced, truthful, and loving. Our lives will find harmony and our hearts will find happiness. As humans we have been consistently living with the absolute intention and will of expanding our evolving consciousness since the beginning of our creation.

As we begin to look at ourself we begin to take ourself out of the dark little boxes of identities and roles that we have created with our beliefs and we let the spirit light of love into our one integrated conscious mind. Our search for self-understanding and knowledge is the most important search ever for our dual soul and spirit consciousness. Without the intention of searching to understand ourself and our relationship to all of earth, we tend to wallow in self-pity without an awareness of our actions. Wallowing in our victimization and poverty consciousness is a method the immature soul uses to expand our awareness of consciousness. After so many, many lives of wallowing in the ignorance of judgement, blame, and self-pity, we begin to see that we are creating exactly what we must live to learn our lessons of independence, freedom, equality, truth, and love.

Fortunately our family, religious, and scientific teachings have supported us in our cause and effect of blame and judgement from the beginning of those specific focuses in our soul descent. We have always done the best that we could as human beings with the information that we were aware of as our current "truth," so there is no one to blame and judge. There are many lessons to be learned by the way that we have lived and wasting time on placing judgement and blame only holds us in our pain and suffering and limits our ability to continue evolving as a soul. We have been stuck in our revolutions of beliefs for thousands of years.

The most challenging change that we face at this time in our soul evolution is releasing the "religious beliefs" that we consider to be "fact." Our religious beliefs are dependent, unequal, deceitful, fearful, and they have removed our soul from an understanding of the personal responsibility for its own journey. The worship of religion or anything physical, such as a person, relationship, or money, is our core behavior of inequality that is learned as part of our physical nature.

When we are challenged to change our beliefs, we trigger the fear of our ego and we feel threatened by all of the beliefs that have created the foundation of our physical nature. We see taking away the foundation of worship and dependency that we have come to rely upon as a fate worse than death. In reality if we don't change while we are alive, our soul will choose death as a method of changing our perception. In the days of the Old Testament we lived six hundred to one thousand years in each lifetime. In our recent past, as we have lived at the very depths of our immature descending soul, our life expectancy has been as low as twenty-eight years. Our soul chooses death more frequently to escape the negativity of our perception of life than for any other reason. At this time in our life we are once again expanding our time on earth and we will continue with that expansion as we evolve into our mature soul thinking and emotions.

As we explore the trinity of consciousness in the pages of this book, it is important to read with the open mind of a philosopher seeking wisdom. When our beliefs are closed and intense, we can become angry and fearful when knowledge goes beyond them. Yet it is important to challenge our ego with new knowledge since it is our ego beliefs that are holding us captive and keeping us from seeking the knowledge that we must have to free the consciousness of our immature soul mind and emotions.

For many of my readers who are lovers of wisdom, the knowledge in this book will give you the sense on a cellular level that you are coming home. You will feel the truth of each word. When we begin to break free of our captive beliefs we feel the truth of ancient wisdom within our heart and in every cell within our body. The singular and linear focus of our intellect on our ancient superstitious beliefs and rituals must come to an end if we want to continue with our evolution as a mature soul.

Without change being accepted within our mind and emotions, we will begin to devolve into our primitive memory and killing will become rampant along with the inequality, abuse, fear, and deceit within our relationships. The behavior that we experience as inequality, fear, and deceit will continue to be the "usual" in our society and life will not be pleasant if we allow our present behavior to devolve. Today we are seeing examples of devolution as our societal behavior becomes more primitive and our worship of inequality and judgement becomes more intense.

If we were all evolving, we would not be experiencing the behavior that we are now living. If our life were perfect and change was unnecessary, we would already be living in a "heaven on earth." No one has to be a genius to recognize that we are living our "hell on earth" and that we have not yet become civilized as human beings. Civilized people do not believe that men and women are unequal, and they do not judge, abuse, cheat, and kill other people.

Once metaphysical philosophy is understood there will be multiple opportunities to do wonderful research that will support us in our soul growth. At the present time trillions of scientific dollars are being spent uselessly because they are focused on the external perception of cause and effect. The space program is a wonderful example of our external physical focus. In our uncivilized state we would probably focus on fighting and attempting to conquer anyone that we discovered in space, and then we could create the reality of star wars as our everyday life.

With new beliefs and a new attitude, we can learn to understand ourselves. Our immature consciousness moves in constantly tighter circles of revolving energy and we have become captured in the terminal revolutions of primitive beliefs and behaviors that can destroy us. Our transitional mind is like "the eye of the needle" as we focus on old, unnecessary judgement and blame, unwilling to praise and respect the good that is inherent in each of us. Unless we change we can and will destroy ourselves not only physically, but we will allow our soul to devolve and we will live our fear all over again.

As you read *The Journey Home: Our Evolving Consciousness* keep your mind open to the relationship of what you are reading to your own knowledge and consciousness about your life. Being open-minded will allow this book to stimulate your feelings and your soul memory, which will help you evolve into another level of consciousness without pain and suffering as you begin to consciously live the beautiful pattern of your own soul as it is being created.

Note: Metaphysical definitions and spelling of words are frequently different from the habitual definition and spelling we may find in our modern usage and dictionaries. These words in this text are defined in the glossary at the end of the book.

OUR TRINITY OF CONSCIOUSNESS

We are a trinity of consciousness. The foundation of our trinity of consciousness is a chemical consciousness. We are chemicals that came together to form a physical body, a dual soul, and a spirit consciousness aeons ago. We began as spirit consciousness. Our spirit consciousness is the chemical seeds of a universal Spirit Consciousness. Our spirit consciousness created our dual soul consciousness of male and female. Our spirit consciousness and our dual soul consciousness created our physical body as a fractal pattern of the universal design. Our physical body is finite. Our trinity of consciousness is *enfinite* as a spirit consciousness. Our dual soul is infinite as a male and female consciousness, and as the "Lord" it has dominion over our physical reality. After aeons of expanding our male and female consciousness, we will once again integrate into a spirit consciousness. We will continue to live eternally as a spirit consciousness. Our physical body is a reflection of our trinity of consciousness. The matter of our body is and always will be finite, serving the "Lord" of our male and female consciousness as a tool known as the miracle of life.

In our evolution and revolution of consciousness through our multiple physical lives, our dual soul of male and female consciousness is transitioning into one integrated soul consciousness. We have been in the throes of our soul transition for

1

aeons of time as evolution and for fourteen thousand years as an event of transitional revolution. We are at all times integrated as a trinity of dual soul and spirit consciousness living within a physical body. Our dual soul has an inherent form, structure, organization, discipline, and freedom of choice, will, and intention. As we have lived in our male physical nature, we have been the child of our soul. We have been learning to be aware of our consciousness as we live our art of creation as our physical experience. Our consciousness exists in a trinity of consciousness as male, female, and spirit. In our male consciousness we have lived more through an automatic belief reaction than we have through our sensory stimulation. In our female consciousness we will respect our sensory response and expand our consciousness.

Our beliefs are the conclusions that our intellect has reached in its journey of evolution. Because we found ourselves without memory, we looked externally at everything that existed around us and tried to reach a conclusion that would explain us and our presence on earth. As we explored our surroundings, we created observations as symbols that became our superstitions and beliefs that we created various rituals to support. Some experiences were not pleasant and we developed fear and superstitious rituals in our attempt to prevent a reoccurrence of the event. Other experiences were pleasant and we created superstitious rituals to protect the repetition of the event. As our beliefs, superstitions, symbols, and rituals expanded, we suppressed our inherent emotions and feelings through our fear and self-judgement.

The developing consciousness of our physical nature has focused upon learning by creating every thought, word, emotion, and feeling as our external physical reality and relating each creation to our superstitious fear beliefs. As we have lived the physical experience of our physical art of creation, we have been creating an awareness of ourself, nature, earth, and the universe. By exploring the external world around us, we are becoming conscious of how nature, earth, and the universe are supporting us in our evolution and we continue to try and discover the source of our physical body and mind.

To grasp the reality of who we are as a consciousness so that we can begin to understand ourselves is the most flamboyant opportunity that we have faced as an immature, childish soul. Learning about the physical power that we can use to create our reality is insignificant next to the mind power that we can use to create our reality. As a trinity of consciousness we are living our dual soul evolution, and at this time we can observe our own change within our society as we move from our physical creation to our emotional creation. The transitional level of our revolution is changing our emotional consciousness. The primary lesson for our dual soul as it lives our normal transitional emotions of depression is to expand our consciousness and change our emotional perception from fear to love.

As a trinity of consciousness we live with enfinite levels of consciousness in each of the trilocular dimensions of our brain. The three brains are our three minds and emotions, and they are locked together with a network of neurons. It is the neurons that provide our sensory feelings which stimulate our emotions. The *callosum commissura* acts as a bridge to connect our dual soul mind and emotions. Our dual soul is seated in the left and right hemispheres of our brain as our male and female consciousness. Our spirit consciousness is our ancient or posterior brain as our universal mind.

Our dual soul is dual in every aspect. It is dual as left and right, male and female, negative and positive, external and internal, fearful and loving, mind and emotions, dark and light, action and reaction, creation and motivation, physical and divine, unhappy and happy, descending and ascending, matter and energy, thought and words, equal and opposite, electricity and magnetism, inhibition and excitation, and this duality is also the design that created us as twin souls.

Our twin soul design of opposites is how we became physical males and females as we began our dual soul evolution. The same design tells us why both the male and female were placed within the physical nature to live our evolution equally. Learning to create equality has been the major lesson for our physical nature as males and females while we have lived our art of creation. Religion was created as the symbol of our revolutionary path to remind us of our lesson of equality as males and females. Because we are dual as a soul, we create what we don't want in our physical nature to become conscious of what we do want in our Divine Nature.

Our left brain symbolizes our male physical nature and it has been the immature intellectual and ego brain that we use as a gatherer of information. Both the male and female physical being have been focused on learning through the male physical nature of the left brain. Our left brain has perceived life as negative, fearful, and external to our physical body. Throughout the path of our physical nature we have not related our external world to ourself, but we have believed ourselves to be victims of the external forces of life, nature, earth, and the universe.

Our immature left brain intellect and ego is our descending and ascending soul. We have moved two steps forward and one step backward both mentally and emotionally because of the resistance and denial of change that we experience at different levels of our evolution. At this point in our immature soul evolution, we are living the duality of our descending and ascending soul. As we have gathered information and ascended our mind, we have suppressed our emotions, allowing them to accumulate as they descend.

As we have become unequal in our emotional growth, we have accumulated our fears and now we are living our emotional descent. The diversity that we feel from the ascending accumulation of knowledge in our mind and the descending accumulation of fear emotions allows us to feel emotional depression as we face the change in our soul focus. Depression is good because the desperation of the inequality of our mind and emotions acts as a sensory stimulus to our feelings, which triggers our emotions and expands our sensory consciousness. Because we are comfortable suppressing our emotions, we become uncomfortable when we begin to feel our emotions. If we have a belief that depression is a form of mental illness, we will get stuck in our beliefs and fear, instead of laughing at our emotional stimulation and enjoying the change. We must balance our mind and emotions if we want to continue our evolution as a soul.

The pattern of our evolution is inherent within our consciousness. Because we have not learned how our consciousness functions in the trinity of our minds and emotions, we have lived the design of our aware consciousness without a consciousness of the interaction of our minds, emotions, and feelings. Our dual mind and emotions represent our dual soul as opposites as a male and female consciousness. Males and females are opposite because the male focuses upon the mind and the sexual core of his physical nature, and the female focuses upon the emotions and love as the core of her Divine Nature.

The opposite focuses for the male and female while living in the same physical nature created the magnetism that is essential to our survival. The magnetic arc or "rib" of opposites that has separated the male and female has assured constant evolution for the human species. The opposite of the male and female also gave us the perfect pattern for procreation to continue with our eternal soul. The opposite focus of the male and female also provided the magnetic attraction and procreation as a sexual magnet that would provide pleasure as the total sensory stimulation of all three dimensions of our senses to expand our consciousness. Our soul design is pure genius and unconditional love because it has kept us evolving and expanding our consciousness without our being aware of what we were creating or why we were creating new life. The female persona has always been the sensory stimulus for the male persona.

Our spirit consciousness is a trinity of consciousness within itself as a universal mind, unconditional loving emotions, and sensory feelings. Our spirit consciousness is the inspiration for our intellectual mind, the motivation for our emotions, and the sensory stimulus for our feelings. Our male and female soul consciousness has only the dual mind and emotions as the physical living soul of the spirit that is guiding it. Our soul is dual and our spirit is a trinity. As a dual soul and spirit, we become a trinity of consciousness in our physical nature and our physical body by sensing.

The pattern of our physical body, dual soul, and spirit consciousness is the DNA. As the DNA, our soul and spirit is embedded in every cell of our physical body. The dual soul is our dual electromagnetic energy. The electricity symbolizes our male mind and the magnetism symbolizes our female emotions. When our mind and emotions are living in inequality as an electrical and magnetic force, we will be living in depression. We will unconsciously create an imbalance within our brain's electromagnetic energy by creating an imbalance of chemicals within our body. Our mind and emotional imbalance will be supported by our physical behavior. When we interfere with our biological need for fresh foods of nature, pure water, and pure air to restore the chemicals within our brain, we create a chemical imbalance. The reflective energy of the soul allows us to create the supporting physical behaviors in our lives to capture our attention and expand our awareness of the internal inequality and imbalance.

We have been living in the immature childish soul of our physical nature and we have been collecting information to understand the relationship between ourselves, earth, nature, and the universe. As we have been living our finite journey of one physical life after the other, we have been collecting information and learning lessons as the art of creation. As we have learned, we have stored the wisdom in the memory nodes of our mature soul of love. Those lessons that we continue to work with as our superstitious beliefs and fears, we have stored in the subconscious intellect, which we call our ego. Our ego acts as a cosmic shell that surrounds our intellect and limits it to linear thinking. Only our intellect has a focus on a linear consciousness. As we transition we remove our cosmic shell of beliefs that has limited our intellect by distorting our spirit inspiration, and we open our mind to the integration of our immature soul with our mature soul. This allows the trinity of our minds and emotions to function as a cyclic whole mind, giving us access to our spirit inspiration in the intellect, our mature soul motivation from the wisdom of its memory nodes, and our universal mind of enfinite knowledge and unconditional love. Our intellect remains as the creative mind that continues to seek new knowledge, but as a whole mind we think in a complete cycle and we become enlightened by our spirit consciousness. True enlightenment is still aeons away but the consciousness of equality, truth, and love as we integrate our dual soul will provide us with a new level of spirit consciousness that will bring light and openness to our intellect and balance our soul with loving emotions.

To think in terms of completing the transition from our level of revolution into living the consciousness of our mature soul is our next step in evolution. When we seek the knowledge to live the miracle of our life, we will create such a loving, beautiful place on earth that we will astound ourselves. Hell is the symbol of learning the art of creation from the immature soul of emotional fear, addictive beliefs, superstitions, and our ritualistic approaches to life. Heaven is the symbol of learning the power of creation from our mature soul of loving emotions and wisdom. Our dual soul of male and female consciousness is preparing for the eternal embrace of being equal as like mind and emotions of love, while continuing in the opposites of physical gender. The beauty, love, and comfort zone that we have always searched for in relationships will be the normal relationship of our mature soul.

Our spirit is a higher vibration of electromagnetic energy and sensory feelings as a higher level of consciousness. Our spirit consciousness is our universal mind. Our universal mind contains all memory of our creation and our journey of evolution that is stored in memory nodes or neurons within the posterior brain of the cerebellum. This part of our brain is frequently referred to as our mammalian or ancient brain. This is a beautiful description, as it is the eternal lifeforce within us. Our ancient brain is the true spirit consciousness within us that is the eternal memory bank of our creation, eternal dual soul design, and our infinite journey as a living soul in physical nature. Because we are spirit consciousness at the core of our trinity of consciousness, we stay out of physical matter for a maximum of three physical days. When our body dies, our soul and spirit that has been living as chemical gas, liquid, and solid matter within our body returns to the state of chemical gas and leaves our body. In the ethereal state of gas the electromagnetic energy of the soul and spirit travels with the speed of light at 186,000 miles per second. The vibration of the dual soul and spirit in ethereal form is extremely fast. In three physical days the soul and spirit lives aeons of time as we understand physical time.

Our soul and spirit contain total memory of our unique DNA as the pattern of our physical body, dual soul, and spirit consciousness. The soul and spirit will return to a new physical life with the precise pattern of lessons that are embedded in the DNA. The dual soul is learning, as a child of our spirit, to expand its consciousness. When we began our path of expansion as a male physical nature with an immature soul of intellect, ego, and physical body, we began our journey home to our mature soul and spirit as an evolving consciousness. As we reached the transitional level of our soul and began to tighten the revolutions of our fear beliefs as our remaining lessons, we were following the stasis pattern that is designed into our eternal soul. In our physical nature, we were learning from the negative, external, fearful side of our mind and emotions, but our indwelling spirit has always been guiding us. We began our immature soul focus by ascending our intellect. As our knowledge expanded, we began to descend our emotions. As our mind and emotions were opposites, our fear emotions began to stimulate our feelings and expand our consciousness. The more we expand our consciousness the easier and happier our life becomes as a living soul in a physical body.

Our journey shows us the fractal pattern of our three-dimensional energy as our trinity of consciousness and the smaller fractal pattern of thoughts, emotions, and feelings of our immature soul. When we began our journey as a living soul we began without intellectual memory or emotions, but we did have our spiritual senses in all three dimensions of our energy. All that we have learned began initially as the sensory response to our physical senses. We expanded our intellectual mind and our emotions one step at a time. We reached a point when we began to form beliefs that we brought back into each new physical life as our cosmic shell of subconscious or karmic beliefs. Our beliefs began to limit our thinking and suppressed our loving emotions as we became addicted to our fear emotions. During our journey of suppressing our emotions, we also learned to suppress our senses as our feelings. The suppression of our emotions and feelings began the suppression of our female Divine Nature and the physical female in our society. With female suppression we entered the major lesson for our immature soul as the lesson of inequality.

As we created the fractal pattern of inequality from our male to our female soul and from our physical male to our physical female, we also created the ascension of our intellectual mind and the descent of our fear emotions. This has allowed us to live all three dimensions of the fractal pattern of our mind and emotions at one time as we learn the lesson of inequality as a male and female soul, a male mind and female emotions, and a physical male and a physical female.

Our fractal pattern is always repeated within every aspect of our physical lives, our physical body, our dual soul, and our spirit. The clever design of our soul, which changes its physical sexual gender with its twin soul in an equal number of lifetimes, makes certain that we reap what we sow. If we are male and abuse the female, we will be abused when we are female. Many times the lesson of the soul will be lived with the identical soul family members. Our soul families are our safety net of unconditional love and they are always willing to help us live a lesson.

Our dual soul and our spirit are functioning within us to expand our consciousness as we live each level of our soul growth by learning to create our lessons as physical experiences. Our seven senses exist in three dimensions of energy. We have our physical senses, our mature soul senses, and our spiritual senses. As we use our senses in their different levels, we experience a conscious sensory response that expands our consciousness of the physical experience to expand our perception of life, ourself, and our spirit consciousness.

As we expand our consciousness, we are now becoming consciously aware of all three levels of our senses. We not only hear physical voices but we also hear our mature soul voice and our spirit voice speaking to us. We can hear, see, smell, taste, touch, think, and speak in all three dimensions of our senses. As we use our mature soul and spirit senses the sensory stimulation is far superior to what we feel with our physical senses and each of our senses will be using various components. As an example, we may physically see a light bulb and have simply a casual awareness that the light is on. Our soul senses pick up the electricity, magnetism, vibrations, tones, the interchanging colors, the smell, the temperature, the weight or density, and these sensory interactions will change our thinking as they speak to us in different languages, such as mathematics, physics, or some universal law that our soul wants us to understand. Our mature soul senses are much more expansive than the immature soul senses. As we spiral into the spiritual dimensions of our senses we use all seven of our senses at a still more expansive dimension, which again contains an enfinite number of levels of sensory stimulation.

The awareness of our consciousness is much, much more expansive today than it was when we began our immature soul journey. Our consciousness is moving more quickly now as we work intensely with our emotions. As we have focused upon expanding our intellect, we have suppressed our emotions and our feelings because we have stayed in ignorance of the sensory stimulation of our physical experiences.

All of our consciousness expansion follows the same spiral path of growth that our soul, our body, and our nerve cells follow in our brain. This same fractal pattern can be found throughout nature and it is showing us the pattern from which we too were designed. Once we understand ourselves, we will understand the universe.

All patterns within the universe come from the universal pattern of life. The patterns differ in size and therefore in complexity but the basic pattern is the same. Chaos is a prototype of the pattern that is always changing and finding its balance. As humans we have lived in chaos as we have learned inequality. With the balance of equality we will no longer experience chaos. All systems live in chaos as a primitive but constantly changing pattern. The universal laws apply to all systems of life. Chaos is the law of action and reaction which occurs without consciousness. Once we learn to use our trinity of consciousness, we live through our conscious sensory response. As we become mentally and emotionally balanced, chaos is no longer part of our personality.

Our dual soul and spirit have the internal power to make the transition from our descending emotional soul to our ascending intellectual soul and balance it with our ascending mature soul. If we are willing to look carefully at the truth of our beliefs and whether or not they are continuing to serve us today, we will see the logic of change. We have created our addictive beliefs and our obsessive habitual behaviors throughout our descending emotional soul because we are afraid to change.

If we can understand our trinity of consciousness as three minds and emotions which we are evolving within, we can understand that we have evolved through one third of the whole of our consciousness when we transition into our ascending female Divine Nature by balancing our mind and emotions. To deny changing the way that we think, our emotions, and our feelings is to deny our mature soul and spirit consciousness. If we had created a Utopia in our physical nature our reluctance to change perfection could be understood. Fortunately our soul is much too clever to have created perfection in our physical nature. As a soul we would have created a true resistance and denial of change if we had learned to create perfection as our art of creation. Our reluctance to change from our physical nature comes from our fear of change. Our fear of change shows us the power of our ascending intellectual soul to become addicted to ancient beliefs and behaviors through the fear of our suppressed emotions. When we deny all change of thinking and emotions, we show no respect, honor, or value for our dual soul and spirit consciousness. Denial and resistance are both symbols of the suppression of the sensory response of our spirit consciousness.

We are a dual consciousness as a soul. The electromagnetic energy of our dual soul of male and female consciousness is seated and functions within the dual mind and emotions of the left and right lobes of our brain. The consciousness of our dual mind and emotions gives us the picture of opposites that we have been living. We have been learning to grow within our negative per-

ception before we can evolve into our positive perception. This
was a clever design for our dual soul consciousness because it
had to allow us to see what we don't want so that we would
learn to appreciate what we do want. If our spirit consciousness
had given the physical nature of our dual soul the absolute
power of creation at the beginning of our journey, we would
have totally destroyed ourselves by the misuse of our power.

When we were created as a male and female consciousness,
we were given power over our own evolution on earth. Our
power is our personal responsibility of creation. When we began
as a living soul we began with our focus of consciousness in our
male physical nature. Both the male and female were focused
within our physical nature, with the male having the precise
focus of the mind and the female of the emotions. This design
gave us the eternal image of the dance of life that we must consistently live in our physical experiences as a way of balancing
the double helix of the mind and emotions of our physical
nature. Creating the balance of life within our dual soul is our
personal responsibility and no one else can do it for us. Our ego
has created multiple illusions of others saving us, such as Jesus,
gurus, medicine, relationships, and money. As a trinity of consciousness we are totally responsible for seeking the knowledge
to save ourselves. Evil is the symbol of ignorance. Evil is implied
in the use of other words, such as the devil, sin, darkness, pain
and suffering, mystery, and various other names. All of these
words are images of different levels of ignorance. Ignorance is
the opposite of knowledge. "Evil spirits" is an oxymoron. No one
can be ignorant and living a spiritual life at the same time.

Our male and female consciousness formed a trinity of consciousness as it became the living soul of our spirit consciousness, which is the core or seed of us. We are a child of the eternal Spirit Consciousness and we are a living soul that was created as a child of our spirit consciousness. As a living soul consciousness we are both male and female in our physical body.
We have both a physical nature and a Divine Nature as a male
and female soul, and as physical beings we have both a male and
a female nature as our mind and emotions.

The perception that we have lived of the male and female being dramatically different, separate, and unequal is secondary to our addictive religious beliefs that are the foundation of our revolutionary consciousness. Our religious beliefs are the prima- ✳ ry source of the collective consciousness that is now creating a dramatic stasis that could act as the strongest force of motion to create devolution within the human species. The fear of change is obsessive in the immature souls that are addicted to the superstition and ritual of religious beliefs. Religion means a cult worship. Worship means inequality. Inequality is the lesson that our immature soul must learn before the transition into our mature ✳ soul can take place. The inequality between the male and female is the core of religious belief.

The physical gender that we choose in any one life is judged by our religious beliefs about the identities and roles of the male and female. Advanced souls will not be comfortable with the religious roles and identities that are chosen for them to live. The expected inequality of the male and female is the primary issue in all relationships. The focus of our consciousness is now changing and interpenetrating itself as both a male and female consciousness, which is creating confusion in terms of our physical gender. The interpenetration of our male and female consciousness is essential to our growth to show us that we are both male and female. Our religious beliefs that assign identities and roles to the male and female in our physical lives are being challenged by our mature soul to show us the independence that is within us as a trinity of soul and spirit consciousness.

To relate the words of religion to the spiritual understanding of ourselves as a trinity of consciousness, we would see ourselves as "a child of God," with our connection to God being an internal chemical connection and an internal chemical cellular/DNA connection, rather than an external connection. Our spirit consciousness is our lifeforce, internal inspiration, and our sensory response that is at all times guiding our expansion of consciousness as a living soul in physical matter. Our living soul, as a male and female consciousness within one physical body, is our mind and emotional consciousness, the chemical pattern of our life as the DNA and RNA, that is designed to embed our male and female consciousness into physical matter. We use our body as a tool for living in our physical nature as a true physical experience of our art of creation for our dual soul and spirit consciousness.

The living soul of our physical nature as both males and females has always been motivated by the memory nodes of knowing that are stored within our mature soul Divine Nature and inspired by the universal memory of our spirit consciousness. Our soul and spirit memory continues to be a significant pattern in our physical relationship experience as the male frequently looks to the female as his loving anchor and motivation for living his physical life.

The female, as the symbol of our Divine Nature, is the creator of new life. The art of creating new life is at all times sending a message to society that defines our power of creation. For many years during the journey of our immature soul the semen of man was considered to be the microscopic version of the human body. Woman was considered to act only as the incubator to help the "seed of man" that was "made in the image of God" grow into human form. This belief came to be because man saw himself as "made in the image of God," as the "Creator," and "woman" as being on earth only to serve man. It is our focus on this unequal Antichrist belief that is the focus of religion in our human experience.

We are each male and female because we were created equally by our spirit consciousness. Before any individual can truly transition from the immature soul to the mature soul he/she must learn and live the lesson of equality at the physical and immature soul level of consciousness. Learning a lesson does not mean that we store it in our intellectual memory and from then on we can discuss the theory intellectually. Learning a soul lesson requires that we live the soul lesson as the love of our immature soul within every aspect of our physical experience. When we learn the lesson of equality of the male and female, we will also learn the lessons of truth and love. These three consciousnesses are the mental, emotional, and behavioral lessons of our immature soul consciousness. We must consistently live our

14

equality, truth, and love to become spiritual beings. Living our equality, truth, and love allows us to be spiritual. If we are religious we are not living our equality, and therefore we are not living our truth or the love that we feel for ourselves. Religion was created from the ignorance of ourselves. Spirituality can only be created by living the knowledge of equality, truth, and love. The consciousness of our physical nature experiences life from our descending emotions of fear. We can only live our spirituality when our intellect and emotions are balanced and equal as the love and truth of our male and female consciousness. As our mind and emotions again move in the ascending dance of life, our integrated male and female soul will continue the journey home.

As a trinity of mind and emotional consciousness, we have an enfinite number of levels of consciousness within each mind and emotion. Our path of growth through these multiple levels of consciousness is designed as the art of creating and living the physical experience that would capture our awareness and thus create a forward evolution into a new level of consciousness. Our immature soul journey has been focused on becoming aware through the stimulation of the three dimensions of our seven senses, which expands our level of consciousness. At this time in our evolution of consciousness, we are more advanced than we have ever been since the beginning of our creation as a dual soul and spirit consciousness that has the intention of change as ascension.

Our religious belief that we have "only one life" has been a form of denial for our immature soul that has limited our consciousness of understanding ourselves. When we look at the role that religion has played in attaching us to denial beliefs, we can see how desperate we are as a soul to get through our revolutionary cycles. There are many mansions of our mind still to be visited in our journey and our consciousness is becoming paralyzed with its stasis beliefs and behaviors. The religious beliefs that our fathers have passed down to the generations of the sons are the karmic beliefs that act as our subconscious ego cosmic shell. As we have lived our journey over aeons of lifetimes, we have accumulated multiple karmic beliefs. Our soul journey has not been wrong or sinful and God is not judging us, angry with us, or punishing us. Our soul journey was designed as a pattern for our soul to live as a way of expanding our aware consciousness of what it means to have a closed mind. Our journey was not predetermined or predestined. The details were left up to us as our creation of personal responsibility. We are our own ancestors. We will continue with our immature soul life until we begin to understand ourselves.

Biblical prophecy explains our pattern of revolution to us by "the sins of the fathers will be passed down through the generations of the sons." As a soul it takes us many generations of lifetimes to see that our beliefs and behaviors must be changed. When we change we do so by taking one step at a time. There is no destination, no line to cross, there is only the opening of the mind very gently to let in the light and reveal to our mind and emotions a new way of living through an expanded thinking, loving emotions, and feelings. When our change occurs it must occur in our living for us to become spiritual. When each individual lives the equality, truth, and love of the mature soul, our society will at last become civilized.

As long as we are dependent upon someone else saving us, we will never learn to accept personal responsibility for the wisdom and beauty of our spirit consciousness that saves us from within. Being dependent takes away our power and freedom. We have acted out the immature soul lesson of dependency and control by living for multiple physical lifetimes with the female being dependent upon and unequal to the male. Dependency and control are the behavior of inequality that is supported by our religious beliefs. Our focus on making the Divine Nature dependent upon and controlled by our physical nature was important to help us learn the lesson of inequality. Our soul journey is bringing us further along within our eternal life cycle and we are discovering the excitement of change.

As we are transitioning into our ascending emotional soul we are rebelling against inequality and we are seeking equality, love, and truth in which to continue our soul journey. Equality gives us the power to know who we are. As we ascend emotionally, we are learning to love ourselves. We will live the magnificence and freedom of our trinity of consciousness through the love that we discover within ourself for the rest of our journey home. We will no longer "need" to create fear and inequality as our physical lifestyle. We will no longer need to control or to be controlled. We will no longer need dependency as our savior. We will become passionately independent and free.

The religious mission of Paul as the Antichrist was a stroke of brilliance for our spirit consciousness. As a spirit consciousness we can only accept dependency, inequality, deceitfulness, and fear for the period of our immature soul. Our time to live with that consciousness focus is running out, and our soul change is synonymous with our physical survival as an evolving soul. By creating the dependent revolutions of our addictive religious beliefs as the stasis level of our transitioning soul, we have forced ourselves to look at our unequal beliefs and behaviors in our physical experience. In living our addictive religious beliefs of inequality, we have lived what we no longer want as a soul. Many males and females are no longer comfortable with the inequality, dependency, control, and fear of religion and are opening their minds to change. For our male and female soul consciousness to become one ascending soul consciousness, we must learn to live our equality, truth, and love as our thinking, emotions, and feelings moment by moment in our physical lives.

Religion is synonymous with a mental and emotional worship which creates our behavior as totally dependent, controlled, and unequal. To worship anyone or anything, we must have a belief that the person or thing that we are worshipping is superior to us. The changing of our beliefs has affected our male and female relationships, because women are choosing not to worship the male as superior but to live equally with the male.

As females rebel against the religious identities and roles that are predominant in our society, we gradually bring change into society as a new perception of thinking, emotions, and feelings. If females are willing to be controlled, they act as opposition to change, which reflects their male persona. If males are willing to change and cooperate with females in change, they reflect their

their female persona of the Divine Nature that will support our soul in its journey home. It will be the males and females who are living their male persona that will act as the Antichrist opposition to the soul continuing its journey home.

When Paul created Christianity he used the laws of Judaism, Hinduism, and the pagan Persian God Mithra as the core of his Christian belief. To be ruled by the "law" of inequality between the male and female, the untruth of superstitious beliefs and rituals, and to live in fear of judgement and wrath is no longer acceptable to our Divine Nature. If we are truly ready to live our equality consciousness, worshipping laws that hold us to identities and roles of inequality, judgement, and fear is no longer appropriate.

Some people are living a soul level of consciousness that is ready to move beyond the primitive consciousness beliefs and behaviors of our descending emotional soul. Some individuals with an ascended intellect can find little if any logic in our ancient addictive religious beliefs, but they adhere to the charade because of their descended emotional soul, which makes them terrified of change. Other people are obsessively attached to their addictive religious beliefs and behaviors of inequality and fear. Many of these people will create sexual and food addictions within their lives and not understand the karmic connection of their biological needs trying to support them with a chemical emotional change and sensory stimulation.

The sense of inadequacy and worthlessness that lives in many immature souls creates the "need" to feel superior through judgement of others but internally they know they are living a lie and "need to be saved." Those who see themselves as unequal will judge and blame others as a reflection of the judgement and blame which they feel towards themselves. The immature soul that is addicted to religious beliefs is also addicted to an extreme fear that can send shock waves through the subconscious ego when the intellect is threatened by different perceptions of thought.

Our society is overflowing with and burdened by countless people with the negative, external, fearful, and judgemental consciousness of our physical nature. When the awareness of how truly destructive our external judgement is can be seen on a mass scale, people will begin to see the importance of change. The behavior of our physical nature has left much to be desired when it attacks a spiritual consciousness based upon its addictive religious beliefs that limit the conscious awareness of its intellect and suppress its emotions and feelings. The cult of religions has "brainwashed" our thinking and emotions and focused us on external, negative, and fearful beliefs for fourteen thousand years of our immature soul journey. Because of the duration of our habitual repetition of these addictive religious beliefs, we now feel fear and anger with any perception of change. Once these same souls begin to act out the physical experience with rage, the soul is getting very close to beginning its lives of rebellion and change.

Our world is living the duality of its collective immature soul consciousness as the reflection of all souls upon earth that are searching for balance without understanding. Until we understand that we are a trinity of our dual soul and spirit consciousness that is seeking the knowledge of how to live our equality, truth, and love, the acting out of our judgement, blame, and fear will overwhelm us as we design our physical experiences as the "pie in the face" exposure to our soul lessons. The emotional suppression, the revolutions of our addictive religious beliefs of inequality, and the suppression of our sensory feelings must change for our society to evolve out of chaos.

Many of the prophecies of old are wonderfully revealing when they are interpreted from the Divine Nature. One such verse is "he that is without sin among you, let him first cast a stone...." (John 8.7). There are no souls on earth who are free of our religious concept of "sin," which is the emphasis of this verse. The verse means that our ascending intellectual soul should not accept blame, judgement, and fear as the appropriate behavior of the descending emotional soul, but that we must continue our journey home to our mature soul by balancing our mind and emotions and opening to our mature soul. If we maintain the love, respect, and dignity for ourselves and not allow ourselves to be magnetized to the negative energy of judgement, our soul will evolve more quickly. Only ignorance creates the "sin" of judgement as an "evil" fear behavior. Our ego will attempt to magnetize us back into our descending soul emotions. It is our freedom of choice not to participate in negative and fearful behavior that will motivate us to become equal, truthful, and loving. Changing our beliefs, as our focus of thought, allows us to emotionally ascend as a soul. Religion is an emotion of fear worship. We have created religion as an intellectual function of our physical experience and we have used our religious beliefs as the foundation of our societies. Religion has never been a true thinking man's elixir because it has no logic and it controls our imagination and ideas as well as our emotions and feelings.

The infinite levels of our immature soul consciousness are being shown in the extremes of society today, giving the mature soul the opportunity to live its freedom of choice of equality as its spirituality. Our immature soul mind and emotions is jammed with memory nodes of our primitive beliefs and behaviors that remain as lessons for the descending emotional soul. When the ascending intellectual mind is brimming over with knowledge it can no longer accept religious beliefs. Our primitive memories of religious beliefs will be revisited by our ascending mind and descending emotional consciousness and acted out in our behavior if we do not consciously choose to focus our mind and emotions on the positive, internal, loving perception of life.

As our ascending mind flirts with its next physical creation, we have enfinite levels of emotional consciousness that are recorded in our mature soul memory that begin to tease our loving emotions into wakefulness. As our focus of consciousness begins to change and balance our ascending mind and emotions, we can access any node that we are magnetized to by a sensory stimulus of our dual subconscious soul memory. In that nanosecond, we can relive that memory node with total clarity. If it is a mature soul memory node, we will internalize the soul memory and learn from the relationship that we find to our present physical experience. If it is an immature soul memory node that we access we will act out the physical experience externally in our physical life without any understanding of the relationship of the memory node to ourself.

The more open our mind becomes the more memory we can access and the more clarity we will have in relationship to the memory. When our soul magnetizes us into the past memory it will always have a profound relationship to our present physical experience. Our ego will create the illusion that we have fulfilled our expectations and reached our destination in our life by acting out the physical experience as our physical reality. The ego intention will be to keep us from understanding what is happening within our trinity of consciousness. Our ego consciousness will do all that is in its power to keep us focused upon the negative, external, fearful, and judgemental emotions that give our ego its beliefs of superiority. When we begin to access memory nodes at other levels of our mind and emotional consciousness it is extremely important that we seek the true knowledge of what is happening in our trinity of consciousness.

As we review our present life and the societal dramas of others, we can clearly understand exactly how we are choosing to live our lessons and we can become conscious of the importance of changing our level of consciousness. As a consciousness we are never shooting stars. Our soul journey is a gradual expansion of our consciousness through the sensory stimulus response to our thinking, emotions, and feelings. Each soul must accept personal responsibility for the journey of our soul and we must walk the journey one step at a time. It is the accumulation of our physical experiences of consciousness expansion that is responsible for our soul evolution.

To transition from our descending emotional soul to our ascending emotional soul is what we are attempting to accomplish. As we ascend into our emotional soul consciousness we will be balancing our ascending intellectual soul consciousness with our ascending emotional soul consciousness. Our intellectual mind symbolizes our male consciousness and our emotions symbolize our female consciousness. The mind and emotions of our physical nature symbolize our male and female consciousness. Until we can balance our mind and emotions, we cannot

21

bring the male and female consciousness of our soul together in
equality.

The normal emotions of our transitioning soul are multiple
levels of depression, which have a range from our consciousness
of separateness and unhappiness to our consciousness of being
dispirited with hopelessness. It is the sense of depression that we
feel as we resist changing the focus of our thinking and emotions
that is encouraging us to look internally and love ourselves. The
levels of consciousness in between unhappiness and hopelessness are infinite and will bring us to the depths of depression,
anxiety states, phobias, addictions, and stress-related diseases.
The way to give up depression forever, at all of its various levels,
is to gain the knowledge to understand ourselves. Once we realize that we have total freedom of choice in the focus of our consciousness, the easier it is to focus internally and the happier we
become in our daily lives. When we can understand that depression is normal in a changing soul consciousness, we begin to
immediately feel better about ourselves and we begin to seek the
knowledge that will help us evolve into the ascending emotional soul.

Our trinity of consciousness lives in the three dimensions of
consciousness that exist as our immature male and mature female
soul and our spirit consciousness. Our spirit consciousness always
makes certain that we have examples of what is going on in our
mind and emotions in our physical experience to support our soul
growth. We routinely create our thoughts, emotions, and feelings
as our physical experiences as we learn our art of creation.

Computers are the analogy of our trinity of consciousness.
Our left brain of male physical nature consciousness is our floppy drive. Our right brain of female Divine Nature consciousness
is our hard drive. Our posterior brain of spirit consciousness is
our main frame or server unit. Computers are showing us the
path of our trinity of consciousness and the loop of communication that is always present within our trinity of consciousness
through our memory nodes.

Science, and especially medicine, is an example of our left
brain external, negative, and fearful consciousness. Our society

lives in fear of some external organism destroying our life. If that happens, we will be the organism that creates the destruction. Medicine looks externally for negative cause and fears the effect of disease on society. It has overlooked the power of our mind and emotions to internally create disease and to heal disease. Medicine has overlooked the logical pattern of how we were created and the relationship that we have to nature and earth as our inherent support system for health.

Medicine is in competition between life and death because of the religious belief that we have only one life. When we add our fear of death to another karmic religious belief that "death is a sin," we begin to understand the intellectual and emotional consciousness of medicine. Our religious fears focus our thoughts and emotions externally and we spend more time in competition with death and we fail to accept death as a valuable experience of life. Birth, life, and death are a continuous cycle of expression for our dual soul as we return to continue with our journey home to the spirit.

Many scientific medical programs are literally a waste of money because the external focus does not enlighten us and does not heal us. When we understand ourself we will understand the universe. Since we do not yet understand ourselves, the space program is a wonderful example of looking externally and how we can create destruction for ourselves and earth. It would be more advantageous for us to learn to understand ourself and earth than to figure out methods to inhabit other planets or exercise our curiosity about whether we are alone as a universal form of human life.

It is earth that supports us and will always support us in our present form. Our space program has managed to trash space, which has the potential to create more problems than it will ever solve. Because we do not understand ourselves we do not see the relationship of earth, nature, and the universe to us and we do not see the fractal pattern of us that explains the universe. As we change our thinking, emotions, and feelings, we will also change our research and learn to understand and support ourselves in our physical experiences of consciousness expansion upon earth.

We are not the only trinity of consciousness that lives within

the universe, but as long as we are living the external, negative, and fearful perception of our immature soul we have to wonder if we would relate to another being on another planet any more lovingly than we relate to each other on earth. There are no "aliens" within the universal system of consciousness, although there are multiple levels of consciousness that are being focused upon at this time. We are all children of the same consciousness and equal in our potential for which we were specifically created.

Since we are a fractal chemical pattern of the greater Spirit Consciousness, we live with the Christ Consciousness within us. Our Christ Consciousness gives us the inalienable right to save ourself as we expand into a higher spirit consciousness of equality. When Paul began his mission as the Antichrist his focus was to make us dependent upon someone else to save us, thus removing our personal responsibility to save ourselves. As religion has taught us the perception of the Antichrist consciousness it has taught us our personal responsibility to seek new knowledge that will allow us to ascend emotionally into our mature soul. Paul and his religion were gifts of learning for our immature soul.

By living the dependency, control, and fear of our mind and emotions through our religious beliefs, we are learning what we don't want so that we can change and balance our ascending mind and descending emotions. When we accept our freedom of choice to live what we do want as truth, equality, love, independence, and freedom, our evolution as a soul will be assured.

To understand ourselves we must shift our focus of consciousness away from our external physical image as the superior perception of ourself. Our society, business, medicine, and the media have played a dramatic role in focusing our consciousness on the worship of our physical sexual image. Our intellect and ego have created our "expectation" of the prototype physical-sexual image as being the perfection of health, sexual attraction, and our identity and role. As both the male and female have focused into the intellect and ego consciousness of our male physical nature, we have lived our control, inequality, and fear so that we could understand that we want to live our freedom, equality, and love. We have lived in our physical nature with a sexual focus. We will live in our Divine Nature with a loving focus.

When we began with our focus on our male physical nature as a living soul, we soon lost our memory of creation and our memory of ourselves. As we begin our transition into the ascending mature soul we will restore our ancient memory and we will begin to take all of the knowledge that we have learned and we will relate it to ourselves. As our consciousness expands we will see ourselves in all of our power, wisdom, and magnificence and we will love being human.

It would never have worked for us to be aware of our power when we were functioning from our ego belief systems. We have abused our physical power, which allows us to see how sadly we would have abused our spiritual power. As we begin to live the humility of our mature consciousness, we will have the wisdom to use our power with equality, love, and truth.

As a spirit consciousness we are a fractal chemical pattern of the universal consciousness and we have absolute memory of our creation. It is this inherent universal memory that allows us to return into enfinite physical lives to continue the physical experience of expanding the male and female consciousness of our living soul. The expansion of our dual soul consciousness accumulates and becomes the expansion of our spirit consciousness. Our spirit consciousness is at all times the lifeforce energy of our physical body and our living soul.

We are a trinity of soul and spirit consciousness and we have been given the miracle of life. In understanding ourselves we can live in the joy, passion, and ecstasy that we were meant to live. We can create a "heaven on earth" as we acknowledge and understand the equality of our internal male and female consciousness as our dual soul that is living its journey home to our spirit.

OUR CHEMICAL CONSCIOUSNESS

All of my life I have been an avid reader and I sometimes feel that I have searched so intensely through books because I have known that somewhere, in some book, is hidden the information that I am constantly being taught through my universal mind.

I have yet to find what I am looking for spelled out in simple terms, but I have found the pieces of what I am taught in many different scientific disciplines. My spirit has constantly and consistently told me from the age of two that we are a chemical consciousness that must be supported by the foods we eat to maintain our physical bodies. This philosophy was explained to me as a child when I was very ill.

When I wrote this information in my first book, *Joy of Health,* in 1988 I truly thought that our societal mass consciousness was open enough for us to begin to understand this logic. I think some people understood it and other people certainly didn't understand, but I have continued to say it in multiple ways, hoping that it will make a difference in the lives of those who hear.

The secret to our happiness and health is understanding that we are a chemical consciousness, and understanding that we were created with a very precise pattern that allows us to continually support our mind and emotions as a chemical consciousness and the cellular structure of our physical body as a chemical consciousness. Becoming conscious that it is our beliefs that are leading us down the primrose path to disease is the personal responsibility of each and every individual as an evolving soul and spirit.

Hippocrates came the closest to defining our inherent chemical consciousness when he said, "We are what we eat." These words could not be more accurate. But our food sources are more polluted today than they have ever been. Our polluted air, water, and foods are the basis of our diseases.

Medicine is now absorbed with genetics, which is the chemical pattern of our eternal soul and spirit. Physics has defined the Universal Laws that organize the evolution of our soul as it has discovered the physical laws. Mathematics defined the fractal pattern of life which is easily revealed in numbers. But chemists and biologists are the real jewels of science because they hold the key to putting all of this information together to see how we are made from the elements of the universe, earth, and nature. We are what we eat, and the chemicals that we eat restore our body, soul, and spirit, or they make us sick.

We have been given in nature every element that we need to maintain our health and our growth. When we choose not to believe that we create our own reality of life, we will continue to ignore the obvious. Not only will we hide behind our beliefs as a wall of resistance and denial, but we will innocently do everything that we can to sabotage our health as we try to wake up our consciousness to its ignorance. Because most people do not understand what our consciousness is or who we are, our chemical foundation is a good place to begin our understanding of self so that we can be open to change.

We have a trinity of consciousness as male, female, and spirit. Each trinity of our consciousness is chemical and lives within us as the trinity of our minds and emotions. Our three minds have multiple mansions, which are different levels of consciousness. We must evolve within and live through each level of consciousness that lives within us as our male, female, and spirit minds and emotions. Our male and female consciousness is the immature and mature journey of our dual soul mind and emotions as we make the journey home to our spirit. Our spirit consciousness is our universal mind and our unconditional love is its emotion. Our spirit has a third component as our three dimensions of senses that provide the sensory stimulation that expands our consciousness. All levels of our soul and spirit are chemical and we are influenced in a positive or negative way by chemicals.

When we were designing our "living soul" in human form we created a pattern within that design that would automatically support the existence of our chemical consciousness. The "living soul" pattern of us as a male and female consciousness in a human body was designed as our chemical DNA and chemical RNA and our spirit consciousness was designed into every cell with the DNA and RNA as the three dimensions of our senses. Our dual soul represents the dual consciousness of our mind and emotions as a male physical nature and a female Divine Nature. Our senses are our feelings and are designed in three dimensions of physical, soul, and spirit in every cell within our body as a means of expanding our consciousness.

We patterned the care of our chemical consciousness into our biological needs. The natural air, water, and foods of nature were given to us to support our chemical consciousness. Breathing, drinking, and eating stimulates each and every sense within our body and as such it provides the sensory stimulation to expand our consciousness. It was also breathing, drinking, and eating that was designed into our behavior to support the "life" of our physical body, maintain the integrity of our chemical cellular structure and consciousness, and allow us to expand our awareness of ourselves as a spirit consciousness.

Our biological need for sex was given to us as another inherent pattern to procreate new life as eternal souls, for pleasure as sensory stimulation of all our senses, and as the magnetic influence to evolve us unconsciously as a soul, until we could understand ourselves and use our freedom of choice to evolve or devolve. Without our biological needs of air, water, foods, and sex we would not have evolved or survived as human beings. Our biological needs were gifts from our Spirit Consciousness that would allow us as "children of God" to stay in physical form until we could appreciate and honor the power of our spirit consciousness.

All of nature and earth were created to support our biological needs. Our chemical consciousness is made up of the same identical chemical elements that are found within the universe, the earth, and nature as air, water, and foods. Each of our support systems provides us with the identical chemical elements that are the foundation of our own chemical consciousness.

As we have polluted our air, water, and foods, we have changed our chemical consciousness with chemicals that are foreign to our chemical cellular pattern. It is the innocent changes that we have made in the chemicals that we breathe, drink, and eat that has led us into the path of self-destruction from disease. In following our beliefs that we are only physical beings, we are forcing ourselves to become conscious that we are chemical as we inflict chemical imbalances into our lives.

We are not an accident of creation. We are an intentional creation that has energy form, physical structure, total organization and discipline, and the freedom of choice, intention, and will in our lives. We are a miracle of creation, as a seed of the Creator. We are a chemical consciousness that has the potential of living in a physical body with a total consciousness of our magnificence, beauty, and wisdom, when we understand ourselves. Many people are living in absolute fear of change, which attaches them to primitive beliefs that no longer serve our soul in its evolution.

What religion has taught as mysteries is no longer a mystery. Once we are willing to look at these ancient beliefs that capture our thinking and limit us to the expectations of our beliefs, we can release our fearful beliefs and get on with discovering the beauty of us as human beings. The theories of science that focus us upon physical evolution also limit our thinking and expand our religious fears that are embedded in our karmic beliefs, which are not consciously understood.

Opening our minds to a new focus of internal thinking and emotions of love is not something that we have been taught. Instead we have been taught to be obsessive in our external and fearful attachment to "what has been." If we look at what is going on for us in society and in health we have to question the wisdom of such teachings.

If our teachings and behavior were perfect, we would have a perfect world. When our immature soul mind is full of knowledge, we will automatically begin to cross-fertilize our right brain, which cracks the surface of the cosmic shell of our beliefs and takes away our limitations as it opens our mind. This works because of the chemical electromagnetic energy that is the core of us as a soul and spirit consciousness.

It is our beliefs that allow us to eat foods that paralyze the chemical consciousness of our spirit senses and allow our soul mind and emotions to live in an alphabet soup of unwanted chemicals that creates a roller-coaster ride for us physically, mentally, and emotionally. We are living our lives as a reaction to misinformation and greed rather than looking within ourselves for the truth. It is this misinformation that allows us to pollute the air, the water, and our food supply.

We are a trinity of consciousness as male, female, and spirit and we are made in the fractal pattern of the Creator. God is not male and he is not external to us. These beliefs were normal in the male consciousness of our immature soul mind that was captured by fear and controlled by its ego beliefs. We took our fear and created God externally in the image of man, who felt superior to woman, and we made God in man's image of fear, anger, wrath, judgement, and punishment because that was our vision of ourself.

Because we are equal as males and females, we have both been living the journey of our immature soul using the "scatter program" of our immature soul mind and emotions, and we have been consistently motivated by the sexual core of our physical nature. As we have been focused upon our physical nature, we have not understood how we were created and the personal responsibility that we have in restoring the elements from which we came. We have abused ourselves as a way of expanding our consciousness by living what we don't truly want as souls.

At this time, as both the male and female are ready to enter into the ascending emotional soul of our Divine Nature by ascending our fear emotions, we are changing our thinking to an internal perception of who we are. We will not trash our intellect or our biological needs, but we will consciously choose to balance our intake of the pure chemicals that can restore us and in turn balance our intellect with love. Our sexual activity will no longer be the illusion of sex as love, but we will seek sex only when we are feeling the emotion of love for our partner.

We have lived the journey of our changing consciousness very gradually over billions of years, because it has been important for us to learn the strength of our power before we could consciously use it in an expansive form. As we have moved from one perception of reality to the next we have lost a large portion of our early memory but we have expanded our knowledge of the universe, earth, and nature. The missing link in the knowledge is our understanding of the relationship that we have as a physical body, soul, and spirit to the universe, earth, and nature and why the relationship was created. We are the same chemical elements from which air, water, and foods are created within the universe, earth, and nature, and these chemicals are essential to support our health and life.

We have evolved without an aware consciousness of our evolution but the magnetic influence of our chemical consciousness has held us in the magnetic arc of the growth of our dual soul consciousness. We have restored our chemical balance from the foods, air, and water of nature for billions of years because we have held the memory of these elements of nature as being essential to our survival as our biological needs. But in the past fourteen thousand years our ancient memory has been lost and we have failed to remember why we eat and why we are motivated to have sex. In our self-centered mind our biological needs are lived because they give us pleasure. It is the pleasure of eating and sex that awakens us to feel the total sensory stimulation of our senses.

The further we have descended into the pit of our fearful emotional soul the more we have denied the memory of who we are, and we have essentially adopted the quick-fix mentality towards food that has led us into disease and devolution as a soul. Our loss of memory has allowed us to trash our environment and pollute our foods, water, and air. This has been a major problem for over two thousand years and now we are reaping the rewards of disease emotionally, mentally, and physically. When disease affects us as an individual it also affects society and the world.

We have sensed that freedom is important to our soul and we have interpreted this sense as sexual freedom because that is the core of our physical nature. We have not realized that our soul is encouraging us to free our mind of limiting beliefs and our emotions from suppression. The interpretations of our inspired thoughts, which are being sent to us by our spirit to trigger our mature soul mind and our body, are all essential because of the ignorance of our beliefs that chain us to our superstitions and rituals. All thought begins as inspired thought and as it moves from our spirit mind into our intellect it is filtered by our beliefs, which act as a distortion to the truth of our spirit mind.

Both mental and physical diseases play a role in getting our attention so that we can take a new look at who we are and why our world is still living in fear, judgement, blame, and killing. Science can never eradicate disease until it understands who we are as a chemical consciousness. It is the personal responsibility of each of us as a human being to learn who we are and how to save our own body and mind. Because we are spiritual beings trying to learn how to live and grow as human beings, no one else has the power to save us but ourselves. Knowledge is the key to opening our immature soul mind and emotions because we are living in the level of knowledge as a soul. The knowledge of our chemical consciousness and how to balance the chemicals within our brain and the other cells of our body is essential. In living and eating as close to nature as possible, we give ourselves some protection from disease.

Saving ourselves is equal to understanding ourselves. When we can understand that we are carbon, hydrogen, oxygen, nitrogen, and minerals we can understand through the laws of chemistry exactly how we created ourselves and how we can clean up our planet and live long and happy lives. No one else is going to do this but us. We have become a dependent society that puts our lives in the hands of corporations, government, insurance, banks, medicine, the educational system, the judicial system, and religion, and we have a grand expectation that someone else will save us. Being saved by someone else is the illusion that we create with our ignorance.

As a soul and spirit we are here to consciously learn the art of healing ourselves and our planet. We are not here on earth to be ignorant of ourselves and our relationship to the planet. We have been gradually gaining in knowledge, which is helping us to understand how we are harming ourselves by many of our choices. As we gain knowledge we are trying to understand ourselves.

Unfortunately we still have the mental and emotional "scatter program" of ego trivia within our immature soul mind that looks externally, with a negative and fearful attitude, which sinks us to the pit of depression. Balancing our chemical consciousness is our way out of this dilemma. Medicine has acknowledged that depression and some "mental" diseases are a chemical imbalance, but they see the answer as adding more external "foreign" chemicals to our consciousness as a method of curing our imbalance.

Medicine is reacting to the scientific belief that "food does not affect disease." The natural unpolluted foods, water, and air of nature are the spiritual way to cure physical disease and to prevent disease because the patterned biological need of our soul and spirit is to support our chemical consciousness that not only lives in the trinity of our mind and emotions but creates the cellular structure of our physical body.

The answers to our life are designed internally within our cellular pattern, but we reflect our beliefs externally to create our physical lives at the level of behavioral consciousness that we are living. We are a fractal pattern of the universe, earth, and nature as a chemical consciousness living in a chemical body. We each have a unique physical structure but we all have the same chemical energy form. Each of us as a soul and spirit live by the organization and discipline of the universe which is also found in the physical laws of nature, earth, and our soul and spirit.

Christian religion came into our lives approximately two thousand years ago to help us get our attention. When Jesus was born as an old and highly advanced soul to teach us a philosophy of understanding ourselves he taught in small groups, until he understood that the human species was not ready to transition into the ascending emotional soul at that time. The next soul that was given a mission to help man was Paul, who founded Christianity and created the revolutions of our savior attitude as a method of helping us see the folly of our limiting beliefs.

Today we have other souls that are playing out roles for mankind to witness until we are so sick of the dramas that we can change the focus of our thinking and emotions. The advantage that we have now is the multiple methods that we have to communicate what is happening to the entire world. When Paul started marketing the Bible and religion it had to be done primarily on a one-on-one human basis. Now, marketing the gossip, judgement, blame, and untruth is being principaled by our judicial system and supported by the mass media. The sensationalism, as judgement, that is being put out to all of the world is showing us the ignorance of our physical nature and its limiting beliefs. We are being given another opportunity to live and grow or to devolve back into the revolutions of fear and judgement.

Our change is an important issue because it creates a collective consciousness of truth or untruth, judgement or acceptance, fear or love. Because we are subject to the law of motion as a soul, we are now facing our freedom of choice in which direction our collective consciousness is going to swing. Are we going to allow the forces of judgement, fear, and anger to rule us or are we going to have the forces of acceptance, love, and growth evolve us out of our ego beliefs?

Our chemical consciousness is reflected into our beliefs, emotions, attitude, personality, character traits, language, and behavior. The choice is ours because we have freedom of choice, intention, and will as a soul and spirit. The "condition" of our chemical consciousness creates our thoughts, beliefs, emotions, attitude, personality, character traits, language, and behavior.

Someday this will be proven because it can be found in our DNA
pattern as specific chemicals.

As immature souls that are moving into our mature ascending soul we must have a strong force of positive, truthful, and loving consciousness to make certain that we continue with our evolution. Judgement, fear, wrath, and punishment is the path of our immature soul, and if we become intellectually attached to this energy within ourselves we will add to the consciousness of devolution. This special moment in our time is of the greatest value of any time since the birth of Jesus. Jesus was born during the time that we were living another chance to live our love and begin our ascension. We have continued to revolve during the past nearly three thousand years but now we are completing that time period and devolution will occur because we have set ourselves up as a chemical consciousness to devolve.

The biblical saying, "Let he who is without sin cast the first stone" is showing us how to lovingly accept the behavior of others because as a soul we have lived the same behavior, if not in this lifetime we have lived it in another lifetime. When we judge another person we are appeasing our own guilt by internally judging ourself. This is our ego's way of distracting us from the positive focus of understanding ourselves. In effect, our physical nature and our Divine Nature are living their tug-of-war. Many souls on earth understand this internally and are not choosing to buy into the judgement of others.

One of the primary reasons that we have everything imaginable that we can experience in life passing through our lives at this time is to capture our attention and make us sick to our stomachs of the whole mess. When the dramas become so intense that we become conscious of the lies, greed, revenge, rejection, judgement, and sense of abandonment that we are being exposed to, we have to stop and consider what message we are sending to the world around us. This allows us to stop focusing on the external and begin to look at ourselves internally because the judgement and anger that we see externally is not comfortable for us internally if our chemical consciousness is in balance.

Our chemical consciousness reflects our level of aware consciousness of the reality of who we are. There are multiple levels of consciousness that are being lived in our society. As a chemical consciousness we create an energy field as the electromagnetic energy of our chemical consciousness, which we reflect outward into the energy space around us. We attract others of like energy as we wear our energy field, which is our "coat of many colors."

People who are negative attract people who are negative and the opposite is also true, as the positive people attract positive people. When we are living our transition our behavior will be dual, or both negative and positive, and we may find that we have a dual life with both kinds of friends. We attract opposites to ourselves to complete soul lessons that we have designed into our lives. The energy of the masses affects everyone upon earth, and the closer the proximity of the energy field the more effect we feel upon our own body and chemical consciousness. It is the focus of the mass consciousness that is important in societal change.

The negative, external dramas of our world are smothering us with their energy and trying to overcome the positive energy. We have contaminated food, unacceptable behavior, wars, genocide, sexual dramas, judgements resulting in everyone suing everyone else, and it is all played out in the media ad nauseam, so that none of us have any place to escape the negativity except to look within ourselves.

It is appropriate that the behavior of our physical nature and its sexual core be in our consciousness at this time so that we can choose which consciousness we want to live within as we feel the pressure of an unacceptable energy force. We can choose to devolve and we will slide backwards into even more intense dramas or we can choose to evolve and move forward into our Divine Nature. The primitive beliefs of worship and "being saved" are also negative beliefs of our physical nature.

Our chemical consciousness must at all times be supported by the air, water and foods of nature in their purest forms. As we become loving of ourselves we begin to change the way that we

tionally to get our attention. This is our soul and spirit's intervention to help us learn that we must change our behavior for our evolving soul to survive. Change is the definition of survival for our soul.

When our beliefs are focused upon revenge, fear, anger, hate, and judgement we are in effect feeling this way towards ourself and we are reflecting our beliefs outward into our behavior. Our perception of reality will be reflected from the relative truth of our personal beliefs. Therefore, multiple people will have multiple versions of "truth" that will be the focus of their specific level of consciousness. Our intellect is the mind of our immature soul and therefore our perception of physical events will be judged in relationship to our ego beliefs. The mature soul within us knows how important it is to release our limiting beliefs and the only way that it has to get our attention is allowing us to create the drama in our physical experience so that we can live it.

As we live out our intentions in each physical experience, we are limited in our perception of reality by our cosmic shell of beliefs. Our immature soul has been focused upon our sexual core, with the emotions and thinking being different in the female and male mind. Therefore, as each person reacts to his/her relative truth they are reflecting the "truth" of the many mansions of their mind and the precise beliefs that limit their level of consciousness. The more emotional stress the body and mind are experiencing the less realistic and logical their perception is, because stress destroys the chemical balance within our intellectual consciousness.

The other focus of consciousness that is opening for many people is the willingness to change their perception of reality. These people will strive with a diligence to begin cleaning up their lifestyle habits, their eating, and their belief systems. As we look at our society we can easily see those individuals that are openly making changes in their lives. We cannot just talk about change. To be spiritual we must get rid of our limiting beliefs and live our change.

Until we change our beliefs we are simply intellectualizing our spiritual consciousness without living spiritual behavior. As we see countless people change their eating habits, stop smoking, stop drinking alcohol excessively, stop using drugs including prescription drugs, and stopping other addictive behaviors, we are seeing people living their transitional change.

Our most intense addiction as a soul is our addiction to beliefs. When we can release our negative and fearful beliefs and begin living happy, creative, and loving lives, we are living the individual ascension of our soul. Many people must ascend before the force of the collective consciousness can pull the entire population of earth into the ascending level of consciousness evolution. When we begin our ascension we become free of old beliefs and we live our freedom of choice, independence, strength, courage, equality, truth, and love. We cannot make lifestyle changes that will endure the test of time without changing the chemical balance of our body and dual soul mind and emotions.

As I have written books to support people in their transition I have explained the utmost importance of our biological need for the pure air, water, and foods of nature to support our chemical consciousness. As we see people seeking organic foods, bottled water, and cleaner air we are seeing those individuals who are changing. Whether or not they understand the motivation and inspiration within them to change, they are willing to live their change. As the chemical balance changes within our cellular structure our mind and emotions begin to change and we create a new and more loving world around us with absolute ease.

Because medicine does not understand the relationship between food and disease, medical professionals do not understand the relationship between food and the DNA pattern of our chemical consciousness. Without an understanding of the relationship between the pure foods, air, and water of nature and our dual soul and spirit we cannot understand that our consciousness is chemical and our body is chemical. In understanding that "We are what we eat" we support our chemical consciousness and all changes that we make in our lives become easy.

As long as we look externally we miss the relationship of our knowledge to ourselves. Yet our entire focus of gathering knowledge has always been to understand ourselves. The relationship of knowledge to the trinity of us as physical body, dual soul, and spirit consciousness is the key element for us to change in every discipline of science. "Facts" are irrelevant unless they can fit one more piece of the puzzle of our life together for us to understand. Every piece of knowledge that we have gathered can help us understand ourself as a soul and spirit living in a physical body if we perceive the information internally rather than externally.

When we believe that we don't have an internal and eternal soul and spirit, we cannot understand the relationship of ourself to anything else on earth and then we hold ourselves as separate and unequal, allowing us to feel inadequate and worthless. Feeling that we are inadequate and worthless makes us angry and we begin to seek revenge through punishment as self-abuse. As we act out our fears in our everyday lives, we wonder why our relationships are not happy. If we are not happy internally, we live with an unhappy perception of ourself and life and we set our course for our relationships to fail.

As we change our beliefs we begin to see that we are all equal because we are all made with the same chemical consciousness and chemical body. It is our perception of ourself that is different and that difference is created by the beliefs that we are living and the chemicals we ingest that create chemical excesses and deficiencies. Religion is the source of our most intense beliefs because that has been the focus of our mind and emotions for over two thousand years. These beliefs did not start with religion as we know it today, but religion was created as a way of intensely living the beliefs to help us discover the importance of truth, equality, independence, freedom, and love.

It does not enter our consciousness to look at what we are chemically creating within ourselves. When we can internally balance our chemical consciousness, we will have a new society and our intimate relationships can be the perfection that we have always dreamed about. It is our personal responsibility to balance our own chemical consciousness and live a healthy life.

40

OUR COLLECTIVE CONSCIOUSNESS

As we learn who we are we are creating a collective consciousness of our dual soul minds, and as we live our internal collective consciousness we will be creating a collective consciousness externally within society. We are constantly reflecting our thinking, emotions, and feelings into our everyday life and into every relationship that we have. As the collective consciousness of our intellect and our mind of wisdom, which is the immature and mature soul minds, join together we change our emotions from fear and judgement to love and communication.

As our collective consciousness becomes the reality of our life we will willingly share our thoughts, emotions, and feelings because communication is the behavior of our loving emotions. When we are unwilling to share any aspect of our life we are continuing to focus on the separate consciousness of our ego, which is fearful of the judgement of others.

The coming together of our immature and mature soul minds is the true meaning of enlightenment. Enlightenment describes the releasing of our old primitive beliefs that have held our intellect in bondage. As our primitive beliefs are released our intellect comes out of bondage and is enlightened by the love of our mature soul. Once our mature soul enlightens our intellect we have no more fear. Our fear is our fear of bondage which we have been living as we have limited ourselves with primitive beliefs.

Our primitive beliefs have limited us to the expectations and destinations of our beliefs that we have created from the superstitions and rituals that have become habitual in our lives. When we created the superstitions and rituals of our primitive beliefs we did so because it was the perception of our conscious mind at that time in our history of evolution. Throughout our journey of evolution we have done the best we could do with the perception of life that we were living. Now, as our knowledge grows, our intellect is expanding and finding itself uncomfortable with our ancient beliefs that are no longer applicable to our lives today.

Our soul is dual in every aspect, and during the time that we have been living in our immature intellect we formed a collective consciousness between our intellect and our ego beliefs that has created our fear of change. Our ancient and primitive beliefs are the wall of denial that we face on a daily basis as we struggle with our fear of change. It is normal for our ego to resist change because it sees our change as its death.

As our ego denies our "need" to change it always begins with the question, "What if?" "What if I am right and everyone else is wrong?" "What if Jesus denies you entrance into heaven?" "What if you change and you go to hell?" "What if this is the devil's work and he is leading you into hell?" If we can look at each question that our ego asks us we will see that the question itself is one of fear and judgement.

The ego feels that the collective consciousness that it has created between itself and the intellect is all there is to the collective consciousness. It refuses to acknowledge that any other mind consciousness can exist except for the intellect and the ego in its dual collective. As spiritual beings who are learning how to be human we have spent the entire path thus far of our immature "living soul" descending into the depths of our physical nature with its sexual core. As we release our ego beliefs we will be free to begin our ascending mature soul.

When we live our ascending mature soul we begin to see life differently, and we appreciate the peace and love that is within us. Many individuals are beginning to live within their ascending emotional and mature soul, and many of these individuals are young children and those who are around the age of thirty. As more people return to life as advanced souls it becomes even more important for society to become advanced as a societal collective consciousness to support these spiritual souls. Children who are not supported in the love and communication that they want will choose to distract themselves from the reality of life by addictions such as drugs, sex, food, and other forms of self-abuse.

When this happens it is because the negative energy of society has affected the positive energy of the advanced soul and created devolution for the individual. Any person that finds himself/herself in the ascending emotional soul journey within an environment of negative energy will feel a sense of confusion, fragmentation, and desperation that they will not understand. This sense of helplessness can lead to devolution because the person cannot find any other way to exist in an uncomfortable world except to move with the majority of the people.

Our soul is organized by the Universal Laws and therefore the law of motion affects the collective consciousness of the individual soul, the societal soul, and the world soul. This means that what we see in the individual as beliefs and behaviors creates the movement of the collective consciousness of society and of the world.

In our descending immature soul we have been collectively focused on the external, negative, and fearful perception of life. In our ascending mature soul we will be collectively focused on the internal, positive, and loving perception of life. To accomplish this feat we need only change the way that we think, our emotions, and our feelings about who we are. We can only succeed in changing the focus of our thoughts, emotions, and feelings when we release the beliefs that hold us in the bondage of our negative and fearful behaviors.

All of society, in countries all over the world, is now seeing the outcome of the behavior of our descending immature soul. As killings, sexual harassment, sexual abuse, homosexuality, pedophilia, inequality, lying, cheating, stealing, self-abuse with addictions, societal abuse with alcohol, smoking, drugs, inappro-

simply living the last dregs of very important immature soul lessons. As we become conscious of and disgusted with our physical behavior, we will be able to accept the wisdom of change.

When we lose our fear of looking at ourselves, we will clearly see that our beliefs and behaviors have not produced a peaceful outcome for us or our children. Because of our fearful societal behavior, we are taking away our personal freedom and the freedom of our children. If our beliefs were beneficial we would have created our "heaven on earth." It is important for us to see what we have done and be willing to change. Until we can reach that point of change within ourselves as a collective consciousness of society, we will continue to devolve into the chaos of the society that we have created. It is our choice to change or to continue with a societal pattern that has not worked in the way that supports us in the freedom of a free society.

We are not separate from society, we are society. But when we are attached to fear and judgement we are not willing to share our thoughts, emotions, and feelings about society. In effect, we suffer in silence because we are afraid to speak, because we fear judgement. As all forms of media sensationalize the negative and deceitful behaviors of society, the collective consciousness is magnetized to that negative behavior which motivates repetition. Conformity is a way of expressing anger in both a passive and active manner.

Violent movies magnetize desperate individuals to the collective consciousness of violence and provide a form of change. Many desperate people suffer in silence and depression, but when they are magnetized to violent behavior it removes the silence and depression because for the immature soul any action is better than no action. Any action can break the habitual belief and behavioral cycle of our soul and change the perception of the thoughts, emotions, and feelings.

It is much wiser if we consciously choose to change our beliefs and behaviors rather than waiting for the immature soul to be pushed over the edge and erupt into violence as a method of getting our attention. If we understood our dual soul rather than relying on ancient and primitive beliefs we could change the negative behaviors that have become commonplace as our collective consciousness finds itself stuck in our habitual fear of change.

Each of us must change for the soul to survive. Our internal dual soul has dominion over our physical body. This allows us to indulge in behavior that is abusive and violent without an understanding of why we have chosen to break the law and create an unwanted change for ourselves. Our immature soul knows that we can sometimes "find ourselves" if we are alone with no external forces to distract us, which allows us to "invite" incarceration with unlawful behavior. This is why many individuals "get religion" while in jail. Unfortunately it is our religious beliefs that are holding us in bondage; therefore, once the individual is distracted by the outside world the behavior will regress once again.

Our evolution depends upon our accepting the personal responsibility to understand ourself. As large numbers of people begin to understand themselves the collective consciousness will move as a mass and we will all enter into the ascending mature soul. If we understand Isaac Newton's law of motion we will understand how the mass collective consciousness is going to move us into devolution or evolution. As a soul we have now reached our awareness of the freedom of choice. Because we have freedom of choice we must accept personal responsibility for the choices that we make.

Religion has played a very important role for us in our immature transitional soul. As we begin our emotional ascension religion must redesign itself if it wants to survive. The word "religion" means "worship," which has been the lesson of inequality that our soul has been living. When we worship we see ourselves as unequal to the person, place, or thing that we are worshipping.

Many people worship Jesus and believe that he alone can save them. Many people worship education and spend many years in school without seeing the relationship of what they learned to themselves. Many people today worship money and

see themselves as nothing without money. Many people worship their work and have no identity except the work identity. Many
people worship relationships and see themselves as unlovable without a partner to love them. Many people worship sex and see their sexuality as their life. Many people worship drugs, food, cigarettes, alcohol, and various other forms of addiction, which becomes their "God" of worship. Many people worship physical possessions and the accumulation of possessions becomes their "God." Many people worship the stock market and are only happy when they are dealing. Whatever we worship becomes our "religion" in life.

As an immature soul we have become a collective consciousness of worshippers. Despite the fact that we are not all worshipping the same "God," we are addicted to our beliefs that we must worship something in the external world. We have not been taught that we are the seeds of God and that the core of our trinity of consciousness is our spirit consciousness.

When we change from our need to worship an external "God" and begin to understand that we are here to grow internally as the seeds of the Creator God, then we will move into our mature soul as a collective consciousness. We are magnificent, wise, and loving as a soul and spirit. Our belief in "only one life" keeps us from recognizing the wisdom that we have stored in our mature soul as we have journeyed in our immature soul.

How did we create such a fearful and judgemental physical world around us as our collective consciousness? We have created our world out of our ignorance, but now is the level of knowledge for our soul and we have all the tools available to us to bring change into our society and world as a collective consciousness of love.

Always, throughout time, there have been people who have access to their universal mind as a means of helping others gain in the knowledge to understand themselves. Despite the wisdom of the prophet the teachings will be interpreted according to the beliefs of the individual. The good thing in reference to prophetic teachings is that they have moved the mass collective consciousness along one step at a time until the information could be more fully understood. Because of this, if we go back into religious history at this time and review the ancient writings, the information will be changed according to the change of beliefs within the mind, emotions, and feelings of the historian.

As an individual soul we move forward in the same manner. The more extensive the knowledge that we gather within our mind today, the easier change will be for our soul. We are now living in the level of knowledge for the soul and we are moving from the awareness of creation to the understanding of creation as our consciousness level. When science began focusing on knowledge of the external it led us into the beginning of change because many scientists stopped worshipping religion and changed to a worship of science as the only answer. The collective consciousness has been gradually changing with science as the new field of worship.

Our immature soul has not been a shooting star but it has plodded along by repeating its beliefs, habits, and behaviors until it can become aware of the wisdom of change. For the past two thousand years we have had an enormous collective consciousness of worship that began billions of years ago. When our collective consciousness became focused into the perception and beliefs of Christianity, we entered into a collective consciousness of worship that we knew as an immature soul that we would change. By living the worshipping beliefs of Christianity, we have been showing ourselves the beliefs of inequality that we are addicted to.

In the collective consciousness of worship we did not all have to worship the same "God," but we have all worshipped some predominant belief within our own mind because we needed to become aware of its presence. We have escalated faster in the past seventy years than we have ever moved as a soul because we are rapidly gaining in scientific knowledge, which is changing many of our religious beliefs within the collective consciousness.

We have an internal tug-of-war going on between our intellectual spiritualism and our true spiritualism. Our belief that our intellect and ego are spiritual because they worship is the basis of our challenge. When we understand that worship is the lesson of inequality for our soul we will be willing to change.

As a collective consciousness we have lived our lesson of inequality as women's suffrage, the collapse of the banking industry, World War II and its ethnic cleansing, the labor union wars fighting for equal wage, civil rights, homosexuality, religious inequality of male, female, and homosexual preference, genetic engineering (a form of ethnic cleansing repeating itself), corporate inequality of both race and sex, all wars, and inequality that deals with control and submission, family abuse, child abuse, and government abuse such as welfare. These are only a fraction of the lessons of inequality that we have lived, but we can see how they have escalated with each year that we live, as we increase our opportunities to raise our level of consciousness of the cause and effect of our beliefs and behavior.

It is important for us to learn how to think with a new focus of mind, emotions, and feelings as a society, which is our collective consciousness. Because we are a chemical consciousness our lifestyle has a dramatic impact on our thoughts, emotions, and feelings. The masses of people that are choosing to eat healthy naturally grown foods, drink pure water, and live and work in unpolluted spaces are the collective consciousness of change. These changes are not accidental to any single being. Since change is the survival of the soul, our soul is constantly guiding us to accept change as the best focus of life for ourself and our families.

As we begin to change our collective consciousness by cleaning up the water, air, and foods that we take into our body, we help ourselves remove the paralysis of our consciousness to the perception of change. Changing our internal collective consciousness requires a personal commitment and personal responsibility that includes our physical lifestyle changes that must occur before we can change the electromagnetic energy of our thoughts, emotions, and feelings. Our mature soul is showing us the integrated being of our physical body, dual soul mind and emotions, and our spirit consciousness as our personal collective consciousness. In making positive physical changes within our lives, we allow our consciousness to change and to affect all of our family, friends, and peers.

If we take the time to open our mind to the changes that are happening within our personal circle of friends at work, our family, and our casual acquaintances we can become conscious of how quickly change is now moving. When we read a newspaper, watch television, go to movies, have casual conversations at parties, or read our mail, we can become conscious of the external versus the internal perception of life.

We will hear people who are quick to judge and others who are quick to praise, some who speak with judgement and fear and others who speak only with love, and we will hear those who speak to create an illusion of their life and those who speak the truth without shame. We have spent the entire journey of our immature soul focusing on concealment and now we are ready, as a mature soul, for revealment. Openly facing our own internal truth will be the beginning of our personal collective consciousness.

We have been learning the lesson of our collective consciousness more expansively in the past one hundred years than ever before, with our mass conformity to beliefs, religion, sports, clothes, education, foods, lifestyles, and various other physical examples. This is an important immature soul lesson because it shows us the power of our collective consciousness. We change different aspects of our society every day through the power of our collective consciousness. We as consumers can make or break a corporation or any business with our collective consciousness if we are willing to actively address societal issues.

When it is our choice to be positive, internal, and loving as a collective consciousness our power will change society for the good. As we have used our collective consciousness to expand our physical reality, we have triggered the memory within our immature soul of the beauty, wisdom, and love that lives within the collective consciousness of our trinity of minds, emotions, and feelings. It has been essential for us to gradually move into an understanding of our collective power by experiencing the supply and demand of our economic structure.

Once we begin to understand ourselves and realize that we

didn't evolve from monkeys but from the chemical consciousness
of the universe, we will understand that we are constantly evolving as a triplet of consciousness (male, female, and spirit) that is
each designed as a triplet of mind, emotions, and feelings that are
the invisible energy that we use to create our lives, society, and
our world.

We are experiencing a dramatic shift throughout our society
and we do not have a collective consciousness of how our
thoughts, emotions, and feelings are affecting all of us. We
choose to look at each event as a separate "accident" or "personal
drama." When we see each event separately, we miss the relationship of all the events to our shifting consciousness.

As we focus our collective consciousness on our sexual core
we are seeing that our sexual core is not our power. During the
journey of our immature soul through our physical nature we
have thought that our sexuality was our power and that man was
superior to woman. Because we see our sexual core as our sexual image we have spent many years focusing on the physical fitness and weight perception to support our belief that we would
not attract love unless we had a specific physical body image that
enhanced our sexual attractiveness.

We have lived with an obsessive belief in our physical image
being the definition of our health. Death is a choice of the mature
soul. We can die at any stage of life: young, middle-aged, old, fat,
thin, anorexic, or "normal," and this happens to both men and
women. Because we have been in competition with death, we
have a collective consciousness that attaches our physical image
of health into a belief about the avoidance of death. Our mature
soul chooses death and disease as a soul lesson of chemical balance. We are a chemical consciousness, and when our collective
consciousness understands this, we will have made dramatic
progress in our shift in consciousness.

Our shifting consciousness is moving us from the perception
that sex is love into an understanding of love as our power, from
our perception that all food is good food to an understanding
that nature's foods support our chemical consciousness, and from
our perception that we are nobody unless somebody loves us to

the understanding that we are learning how to love ourselves. As our collective consciousness becomes aware of how we are showing ourselves the fallacy of our beliefs, which have their roots in religion, we will be more accepting of shifting our mind, emotions, and feelings into our internal loving self rather than our submissive "worship" of the perception of inequality.

It is the shifting of our collective consciousness that is the survival of our dual soul. We were evolving as a trinity of consciousness long before we embarked on our human experience as a "living soul." When we have a collective consciousness that we are eternal as a soul and spirit and that life is about learning to be human, we will have a much greater appreciation for who we are, why we are here, and what our purpose is in life.

Our collective consciousness as a human species is supported by the collective consciousness of nature, earth, and the universe. We all exist in the same chemical consciousness. When we experience earth changes, weather dramas, and our personal fear, we are experiencing the expansion of the universal pattern as we are being given a message that is important to our collective consciousness.

In the past I have written about these earth changes, weather changes, and some universal changes in several of my books. All changes are important for us as a collective consciousness because we are now living these changes as the earth and nature makes every attempt to help us understand ourselves.

The universe, earth, nature, and the human species are all formed from the chemicals around us. These chemicals create an electromagnetic chemical energy of consciousness for everything that we know as our world. When our energy is negative, we attract negative energy on all levels. When our energy is positive, we attract positive energy on all levels. We must reach a specific level of consciousness within our thoughts, emotions, and feelings before we have an awareness of our energy and the energy that surrounds us. Once our collective consciousness reaches this important level, we will shift into our mature soul, which will be a new level of collective consciousness for the human species.

The collective consciousness works on the same principle as

the "hundred monkey theory" or Isaac Newton's law of motion. We must all make the shift forward as a collective consciousness

or, if the negative force is predominant, we will all shift backwards as a collective consciousness. Never before in the history of our living soul have we understood that we have freedom of choice.

Once our freedom of choice is understood as a collective consciousness, we will move as a majority and continue our evolution. Devolution will not be just pain and suffering for the human species if that is the way of our collective consciousness. When we focus upon the stasis of our ego beliefs we are inviting chaos as it has occurred several times before in our immature soul path. When I look at this chaos it can only be related to climbing Mount Everest with only your naked body in competition with the mountain. This is why each of us has a personal responsibility to be committed to our internal growth and our freedom of choice.

It is no longer good enough to just focus on knowledge as an external factual concept. Now we must take all of the knowledge that we have gathered and relate it to ourselves and consciously choose to continue with our evolution. We now have access to the information, which is scattered in bits and pieces among various disciplines of science, with the proof of who we are, why we are here, and what our purpose is.

Science itself is at odds, especially with the concept of the evolution of biology and the creationist theory, which reflects the dual thoughts of science and religion. Only Metaphysics shows us the third reality of our chemical consciousness that has been the path of our evolution as our truth. In the beginning was "the word" should read that "in the beginning we were thoughtform" as spirit consciousness.

Our form as a chemical consciousness is energy. We are energy as thought, emotions, and feelings, which will fluctuate with the chemical balance in our cellular structure. As the collective consciousness becomes aware of the evolution of our energy form, we will shift our physical behavior to support our continued evolution.

As a human species it is essential that we create a collective consciousness within our thoughts, emotions, and feelings of the magnificence, wisdom, beauty, and unconditional love of ourselves. It is our collective consciousness that controls the law of motion within our dual soul personally and as a society. Knowing that we are an eternal soul and that we live as a collective consciousness as souls helps us to understand our power of unity.

Understanding Energy

When we think about energy we think about the energy that runs our house and the cities of our world. The power of electricity lights our cities and homes, turns the dark into light, and keeps us in touch with the world through the communication of television, computers, radios, and telephones. It would seem that electrical energy is the very foundation of technology that keeps our society constantly in a state of expansion.

Seldom do we relate who we are to energy. As a physical body, dual soul, and spirit, we are energy as human beings. It is the energy of our dual soul and spirit that turns dark into light within our consciousness and creates an enhanced awareness that allows our mind, emotions, and feelings to change and grow. It is the magnetism of our dual soul that attracts one person to another and allows the energy of the male and female to create the energy of new life.

If we ask the question "What is energy?" we expect an external, technical, and scientific answer. Energy is the work that a physical system is capable of doing. It is our power of life and it is our vitality and excitement. Energy can be electromagnetic, chemical, mechanical, thermal, electric, or nuclear, and it is always measured by the work that it does. Each type of energy is used within different levels of our physical body in the same way that each type is used in different physical systems within our society. Light is a combination of electricity and magnetism that produces energy.

Our trinity of consciousness is a chemical electromagnetic energy that works as a trinity of mind and emotional energy during our sleeping period, and as a focused and separated intellectual mind and fearful emotional energy during periods of wakefulness. This is why sleeping is essential to our mind and emotional balance. There are many mansions of consciousness within our trinity of minds and we create our reality from the precise level of energy, as thought and emotions, which we are focused into as a consciousness. Our level of consciousness reflects the beliefs and behaviors we are actively living as a physical experience of energy. Our life is an expression of energy in every movement, cellular activity, thought, emotion, and feeling that takes place within us.

As a trinity of dual soul and spirit consciousness we are designed as a fractal pattern of the universe. The fractal pattern of our dual soul has form, structure, organization, discipline, and freedom of choice, will, and intention. The form of us is energy. The energy that creates our form exists in three dimensions and is made up of chemicals, electricity, and magnetism. Energy is not only a part of our design but it is the lifeforce of us as human beings. Without the various kinds of energy that interact and create our soul, spirit, and matter we would not exist.

When we become mentally or physically ill our energy is in a state of imbalance. We always look at ourselves and believe that the illness drained our energy. This is an external perception. We become ill when our internal cellular, mental, and emotional energy is out of balance. We created ourselves as a chemical energy. When the chemicals interact within our body, electrical and magnetic energy are created. The function of our brain, nerves, endocrine glands, and the complete cellular structure of our body is dependent upon the interaction of the chemicals to give us life. The chemicals that provide our energy all come from the universe, earth, and nature to restore and rejuvenate our body, dual soul, and spirit.

The universe is energy and we are a smaller and more compact version of the universal design. Nature is energy. The earth is energy. When the earth and nature get together to create volcanos, earthquakes, tornados, hurricanes, electrical storms, wind storms, snow storms, or floods, we physically experience the powerful energy of nature.

Our spirit moves with the speed of light because it is pure as the chemicals from which we are made. Our spirit chemicals remain in the energy form of gas as the air that we breathe. Our soul is formed by the interaction of chemicals that produce an electromagnetic energy that we use as our mind and emotions. Our soul and spirit are a chemical electromagnetic energy of consciousness that creates thoughts, emotions, and feelings. Our dual soul is our dual mind and emotions that has evolved in consciousness through the energy of physical time as a way of learning for the energy of our immature soul.

Our dual soul is conscious of the energy of our physical nature, but our immature soul denies the subconscious mature soul energy of its Divine Nature. As we transition into our mature soul journey we are choosing to open our intellectual mind and fear emotions to our subconscious mind of wisdom, as an accumulation of mature soul memory, and the loving emotions of our Divine Nature. At each level of energy consciousness, we live, work, and reproduce at a new and different level of energy. Our immature soul has lived with a fearful physical energy. Our mature soul will live with a loving Divine energy that will be in perfect harmony and balance. Light is an electromagnetic energy that is formed by the interaction of electricity and magnetism.

We can compare our immature soul consciousness to the lens of a camera with a physical shutter that we consciously open and close. With a camera we control the light that passes through the lens with the shutter. While we have lived through our immature soul journey, we have controlled the light of our spirit that we allow to enter into the lens of our immature soul by the beliefs that we have. Our beliefs act exactly like the shutter of a camera for our immature soul.

Our physical perception of life is developed by the amount of spirit light or energy that we allow to reach the lens of our immature soul. We control the light in our soul mind and emotions by shutting out our spirit consciousness with our ego cosmic shell or beliefs. When we perceive or view ourselves, earth, nature, and the universe through the murky darkness of our beliefs, we distort the clarity of the image that our mind records as our physical reality because we are limiting the light energy that we are using as part of our mind, emotions, and feelings. Light is created by electricity and magnetism, which controls the activity of our mind, emotions, and sensory stimulation.

The energy that we use to create darkness is minuscule compared to the energy that we use to create light. We have gently eased ourselves into stronger and stronger light energy as we have become prepared to view the picture of ourselves with clarity. We act out our need for more light in our soul by our obsessive feelings that we need sunlight upon our body. Sunlight plays an important role in the body as it interacts with cholesterol to create Vitamin D, which is an essential chemical nutrient for our body, and with our nerves as it affects our sensory response.

As we have been busy creating our perception of the world as an immature soul, we have created our definitions of reality out of the murky vision of our limited consciousness. As humans we have been in the process of expanding our consciousness of reality throughout our immature soul. The definitions that we have created, especially in the last seven thousand years, have been inhibited by the dark, negative beliefs of our cosmic shell, which is still occluding the lens of our mind camera. Our cosmic shell has captured the energy of our immature soul mind in the cave of its beliefs, and we have stayed in our cave and grown in the dark just as a mushroom grows. The darkness that we have lived within has limited our perceptions, which we have accepted as "gospel" or fact. The shadows of our dark soul energy have created superstitions, rituals, and worship as our accepted perception of ourself, earth, nature, and the universe. As our immature soul mind and emotions ascend into the light of our Divine Nature, we will learn to laugh at our primitive imaginings. As we have perceived so have we interpreted, taught, and believed. The more our superstitions, rituals, and worship have grown from billions of years of dark energy accumulation, the more we have crucified ourselves with the thought and energy of emotional judgement and abuse.

With our obstructed and dim view of life we have done the very best that we could to define our reality. Our definitions were perfect for the immature soul but they no longer work for the higher vibrations of energy within our mature soul mind and emotions. Our primitive need to worship is pulling us backwards into the decaying energy of devolution.

We live from the precise level of aware consciousness that we have reached in our immature, transitional, or mature soul. Our conscious awareness creates the physical energy of our body and the energy perception of our mind, emotions, and feelings, which creates the physical life that we live. The energy focus of our beliefs creates the activity and attitude of our daily lives. The level of consciousness that we use in our thinking is our conscious intellectual mentality. The energy of our mind is connected as a double helix to the energy of our emotions, which creates our attitude about life as we perceive it. If we choose to use only the energy of our intellect and we suppress our emotional energy, we put half of the double helix of our soul mind and emotions out of commission. Physically our suppressed emotions could be symbolized as the loss of both legs. We can be paralyzed or lose the use of our legs, but we can still think, have emotions, and use our senses which allows us to feel. We inhibit our mental function when we inhibit our emotions, even though we have the full function of our physical body. This allows us to use only a small portion of the energy available to our body.

Our attitude creates our level of speaking the language that we perceive as our level of communication. The energy of our language and communication reflects the energy of our feelings about ourself and our life in general. The lower our emotional energy, the more inhibition we live. The higher and more balanced our mind and emotional energy feels, the more excited we become about our life. If we do not respect, value, and honor ourselves, we will not respect, value, or honor others with posi-

soul lesson of respecting our self-image and our mature soul power. We live the external reflection of our internal energy fields as our external consciousness. When our immature soul mind and emotions are unbalanced the chemical energy within our brain will be inhibited and we will feel and live our fear. When our mature soul mind and emotions are balanced we will experience a chemical energy of excitation and we will feel and live our love.

Our feelings are the sensory stimulus to the chemical response that we feel from the energy of our seven senses as we think, experience our emotions, and feel from the physical experiences of our life. If our emotions are chemically unbalanced we will shut down our ability to live our emotions and we will paralyze our senses as our feelings. It is our thinking, emotions, and feelings that create the sensory stimulus that expands our consciousness. If we do not have the chemical energy that is required to think, have emotions, and feel, we will not expand our soul consciousness in any lifetime.

Our personality and character traits reflect the pattern of energy that we have triggered within our mind, emotions, and feelings. As our attitude, personality, and character traits are developed by our internal consciousness they are reflected into our external physical behavior as energy and become the physical creation of our life. Our physical behavior is always our personal energy creation, which reflects the precise level of consciousness energy that we have grown into as a soul. If our thinking, emotions, and feelings are inhibited by our beliefs we cannot evolve the energy of our immature soul into spirit consciousness. As our energy breaks down, our journey home stops because we lose our inspiration and motivation to continue our change through the energy of forward movement.

As an immature soul that has been living its unconscious journey of evolution, we have been unconsciously moving from darkness to light. Our movement has occurred as we have expanded our knowledge as a soul. Knowledge is the lens of our camera. Beliefs are the shutter of our camera. We have remained primarily unconscious of our lessons as a soul because of our belief in conforming to blind faith and our belief that we have only one life. These two beliefs have inhibited our soul mind and emotional growth and the expansion of our spirit senses. Once we consciously accept that we are a soul and spirit living an eternal life by using the tool of our physical body to experience each life, we can consciously move forward with our soul lessons and remove ourselves from our cave mentality of inhibiting and limiting beliefs. Our soul movement has occurred because of the Universal Laws of gravity and motion which are accepted as physical laws. Our Universal Laws were created as we were created to help us with our energy expansion until we could consciously understand ourselves.

Our human energy has its source in our trinity of consciousness energy of dual soul mind and emotions and spirit consciousness, with the core of our trinity being our spirit consciousness. The unity of these three energies consistently lives in our physical body and is reflected out from our body in a protective energy field. We are always one as a dual soul mind and emotions and our seed of Spirit Consciousness. We are never separate as a physical body that is dependent upon external forces of energy, except for air, water, the foods of nature, and sexual procreation, which are the eternal biological needs that are inherently designed into the human energy form.

It is only our fear beliefs that create our energy of dependency upon being saved by an external God. As a dual soul we have been given total personal responsibility for saving ourselves through understanding our own consciousness energy. Our consciousness energy is the power of our creation. We have consistently created externally through the consciousness energy of our immature soul as we have learned the skill and knowledge of our art of creation as our physical experiences of life. As we begin to use our consciousness in an internal creation it is because our soul is evolving into the mature soul energy of excitement and passion. Disease will frequently be the first internal energy lesson that we create as a soul in our attempt to gain insight into the

can choose to learn the lesson of our power of creation in death.

To use our unified energy we must be aware that we have a trinity of consciousness as a trinity of dual soul and spirit mind and emotions within our physical matter. We are three dimensions of energy and matter as a body, dual soul, and spirit. Each dimension is created in three dimensions. The three-dimensional pattern is repeated in all of nature and within us. Until we understand ourselves as a trinity of consciousness, we will resist and deny our ability to release our old beliefs and to move into our mature soul mind and emotions. In the consciousness energy of our immature soul we have believed that our intellect and ego are the superior mind within us and we have reacted to the fear emotions of that belief because we have lived the experience of dependency in our fearful, external, and negative intellect and ego. As we have lived with this cold and fearful energy approach to life, we have created our hell upon earth with an accumulation of superstitions, rituals, and worship which has limited our consciousness energy.

The seven levels of soul consciousness energy for our immature soul mind and emotions have been external, negative, and fearful. Because our consciousness energies are invisible, we have not understood how we create our external lives from the energy of our thoughts, emotions, and feelings. The seven levels of our negative, fearful, and externally focused consciousness energy have accumulated and provided a tremendous external energy source which we have used as the energy power of our immature soul. Because our thoughts, emotions and feelings are invisible, we have not been conscious of their hidden power in our daily lives, and we have not been conscious of the effect of external energy on our internal trinity of soul and spirit energy.

When energy is invisible we frequently fail to validate the power it has in our lives. As an example, we take the electricity that provides the power to operate our society for granted until it fails. Once the electrical energy fails to perform for our physical needs, we become conscious of the power it has over our daily lives. We use electrical energy in every aspect of our lives, such as our homes, cars, telephones, televisions, computer systems, trains, airplanes, schools, and every other facet of our world. We take the electricity and the magnetic energy in our physical body for granted and we are often unconscious of the power that swirls around us from our various physical sources of energy. We also remain unconscious of the energy fields within us which we use moment by moment to live. When our internal energy begins to fail or it shuts down, we define our loss of energy as disease.

Our physical energy has reflected the sexuality at the core of our conscious physical nature. Designing our descending physical nature with an external focus upon our sexuality has served a wonderful purpose for our immature soul as it has provided magnetism, procreation, and pleasure for a total sensory stimulation as the three ways of fulfilling the law of continuation for our soul. Because of the magnetism of our sexual attraction, we automatically followed the magnetic arc of gravity for our soul to evolve unconsciously through our biological instincts for procreation. Procreation has allowed new life to support the soul and spirit in its return to a physical body. The magnetic energy of our sexual attraction allowed our soul to continue with procreation without our consciousness of evolution being understood. Our sexuality has also created the opportunity for us to experience the pleasure of sex which acted as a sensory stimulation of all seven of our senses in all three dimensions. Without our belief that "sex is love" we would not have evolved normally with our sexual focus. Our belief in sex as love kept our consciousness focused upon the value of love even when the sex itself was disrespectful, dishonoring, abusive, and unequal. Our physical nature has always been attracted to our Divine Nature because of the embedded memory of love as our soul purpose.

We were designed as electromagnetic energy that is rejuvenated by the foods that we eat which restore the carbon, hydrogen, oxygen, nitrogen, minerals, amino acids, and fatty acids within our body that can continue producing the hormones, enzymes, and other chemicals that are essential to the internal

ture soul, we have forgotten that our life design is part of nature, earth, and the universe. Instead we have focused upon the external processes of life that make work quicker instead of creating a healthy life. Dead foods and chemicals added to foods destroy the integrity of our internal energy.

As a soul and spirit we created automatic breathing that took no thought by our physical body, while it provided the foundation of our constant energy source. We usually do not remember the value of breathing and the energy that it gives our body, until we can no longer breathe easily or automatically. We designed instinctual drinking of water and the grazing for food as the body felt the instincts of hunger as another constant energy source. We appreciated the energy of silence because it allowed us to use our senses to warn us of impending danger. We automatically used the energy of our spirit senses because they provided us with both our survival and our growth of consciousness. In the beginning we heard the guidance of our soul and spirit and we consciously listened as the integrity of our cellular energy caused an acute communication within our senses.

Listening has always been the way to connect with our spirit consciousness, but if we believe that "God" is external to us we will not hear the voices of our trinity of consciousness within our own head. Our belief that hearing voices means we are mentally ill has held us back from trusting the energy responses of our internal senses. The scientific beliefs in fact, which are devoid of emotional energy, can create an attitude of coldness toward our internal consciousness energy that denies our trinity of consciousness. Many old and advanced souls are living on earth today and our external focus is creating dramas of great magnitude. If we hear voices and we believe that hearing voices is a symptom of mental illness, we will become disoriented and live bizarre behavior to create our belief as truth within our intellect and ego. The trinity of energy within us is always communicating with us. When we change our focus from the external energy of life to the internal energy of life we will have a new and different perception of who we are and the power that we exercise on a moment-by-moment basis.

To use our internal energy as one energy in healing ourself or in facilitating healing with others, we must use our integrated mind energy as one powerful, internal consciousness that is open to the stimulus of each and every sense within our body, dual soul, and spirit. Our physical body must be clear of all pollution to allow our nervous system to feel the energy within every cell of our body. We have a cellular sensitivity that is inherent within our autonomic, central, and cellular nervous systems as the energy of our internal spirit consciousness. All seven of our senses live within the three dimensions of us as physical, dual soul, and spirit. Our belief that we have only five senses that exist as our physical senses limits our understanding of our consciousness energy expansion and holds us captive within the cosmic shell of our ego. It is our spirit senses of thinking and speaking that show us that we have an evolving consciousness.

Our spirit consciousness energy created the dual soul as a male and female consciousness energy and the spirit and dual soul created our physical body. We are at all times a trinity of energy. We consistently live from the energy of the level of consciousness that we are evolving within. Our thoughts, words, and behavior reflect our precise level of growth into our lives as our energy persona for all to see. If our thoughts and attitude about life are external, negative, and fearful, our words will be accusatory and judgemental and our behavior will be negative as internal self-abuse and external abuse of others. The energy that we use externally in fear is always abusive to ourselves and others.

An example of this would be someone who says they are spiritual but they are not open to growth, they lie to themselves and others, and they abuse themselves with a lifestyle of external harmful behavior. The only way that we can be spiritual is to live our lives from our spiritual energy of love, truth, and equality. Talking about being spiritual is an intellectual approach to spiritual energy that creates the illusion of being spiritual. When we externalize our life, live in fear, focus on physical processes as our identities and roles, live in anger, judgement, and power-

and emotions. If we hold onto judgement, control, abuse, anger, rebellion, or any fear we are not living our spiritual energy.

The energy of spiritual healing begins within ourself as we learn to think, do, and share from our heart in total love, respect, and compassion. Sharing is an essential concept of living our spiritual energy. If we are afraid to share ourselves, we are afraid to share our love. When we are controlling or dependent we are afraid to accept our internal energy of love. Sharing removes the guilt energy of "secrets" and allows us to speak the truth about our own growth without self-judgement, blame, or fear energy controlling us. Sharing and communication are both energies of our behavior that show us we are willing to look within ourselves and find the energy of the beliefs that are controlling us in fear energy. Denying that we have any beliefs within our mind is an indication of our fear energy of concealment. Our fear of revealment is the energy of our fear of failure. If we think that by revealing our experiences we will be judged by others it is because we are using our immature soul energy to judge ourself.

The revealing clue of a closed mind is the belief that we express when we say, "I know all of that." Our ego jumps ahead to the point that it is intent upon bringing its superiority to our attention. Our intellect and ego response will not be a revelation as a sharing of experience, but it will be a theory or concept that the ego believes will show its superior knowledge and impress others. If it is our intention to understand ourselves and to transition into our mature soul energy, we must be willing to share without worrying what others will think about our self-revelation. What others think does not matter. What matters is that we learn to accept the lessons of our personal experience as normal for our immature soul energy. Our truth of knowledge is found in living our spiritual energy every moment of our life. When our daily energy is focused on our love, truth, and equality, we will be consciously using our spiritual energy as our life-force energy. Our lifeforce energy comes to us as the chemicals that we breathe, drink, and eat to restore the chemical energy within our body. As Hippocrates (460-375 B.C.) said, "We are what we eat."

The trinity of our consciousness energy is the most clever design that exists within the universal system of chemical energy and it is a fractal pattern of the Creative Energy. Whether we choose to call the Creative Energy by a religious or cultural designation truly does not change the energy of our Creator. We have many names ourselves as we move from life to life. Our physical names have energy but they are not as important as what we learn from our physical experience. If we can remember that we are a seed or a cell of the Creator we can see our potential for creative energy. In recognizing our potential for energy we can also begin to understand our potential as spiritual creators and love ourselves. Understanding the energy of ourself is the freedom of choice, will, and intention of our dual soul as a male and female consciousness energy.

The Immature Soul and Our Art of Creation

As an immature soul we have constantly lived our art of creation by creating our physical lives. Every thought, emotion, and feeling has been created in our physical reality as we have learned the art of creation as an immature soul. We are a human seeking to balance our trinity of consciousness as well as our physical body and life. When we can balance out the dual soul mind and emotions of our immature soul we are then prepared to move into our mature soul mind and emotions with a harmony and rhythm that will affect our physical lives. We have always reflected our thoughts and our emotions into our lives as our physical experience and into our physical body as our sexual image. As we are beginning to learn how we create our reality, we become conscious of how we reflect our thoughts and emotions into our physical experience as our external example of creation. The more our soul evolves and changes its level of consciousness the more we reflect the thoughts and emotions into our internal physical body as disease to get our attention. No one ever has a disease without changing their level of consciousness.

Our ability to reflect into the physical as a way of soul growth has supported us in our immature soul. As we move closer to our mature soul we begin to create more disease so that we learn to focus on the internal effect of our mind and emotions and consciously choose change. We exist and continually function from a cosmic fractal pattern of unconscious and subconscious memory which passes into our intellectual mind as thought. We are spirit consciousness energy guiding our male intellectual mind into the constant expansion of knowledge to further our soul evolution by changing our thinking into our Female Divine Consciousness. As the spirit inspiration of thought passes into our intellectual mind it is captured within the cosmic shell of our belief systems and distorted before it becomes intellectual thought. The more beliefs that we have in our ego mind the more distortion we use in our perception of life. Beliefs act as our limitation to thinking with an open intellectual mind.

Our physical body is a hierarchy of cells, organs, fluids, physical matter, chemicals, and hormones designed by our dual soul and spirit from our remembered genetic pattern from which we create the current lessons of our physical experience. We are a complex pattern of fire, air, water, and earth, and on a chemical basis we are carbon, hydrogen, oxygen, nitrogen, and minerals.

We began as spiritual beings and descended from the ethereal or consciousness state of being into human beings of matter, dual soul, and spirit. We are spirits that are seeking the nature of our own truth by learning the art of creating the love and perfection of our spirit being in physical matter. As we live with our core being of spirit consciousness we are learning how to be human as a spirit consciousness.

Before the time of Atlantis we were sentient beings. We used our physical senses in a wider application than we now use them. With the vibrations of the sinking of Atlantis we lost our memory and paralyzed our senses. Before the destruction of Atlantis we had an awareness of the hierarchies of consciousness that exist around us upon earth as nature consciousness and consciousness of matter, as well as the multiple levels of our dual soul consciousness. After Atlantis our focus narrowed into a tunnel view of ourselves as physical matter and we lost our sentient consciousness, allowing us to relate our being, our life, and our reality only to our physical body as the conscious self that we accepted. When the chaos of Atlantis occurred, we began the extreme depths of our "living soul" as it descended into emotional fear as a consciousness level of our beginning depression.

Now we are seeking to shift our mind once more into an awareness of the realm of Spirit Consciousness from which we came so that we can live the ethical values that we learned as we passed through the spiritual hierarchy. It was from the elements of these universal planets that we chose the chemical elements to form our "living soul" as a male and female consciousness. As we lived as a consciousness within the chemicals, we patterned the ethical values that would sustain us into the organization of our male and female soul consciousness. The planets that we lived within to gather the chemicals of our spirit consciousness also provided us with an opportunity to live our ethical values. As a spirit consciousness, we visited Mercury, the Moon, Mars, Venus, Jupiter, Saturn, and the Sun before we began our journey on Earth.

We have forgotten our connection to these planets as the spiritual forces from which we learned our ethical values before our descent into physical matter. As our intellectual mind is seeking truth it is expanding out of the darkness of ignorance into the light of our soul memory and we find ourselves searching for these ethical values within our behavior and beliefs. Expanding our knowledge is our method of soul evolution. As spirit consciousness reflected into a dual soul consciousness we group together into soul families that are connected by the vibrations of our electromagnetic energy fields of consciousness, forming ethnic and world cultures of consciousness. Our fascination with space has always remained as an integrated memory of our spiritual journey. We continue and enhance our fascination with space as the symbol of our physical, external search for the ethical memories that live internally and eternally within our spirit. Souls group together into physical families as a reflection of our soul consciousness to work through the major lessons of our soul evolution, which strengthens our physical lessons of interactive experience and disease as a lesson for our soul.

Our intellectual focus has not changed for thousands of years as our body and mind, as the accepted "self" of our intellect, has

been analyzed, conceptualized, and evaluated as physical matter
from our intellectual, external perception of reality. Our intellect
has no memory of our spiritual heritage until it is open to the
light of our spirit internally. Without the light of our spirit all facts
are viewed, believed, and interpreted as the perception of our
intellect that is formulated within and relative to the negative
beliefs of our immature soul mind.

Our integration as a living organism of physical body, dual
soul, and eternal spirit consciousness has not been accepted in
our overall understanding of ourself. The linear focus of our intellect does not allow us to see with our peripheral vision the
expanding fields of consciousness of ourself and others. Our
intellect has no respect for and sees no value in our sentient soul
and spirit consciousness because our intellect has not yet discovered the intimate relationship of our emotional soul to our
intellectual mind. Our consciousness level has limited us as we
have created the life that we have lived. We continue to limit ourself by our attempt to understand ourselves from the ancient
interpretations of our primitive minds.

Believing ourself to be only finite physical matter allows us
to envision ourself without power and as a victim of multiple
external forces that control, attack, and destroy us. Our beliefs in
ourself as a victim of unseen forces allow us to play the role of
victim as we separate ourself into beliefs defining our personal
vulnerability, unworthiness, victimization, and powerlessness. It
is the beliefs that we take on as our defense and denial system
that form the cosmic shell of darkness around us as our ego,
which holds our intellect in bondage. Our ego beliefs limit the
perception of our intellect and give us the illusion of having met
our expectations and reached our destination of life.

Accepting our integration of body, dual soul, and spirit opens
our mind to acknowledging ourself, our "stuff," our beliefs, and
our power to change. In changing to the use of our integrated
dual soul mind and emotions we heal our fearful beliefs, our diseased bodies, and our destructive relationships.

Change is initiated by bringing the power of our intellect (left
brain) into integration with our soul memory (right brain) and our

spirit consciousness (posterior brain). In using the power of our integrated soul we create the power within us to heal our past soul experiences, our physical body, and our intellectual mind.

The physical matter of our body is a complex tool that is used by our eternal dual soul mind and emotions to guide us into the creation of simple physical experiences that will allow us to become aware of our magnificent power of enfinite thought. Our male and female consciousness is present in each part of our dual soul. Our soul is dual in every aspect and as we live in our immature soul, our intellect symbolizes our male consciousness and our emotions symbolize our female consciousness.

In using our dual soul and spirit consciousness we expand our thinking and emotions into realms that are at this time essentially unknown and unaccepted. Our consciousness is our original source of healing. Our purpose is not to simply heal our physical bodies, but our purpose is to become aware of the absolute wisdom and power in our trinity of minds and emotions as the many mansions of our consciousness that heals our immature soul. As our immature soul learns the art of creation in our daily physical experiences it is expanding its consciousness.

Our intellect as our immature, childlike mind focuses on our physical aspirations, self-judgement, and fear. Our intellectual focus allows us to create a sense of failure, a poor self-image, and depression, creating our reflection of self as a victim of our own beliefs in absolute and unquestionable external standards. Our facts exist only as the relative truth of our limited perception.

Our soul memory as our mature, adult mind focuses on our common sense (knowing), motivation, and enthusiasm. Our soul memory is aware of all the wisdom and ingenuity of our thought and emotions as the reality of consciousness that comes from our physical experience in our multiple lifetimes. Our mature soul consciousness is aware of the consistency and freedom of choice in the life design of the soul and the growing awareness that is occurring for the intellect as we experience the miracle of living. Our mature soul appreciates the beauty of our immature soul mind and emotional expansion as we learn our soul lessons of each new physical life.

Our spirit consciousness as our eternal mind, emotions, and sensory feelings focuses on our inspiration, creativity, and passion. Our spirit is in love with life and it cannot contain its excitement as it sees our intellect as its soul child growing in conscious awareness of the magnificent energy of eternal consciousness. Our spirit consciousness is our androgynous parent as the mother, son, divine child of our individual physical creation. Our spirit has the same pride in and devotion to us as we have in our physical children. Our spirit also has compassion for our lessons of patience, support, faith, and trust that we live as we struggle to expand into our mature soul consciousness that is reflected into our physical lives as we watch our children grow and mature into a life of their own.

The journey of our immature soul creation can be seen as it is reflected into intellectual thought as the personal level of our beliefs. We allow our beliefs to control our emotional soul, which creates our physical body, intellect, and behavior. Each lesson that we learn allows a greater degree of spirit thought into our immature intellectual soul as light, vibration, tone, color, chemical, and emotion, which changes our physical behavior. We are responsible for expanding our intellectual knowledge, which expands our conscious awareness and in turn allows more of our mature soul emotion of love as understanding into our physical perception of reality. Our dual soul as a male and female consciousness is eternal as a reflection of our spirit, clever as it uses the wisdom of all that we have experienced, and it will never give us a challenge that we are not ready to receive and learn.

Knowledge is the fourth level of our soul evolution and we must understand that all knowledge can be expanded. The current belief in mental disabilities comes from the judgement of the intellect. The intellect does not understand the soul journey of growth. Expanding our knowledge requires that our freedom of choice, will, and intention of evolution as a soul be a part of our daily creation of growth into our next level of consciousness. Where we begin as a level of consciousness is not important. Growth can occur when the consciousness is understood. The focus of our search for knowledge must be consistent with the path of changing our beliefs and behaviors as we open to understanding ourself and our relationship to all that is around us in nature, earth, and the universe. We must be willing to change the reality of our lifestyle if we are seeking the knowledge of our soul growth in consciousness. Our choice to evolve in our knowledge requires a willingness to consistently repattern our old beliefs with new ideas and thoughts. To create a new pattern of thought and emotions we must be willing to change the chemical balance that exists within our body. We must consciously honor and respect our chemical balance on a daily basis if we sincerely want to grow.

Beginning with the physical, biological needs that we were given at our moment of creation, we must breathe fresh air, drink fresh water, and eat the purest foods of nature that we can find. As we change our nutrition we begin to chemically change our body, our dual mind, and emotions more freely. As our body and brain heals its chemical balance internally, we begin to balance our mind and emotions so that we can create the dance of life that is essential to our soul and its growth. We have spent many billions of lifetimes suppressing our female emotions by our beliefs and the chemicals that we put into our body. As we change our emotions and our beliefs our word expression changes, allowing our language to express our emotional response. Our thinking and language response to this change shifts our thoughts and emotions to love and we can release our beliefs of fear, anger, control, and rage.

Those individuals that are stuck in the fear of physical beliefs will find it easiest to focus on the physical changes first, which will in turn support the mind and emotional changes. Our dual soul is dual within itself, having a double helix of mind and emotions which it must use together to be in balance. If the will to expand our intellectual knowledge is intense, we can comfortably focus on all facets of our soul expansion at one time and release the fear that suppresses our emotions and, therefore, paralyzes our soul evolution of consciousness.

Our thinking and emotions are controlled by the focus of our consciousness which is then reflected into our language as our reaction or response, common sense ability, intelligence, personality, attitude, character traits, emotions of fear or love, which becomes our individual persona. Our individual persona is again reflected into our physical body as the cellular structure viability and its behavior.

The most important internal physical approach to expanding our intellectual knowledge is an adequate and healthy blood supply to our brain provided by our oxygen, water, and nutrition, to insure the credibility of the chemicals that are internally operating the electromagnetic energy of our brain as well as our entire body. These same chemicals affect the sensory stimulation that we use to trigger our seven physical senses on all three dimensions of our consciousness, which expands our aware consciousness of the everyday life that we are living.

Our soul has designed relationships into our life to act as the fiber of our physical experience. Without relationships we would not trigger our aware consciousness into its different levels of expansion nearly as efficiently. We also use our environment of family and friends to trigger our growth. As we act out the behavior of our precise level of consciousness, we receive feedback from our family and friends by their acceptance of our behaviors or their challenge of us because of our behavior.

It is always important not to reward bad behavior or the ego consciousness of the soul thinks it has reached its destination of perfection and will try to control the behavior of everyone else in its life to match its own perception of perfection. Positive feedback for negative behavior has been common in the journey of our immature soul and has allowed us to support inequality, untruth, and fear from the beginning of our soul descent. Every facet of our physical lives in our immature soul journey has supported the inappropriate behavior of religion, family, science, medicine, politicians, education, and society.

Our brain is known to have one hundred trillion brain cells with only five to ten percent considered to be developed and used. Those brain cells that we have developed have only a limited number of messenger cells acting as neurotransmitters that connect them. The difference between our actual and potential

brain development is immense. Because we focus our consciousness in a linear direction we don't grasp the reality that our consciousness must function in a clockwise motion, forming a complete cycle. Our immature soul mind functions counterclockwise
as chaos, with a linear focus to the ego. It is the scientific intention to identify the precise point for each function of our body
within our brain. This is impossible because that creates limitations upon our brain and ignores our mind and emotional consciousness. The only factor that limits our consciousness is our
beliefs. Every brain cell has the absolute potential of every cell.

Our brain is like an endless beach of sand where we sit fearfully aware and intensely focused upon a single grain of sand as
our reality. In focusing upon the single grain we worry about our
survival. If we knew the drama that we have lived as a soul we
would laugh, and laugh, and laugh at ourselves. Our fear limits
us and it is one of the most ridiculous concepts that we have created because it denies the joyfulness, beauty, magnificence, and
wisdom of our soul.

To grow as humans we must expand our basis of knowledge
by expanding our intellectual mind. It is our focused, tunnel
belief that we can only expand our intellect by memorizing external processes, which we create as physical behaviors. Memorization by our intellect is a behavior of our immature soul mind.
Unless we first make a conscious choice to use our mind in an
open manner and not stay attached to restrictive beliefs, our
memorization will follow the boundaries that we have created by
our belief system. If we open our boundaries so that we have no
belief restrictions, we can immediately use our soul knowledge
that is stored in the cells of our "unused" or subconscious brain.

When we learn to use our total mind, our intellect that we
are conscious of existing, our soul memory that is subconscious
to our intellect, and our spirit memory that is unconscious in relationship to our intellect, then we have succeeded in expanding
our mind. At this point in our conscious awareness, we have
been focused upon expanding only our intellect because we
have not been taught to understand that we have a magnificent
mind that has no limitations once we use it as our integrated soul

mind and emotions. It is when we can freely use our integrated soul that we heal our mind of all fear. When our immature soul mind is healed of its fear emotions, we find ourself living the love of our mature soul. We create our daily experiences of life from the unconditional love of our spirit. In healing ourself we change our thoughts, words, and our behavior to positive, loving action.

There are ways of connecting our soul and spirit mind with our intellectual mind in which we can consciously use the spirit energy within us to support our mind expansion. Our spirit energy comes to us as chemical, light, vibration, tone, and color, and we feel the unconditional love, truth, and equality of our spirit, which is the behavior that we will live. Because energy is given to us in ways which we can readily assimilate it into our everyday life, we have an opportunity to use the higher frequencies of nature's energy to influence our daily activities. We can use full spectrum interior lighting, lots of windows, skylights, and be outdoors as much as possible. We can become conscious of the vibrations that we introduce into our daily life that affect the vibrations of our own electromagnetic energy field. If we are using a chain saw we will feel a different vibration than we will using a hair dryer, razor, or electric blanket. None of these vibrations can even begin to trigger our spirit energy, but classical music can. Listen to voices and become aware of the effect the vibration of the voice has upon your emotions. Listen to your own voice. We can listen to music that provides us with a vibration and a tone working together either in total discord, as in "heavy metal," or in harmony and rhythm as we hear in Mozart or Beethoven. We will choose music that is in harmony with our own vibration and tone. Our choice of colors in our house, car, clothing, and all personal items will reflect the amount of color that we accept from our spirit energy. Because we have been living in the dark side of our soul, we have traditionally used black hearses in funerals. Now we are beginning to see more white hearses, which reflects our change in beliefs. Our cars now come in multiple colors and shades of colors as do our clothes, houses, and personal items. As our mind opens and we are more comfortable with color we find ourselves more willing to eat colorful foods, which helps to balance the chemicals in our body.

Color, tone, vibration, and light can be consciously used as healing influences to open our mind and to help us find peace in our change. Red is a strong physical color, blue is the peace of our soul, and yellow is the love of our spirit. These are the primary colors from which we create the entire spectrum of color. Each color resonates with its own vibration and tone and can be used to lift us out of depression, to heal physical illnesses, and to help us open our mind to its complete spectrum of energy.

Music is a wonderful healing energy that can open our mind into higher and higher levels of harmony and rhythm. The more dissonance or discord in the vibration and tone of the note, the more primitive the emotional response within us. If we find ourself exposed to music that is not in harmony with our level of energy vibration, we can create disease that will first shut down our physical senses and then begin to break down our cellular structure. Silence is the highest form of vibration and tone that we can reach in our physical reality as we listen to our inner vibration and tone as the eternal music of our spirit consciousness.

Our tone and vibration are consistently reflected in our tone of voice and our electromagnetic energy field. When we are in the presence of a voice or body energy that is not in harmony with our own, we can begin to feel uncomfortable. Living with someone who is constantly screaming and yelling can begin to break down our cellular structure. Fearful or disrespectful words have a discordant vibration and tone that instantly affects our emotional response and allows self-judgement and depression, as physical reactions, to overwhelm us. Anger, abusive language, violent physical activity, and withdrawal all have a vibration and tone that causes fear to expand within us as we participate in these reactions and will stimulate fear in others that are close to our electromagnetic energy field. As we abuse ourself with any fearful emotions we expand our fear energy and attract other people with fear energy to us. Our vibration, tone, and dark color has reached out and magnetized energy of the same vibration, tone, and darkness.

it is by the level of light, vibration, tone, and color that we choose to use in our activities that we subconsciously and unconsciously expand or restrict our spirit light. The level of light that we accept into our intellect controls the chemicals that our body produces which creates our emotions and our behaviors as our physical reaction. The air we breathe, the water we drink, and the foods that we eat provide the chemicals within our cells that balance our inner light, vibration, tone, and color.

Once we can understand how we control and create ourself and our life, we can understand that we also have the freedom of choice to create what we want rather than what we don't want. Understanding that we have the power within our consciousness to expand our intellect into a conscious awareness of our soul memory and our spirit memory is the goal of our human consciousness.

Our intellect can be repatterned to include the memory of our soul and spirit through the conscious awareness and use of our physical senses. Our thinking and our communication are dramatically restricted if we are not consciously aware of the expansiveness of our ability to see, hear, taste, smell, and touch as our path to expanding our intellect. We have suppressed our first five physical senses as we have focused upon our thinking and speaking. Because of our focus upon separateness we do not see the wisdom of using the entire spectrum of our senses, and we have not been taught that our ability to think and speak is part of our senses and is essential to our evolving consciousness.

Our immature, childish intellect perceives life only as the external beliefs and activities of our physical reality and ignores or stays in ignorance of the wisdom, unity, and beauty of our mind as a trinity of consciousness gifted to us as our eternal spirit from our Creator. Our eternal spirit as thought is divided into a childish mind of the intellect, a mature mind of the soul, and a universal mind of our spirit. As a human species we are now face to face with the veil of our beliefs and because of our transitional use of both fear and love in our daily lives, we can feel the duality of our transitional soul emotions as we change back and forth in our thoughts.

As we rend the veil of our intellectual mind, we shift our perception of ourself and our life from fear to love and begin to live as a maturing mind seeking to understand the integration of our male and female consciousness. Our shift in thought as our perception of life is physically noticeable as our emotions and behavior reflect the light of our love in our self-image and activity. Our ability to create within our lives while using our positive thought rather than our negative thought is equivalent to our ability to work in a light room rather than a dark room. When we live within a light mind, we can understand our art of creation as a human species to learn and grow in our journey of soul evolution. If we "work" in a dark mind our limited vision can force us to change the way we perform tasks.

As we increase our exposure to natural light and to nature we will feel the light being absorbed by our skin. Many of us suffer depression during the winter months when the light from the sun is seen less often. Others will worship the sun to the point of damaging the skin in their efforts to absorb light. The light that enters our body through our eyes and our consciousness removes physical sluggishness, stress, mental confusion, depression, the winter blues as our feelings of darkness, and we begin to feel a new hope and excitement about life. Our eyes are the windows to our soul and reflect the three dimensions of our trinity of consciousness.

Light increases our attention span, sense of well-being, ability to relax, improves the acuity of our senses, and balances the vibration, tone, and color wavelengths in our electromagnetic energy field. A loving light mind creates health and happiness.

Fear reflects our being in the darkness of our mind and holds us captive in our sense of being unsatisfied, unworthy, unfulfilled, depressed, inadequate, judgmental, and having a poor self-image. A fearful and dark or negative mind creates a sick body and sick behavior.

The external focus of science had not changed its external perception for hundreds of years until it began researching our DNA, which it continues to perceive as external cause and effect. Medicine has studied our body and mind from the externai concept of our finite physical matter being victimized by organisms that should be weaker than we are. What are we doing to ourselves to change the dominion ratio? How do we create our imbalance that allows us to lose our dominion as a human organism?

Despite our focus on physical processes as our healing strength, we have not reached our full potential in healing even with those physical processes. Because we have focused upon science and technology instead of our own power of change we have bypassed those internal processes that could have been used to enhance our mind and its communication and coordination with the body.

Mental disabilities have been accepted as handicaps and treatment has now been relegated to the external use of chemicals and physical support. We have not focused upon the ways in which we can change the production of our internal chemicals and hormones, which can repattern our brain. Yet science accepts some mental disease as a chemical imbalance. Physical disease is also a chemical imbalance, although we have not been educated into an understanding of how we create disease as the outcome of our chemical imbalance. Our scientific perception of external cause and effect prevents our consciousness from recognizing that our cause and effect are internal.

In expanding our intellect into an understanding of ourself as a trinity of consciousness with a dual focus of minds and emotions, we can begin to see the folly of our ways. As science learned to separate us into body and mind parts, the relationship between our mind, body, and emotions was essentially lost. With the scientific focus of blame being both external and separate, the power of our dual soul, body, and spirit consciousness to function as a whole regardless of our focus continued with less and less awareness of our innocent interference in the nature of our very being. The more interference we accepted from science the more separate and external we became from our dual soul memory and our spirit consciousness. As our intellectual mind becomes addicted to scientific beliefs, we strengthen the cosmic shell that separates us from our mature soul and spirit mind.

Religion and science have both contributed to our resistance to internal growth and have added new beliefs to our cosmic shell, preventing the true expansion of our intellect. Because our cosmic shell is so firmly in place and is limiting us in our freedom of emotion, thought, choice, will, and intention, it forces us to use our intellect in repetitive cycles of beliefs and behaviors until we realize they are not true. The more conscious we become that our beliefs and behaviors are not logical and no longer serve our growth, the more willing we are to begin new patterns of thought within our mind as the source of creating our life.

To expand our intellect we must shift our thought out of the fearful bondage of our beliefs and begin to think differently, using new images of new pictures. We can approach our shift in thought very simply by looking at the positive aspects of the image instead of the negative aspects of the image. This is equal to the glass of water being seen as half full, rather than half empty.

Think of a relationship example. Let your mind begin to imagine yourself walking in the other person's shoes. As you become the other person, be aware of how you relate to yourself. Examine your communication, your history, words, thoughts, feelings, the acuity of your physical senses, life experiences that you know the other person has experienced. How would you feel if you had had the same exposures, dramas, traumas, losses, challenges, relationships, and physical experiences? See if you can find a connection of lessons within the experiences you are imagining and you. How would you be feeling now if you had had the same experiences?

Once you can imagine yourself as another person you begin to open your intellect to your soul. You are not isolated and separate as the physical body that you enjoy today. You are a host of consciousness levels that you lived in other lives. Some are hidden, some you are acting out, some are depressed, some are happy, and from this collage of other lives you are always mirroring your own soul memory. It is your own soul memory that is attracting you into your present lesson. What lesson are you acting out in your relationship? Don't be afraid to look at yourself. Look without blame or judgement. Keep your consciousness open and the images flowing until you can see the lesson in your relationships.

Actors and actresses have old souls that are challenging them
with images of themselves in other lives as a way of triggering their soul memory. If an actor or actress can personally relate to the character they are playing they will see their own image in the lessons of the character. This is an active perception of the soul lessons. We can observe our family and friends in their life dramas and passively learn our personal soul lessons. Learning is synonymous with understanding the relationship to yourself. Our consciousness creates our thinking and emotions and this creates the perception of life which we live. As our internal conscious-ness of truth changes, we change our perception of life and the physical experiences that we create.

Change defines our pattern of growth as a soul. As we change our level of consciousness with knowledge, we release our primitive superstitions and rituals that have created the beliefs and behaviors of our lives. Change reflects our art of cre-ation as our consciousness reality in the immature soul, as it cre-ates the physical experiences of our life, moment by moment.

THE JOURNEY OF
OUR DUAL SOUL

As a trinity of consciousness, we are at all times spirit energy but we live as human beings through the journey of our dual soul with the purpose of expanding our consciousness. The journey of our dual soul has taken us on a descending route into the animal instincts of our physical nature, into the transitioning beliefs of our religious perception, and now we are entering into the spiritual reality of our mature soul as our Divine Nature. Those individuals who are fearful of change will hold on to the ancient beliefs of our revolving but descending emotional soul and the beliefs of our religious period of revolution. If it is our choice to continue with evolution, we must release our primitive religious beliefs and begin to live the spirituality of our ascending loving soul emotions.

In our descending and revolving soul journey, we have believed that our soul and spirit are a mystery. When we are ignorant of reality, we call the missing bits of knowledge a "mystery" because the knowledge is not understood by our intellect. Our ego wants our intellect to believe that the "mystery" is beyond our intellectual understanding. The only reason that any knowledge is beyond the grasp of our intellect is our beliefs, which limit our imagination and our search for knowledge as our beliefs remove our freedom of thought.

Our dual soul and spirit is the eternal consciousness energy of us. Our soul is our dual mind and emotions of male and female consciousness, which is seated in our male left brain as our infantile intellectual mind and our fear emotions and in our female right brain as our soul memory and loving emotions. Our

spirit is the core of us and is seated in our limbic system, cerebellum, brain stem, and spinal cord, which controls all three dimensions of our senses through our cellular, central, and autonomic nervous systems.

We began as spirit consciousness of thought and we developed the pattern of our physical matter through the physical experience of our indwelling spirit consciousness and our male and female dual soul consciousness as Lord. Once the pattern was completed for the temple of our physical body, we began our journey as a dual soul mind and emotions, which was focused on developing an awareness of ourself through the physical experience of being human. As a male and female consciousness, we were made the Lord of our soul and were given dominion or choice over the physical experiences of our creation of life.

For aeons we have been living in the dark and fearful part of our immature soul mind and emotions as we have lived the learning experiences of what we don't want. At this point in the journey of our dual soul, we are reaching the point of transitioning into the understanding of our mature soul mind and emotions. As we have lived the experience of our immature soul journey to become a mature soul, we have chosen to live through the sexual focus of our male physical nature as both males and females. As we live our transition we are entering the positive, loving essense of our female Divine Nature as our mature soul.

From the time that we began our spirit journey as thoughtform, we have had a purpose of expansion of consciousness as our intention as a dual soul. Evolution of our soul has occurred within us without our intellect and ego being conscious of the change because of continuing attrition. Therefore our soul memory has remained subconscious to our intellect and our spirit consciousness has been an unconscious presence for our intellect. This has been no accidental occurrence for the trinity of our consciousness. Our spirit consciousness designed our dual soul mind and emotions to experience through the temple of our physical matter as a method of expanding itself into the essense of "God" from its seed of thought.

In the beginning of each lifetime as a child, we have faint memories of our returning to earth in a new body with a new beginning for the soul. As our belief systems are re-programmed we lose these memories of multiple incarnations and begin to separate ourselves mentally into the "one-life" perception of our physical beliefs. At the same time we begin to externalize our belief in the seed of God that lives within us. As we adopt the current beliefs of each lifetime, we develop the belief that we have total understanding of what life is about. Our religious belief in "one life" and our scientific belief that "we know it all" strengthened our ego and supported our primitive beliefs in our intellectual superiority.

Religion has taught us that we have only one life. This belief acts as our first resistance to change because it keeps us from seeing that what we do in one life affects our next life. As we returned time after time into new bodies, we forgot the relationship that we had to nature. The more confidence we acquired that our intellect was supreme the more separated we became from the support of nature that is essential to our physical health and evolution. As we lost our memory of the effect of natural foods within our body, it became essential to change bodies more frequently to prevent mutating our DNA beyond repair.

When the food that we eat affects our genetic structure the mutation that is created will stay with the soul until the lesson that prompted our eating problems is learned. The more expansive our lesson of eating becomes the more all-encompassing it becomes as it moves from an individual lesson to a societal lesson and then to an earth lesson. As a society we now have more mutations and more diseases because disease is an internal lesson for our soul. Disease gives our soul an opportunity to work with our lessons internally even though intellectually we do not have a conscious awareness of the lesson.

As we have lost respect for the purity of food that we eat and have allowed our quick-fix mentality to unconsciously accept a lifestyle of eating dead food, we are compromising the genetic pattern of our soul. All through the journey of our soul we have eaten without an awareness of the quality of food that we eat or how that food reacts within our cells to restore or to decay our physical body. The ignorance of our relationship to nature and to each other prompted "God" to create the parable of Adam and Eve in the lushness of the Garden of Eden as a symbol to help us remember our biological need for air, water, and nature's foods. In showing us that we are both male and female and that we must eat from the foods of nature to survive, we were shown the fractal pattern that our chemical consciousness of spirit as "God" and our male and female soul as the "Lord" created into the physical design of our body as an inherent memory.

Our lessons of food and eating are present on all three levels, within us, within society, and within the world. We innocently expand our self-abuse through our ignorance of the food that we require to restore and rejuvenate our physical body and mind, the environment, and the balance of earth. As our abuse spreads we innocently share our abusive behavior with other countries and absorb their abuse as our own. We began sharing our beliefs about food as we lived the opposite of the design of our chemical physical body.

The greed that is in the heart of our business executives cares nothing about the abuse they inflict upon humanity and society. Our political and government regulations also reflect this same mentality when, for example, a pesticide such as DDT is outlawed in the United States, and the product is then shipped to foreign countries and used on their crops. As the foreign crops are brought back into the United States, the citizens of the U.S. eat the food that has been sprayed with the DDT. As we innocently feel that we are being protected by our government, we are in fact developing more and more cancer and other diseases as a result of the denial and greed of corporate America. Genetic engineering and irradiation destroys the credibility of our food, as do pesticides. The history of our food industry explains our history of disease. Food and disease are inherently linked in humans as the microcosm, society as the mesocosm, and in the world as the macrocosm.

Because our medical community has not been taught the value of natural food in preventing disease, many physicians feel that food has nothing to do with disease. This is an illusion of great ignorance which indicates a lack of understanding of the chemical connection that we as human beings have with nature and our dependency on nature for restoration of our body and health. Science has been living the belief of "knowing it all." Because of their belief, scientists and physicians have ignored over one hundred years of research and continued with their focus on the external pharmacological side of medicine, which is at all times motivated by money. If we corrected our food intake and prevented the major diseases of the world, we would threaten the drug industry. Instead of our feeling threatened, it is time for us to bring about a change of focus in medicine where the welfare of humanity is more important than the money that is made in the stock market.

The journey of our immature soul is to reach the level of integration within ourselves as a trinity of matter, soul, and spirit that is using our physical experience as a way of learning. Each person on earth is living a personal agenda of soul lessons. Because we are all evolving souls, we are given the opportunity of experiencing each lesson on all three dimensions of reality in the infinite images of each lesson. Integration is an unobtainable goal when we die so young that our soul repetitiously repeats the same phases of life again and again without an aware consciousness of what we are creating. Our beliefs hold us captive in repetition. Science, religion, outmoded family values, and our sexuality are held in such high esteem in our immature soul mind and emotions that we feel guilty and sinful if we dare to think about the possibility of change. Our immature soul mind is the supreme force of our physical nature, which focuses on our sexual energy as our external source of power. Our thinking and emotions must grow and change before our transition can occur. Our beliefs act as our denial and resistance, and they are the ego pattern of thought that keeps us repetitiously living the same experiences over and over again. We cling to our repetitious beliefs as fact and deny

the growth of our consciousness in the identical way that we
deny our lessons of history

Expanding our consciousness brings us to an understanding
of the interpenetration and interaction of our physical body, our
dual soul mind and emotions, and our spirit consciousness. It is
impossible for us to conceive of this intermingling of our energy
forces if we ignore the fact that we have invisible energy forces
that are at all times active within us as our lifeforce energy. We
must recognize our trinity of consciousness to understand ourself. Our beliefs about religion, science, sexuality, and the roles
of the family unit are archaic and obsolete to a soul that is learning the value of balancing its dual soul and physical matter into
the equality of its spirit.

To balance our body we must learn to balance our cellular
structure and the chemicals within our cells as the fractal pattern
of our soul design which is reflected in our DNA. It is our responsibility to maintain the healthy function of our DNA by replacing
the hydrogen, oxygen, carbon, nitrogen, and minerals that make
up the design of our internal and external matter. Our DNA is a
master chemist that understands how to break down these various atoms into an infinite number of chemicals, hormones,
enzymes, and amino acids to provide the exact elements needed
by our body. Unless we provide our cells with the raw material
in pure chemical form this conversion will not occur and our
cells will begin to mutate into a state of imbalance. The excesses
and deficiencies of chemicals within our body are the source of
both mental and physical diseases.

To balance our dual soul we must openly use both our left
and right brain and our emotions equally. We balance our physical nature with our Divine Nature by releasing the beliefs, negativity, fear, and externalization of our intellect and ego. As our
ego transitions into humility and the light from our spirit and
mature soul enlightens our intellect, we reach a state of balance
within our dual soul mind and emotions. If we are supporting
our soul growth with the chemicals that balance our body and
soul we can live longer physical lives. When this transition is
complete we will internalize our lessons, love ourself and other

people equally, and consistently live our truth with a positive mind and loving emotions. With physical nutritional support our soul has the opportunity to change with ease.

To balance our spirit we must consciously use all levels of our senses in our daily life. As we eat the food that balances our physical body, we stimulate all levels of senses within our body which in turn stimulates our loving emotions and positive mind. Acute and positive sensing cannot happen without nature's support of our cellular structure, and the dual levels of our soul mind and emotions being in balance. We are at no time separate as a physical body, dual soul, and spirit. Our thinking, language, and behavior consistently reflects the level of our dual mind and emotional soul balance, physical chemical balance, and spirit sensory balance that we have grown into as our level of conscious awareness.

As a soul we have reached the level of knowledge that can keep our body and mind healthy for hundreds of years if we live through a more complete state of balance. But when our beliefs ignore the knowledge of the intention of our soul journey, and as a society we focus on making money at all costs, we are creating a scenario that will bring us to the brink of disaster as our physical body, dual soul mind and emotions, and our spirit senses are in a total state of imbalance, creating chaos in our lives as our personal creation.

We have now reached the brink of disaster from our own ignorance. Although the knowledge is there it is not put together, piece by piece, until the picture is clearly understood in its relationship to our body, dual soul, and spirit as a trinity of consciousness and accepted by people, science, and religion. We remain ignorant of our trinity of consciousness as matter, dual soul, and spirit because of our beliefs in fear, inequality, and separation. When we stay in ignorance of who we are personally, spiritually, and scientifically, we have little hope of solving the mystery of disease in any part of ourself, society, or the world. When we fail to see ourselves as a male, female, and spirit consciousness, we cannot understand that our balance is our healing.

Having said this we must now look at why the information is not put together and understood by science. Science has been separated into multiple disciplines that do not search for the intermingling of information in relationship to us as human beings. Each discipline has its wealth of facts that are meaningless by themselves because they are looked at only in terms of their external influence on theory. Opening the mind to find each missing piece of the puzzle is essential. Looking at the disastrous condition of humanity today should be the first clue that many parts of our knowledge are not understood in relationship to who we are.

If medicine, chemistry, quantum physics, botany, orthomolecular biology, genetics, environmental sciences, and agriculture all examined their information in relationship to human health as our internal secret of life, great discoveries would be forthcoming. If all of science would then examine the cumulative knowledge in relationship to religious knowledge, many of the limiting beliefs of religion would change. Our beliefs are the limitations of our mind that close the mind to any information that doesn't fit into its belief concepts. Our attachment to old theories as absolute truth has deceived us for many millions of years.

Research could now be done on the DNA at birth and death, providing the information to prove rebirth as well as the mutation of the DNA from lifestyle habits, including food habits. The DNA is the pattern of the journey of the soul as it expands its level of consciousness and it contains the mutations that the soul has created within the lessons of past lives. Choosing the parents to support our mutations gives the soul an opportunity to learn the lesson and to heal the fractal pattern of its DNA. Science has only begun in the past one hundred years to understand some of the internal chemical design of matter. Once the perception of life is changed the technology of the sciences will allow for research that will solve the mystery of physical and mental disease, crime, learning difficulties, and disabilities.

No one discipline knows "all" of the information, although that is the precise belief of the individual who supports separation as ignorance in science. Of all of these scientific disciplines chemistry and biology come the closest to understanding the Universal Laws of the soul and spirit and its relationship to matter. Chemists are the jewels of understanding our chemical structure as a trinity of consciousness living in matter. Biochemistry is the key to understanding long life, as it is the very force that patterns, motivates, and inspires life in matter. Mathematics and fractal geometry can explain the fractal patterns of life. Physics can explain the Universal Laws. Other scientific disciplines add their expertise to the puzzle of creation and can help us understand ourselves.

The information to understand the invisible soul and spirit and its role in physical matter was initially passed down from the energy of "God" to humanity. The greed and hunger for power within man has always interfered with the purity of this information. The belief that "man" was created in the external image of "God" as the mirror image of man has created inequality as an imbalance within the dual soul because our soul is both male and female.

Living the inequality of "man as superior to woman" has kept our dual soul mind and emotions in a continual state of inequality and imbalance since the beginning of time. This belief in the superiority of man has been supported in the family moral value system, religion, and science for thousands of years. Our belief in inequality has convoluted the focus of our mind and emotions and kept our intellect in the dark, allowing our mind to grow through judgement, fear, control, and separateness.

Information was hidden or concealed in prophecy, because to reveal this information would have brought persecution to those who believed opposite to the masses. The Hebrews wanted Jesus crucified because they believed that adapting to his different style of thinking, language, and behavior would have interfered with the economics of their society. They wanted Jesus to be the "Messiah" who would save them and at the same time allow them their errant ways. When he refused they wanted to persecute him and his teachings. Two thousand years later the beliefs remain the same, as people want Jesus to save them without their accepting personal responsibility for changing their thinking, language, and behavior.

Persecution was not only the role that religion assumed with the masses but it has consistently been the role that science has assumed. The fear of persecution drove the true information underground long before the written word was common and it stayed unknown to the masses. As information was passed through the families, it was changed and corroded by the need to control as an adherence to the belief system. The art of writing, interpretation, and bookmaking was first controlled by the Hebrews as their family histories and ancient beliefs were recorded by various religious sects as truth.

It is in these manuscripts that much of the information was concealed by the Kabbalists who became one of the four major sects to go underground to avoid persecution by the Catholic Church. These sects were known as the Freemasons, Kabbalists, Rosicrucians, and Sufis and represented different religious beliefs. The Freemasons were primarily of Christian origin. The Kabbalists were primarily of Hebrew beliefs. The Rosicrucians were primarily of Hindu beliefs. The Sufis were the "mystic" sect of Muslim beliefs as the followers of Mohammed. At the time that these sects were attempting to reveal their beliefs in the word of God, they feared for their lives. The beliefs of the rulers and their version of religion, which was being used as a means of controlling the masses, were an economic windfall for those in power. Money and power were an incentive to hold tightly to the control and to remove by persecution any individual who had the audacity to object to the religion of the kingdom as absolute truth for the masses.

Not only did the sects go underground to conceal the truths of humanity and the true journey of the soul, but they symbolized the information as another level of concealment. As the generations have passed, much of the concealed information has been lost to current generations. The symbols have become meaningless or misinterpreted, leading to the superstitions and mysteries surrounding the true knowledge. Few find the available written materials of these sects intelligible even when they are available. When truth is read by the religious intellect it provokes anger and it is not seen as truth but as heresy. Heresy incites violence toward those who believe differently and sets one human against another in violence, which is a current method of persecution as inequality.

The intellect has become so controlled with pain, suffering, and punishment that the mind cannot grasp the true meaning of creation. The belief in only one life has been comfortable for two thousand years and the wall of denial that this belief has created through the singular power of religion is an example of putrid fear. The intellect does not want to change as it has patterned its own concealment from the soul and spirit by its cosmic shell of beliefs. The fear of revealing the intellect and its ego beliefs to self can bring about self-persecution and self-abuse that fulfills the pain and suffering of the concealment. Concealment is a major lesson of disease in our society today.

Religious fear of the unknown casts the internal "being" as evil and dark, something to be concealed and not revealed to another human soul. At different intervals in the history of humanity, old souls have returned to earth with total memory of the invisible energy of the consciousness of the dual soul and spirit. Because our beliefs are still attached to the persecution of those who are different, these individuals were considered dark and evil spirits and have been beheaded, hung, burned at the stake, and banished from society as guilty of sin against religious beliefs.

As the collective consciousness of evolved souls is gradually expanding within society, the persecution has been tempered with the change in balance of the dual immature soul mind and emotions. More and more of humanity are facing the transition of their immature soul, from the darkness of the intellect and ego that is consumed by fear to the depression of the immature soul's transition. When our beliefs tell us one thing and our intellect finds the belief illogical, duality is created in our mind, which is defined as depression because it descends our emotions into uncontrollable fear, anxiety, stress, and phobias. In our heart we will always feel truth.

This change has been gradually evolving within the masses of souls upon earth for several thousand years. When the spirit consciousness, referred to as "Jesus," made his last physical appearance upon earth nearly two thousand years ago in the body of the man known as Jesus of Nazareth, Jesus clearly saw that the immature soul of man was not ready to change its worshipping and dependent beliefs.

When the energy of "God" became a living soul in human form as each of us and as "Jesus," we became "children of God" created in the fractal pattern of the universal chemical energy of Spirit Consciousness as male, female, and spirit. Old, advanced souls that remember the information of creation have always been on earth as guides to keep the awareness of the dual soul journey predominant in the minds of those who are ready for change. When Jesus came to earth, we had already entered the level of knowledge for the soul and we were living our revolutions. It was Jesus's fervent hope that we were ready to become equal within our male and female consciousness. Jesus saw that man was not ready to change his beliefs, and in his disappointment with man he accepted that he need not stay on earth. We were revolving in the transitional level of our immature soul evolution and were being challenged to open our mind to the Christ Consciousness within us. Our challenge to complete our soul transition into the equality of our integrated male and female consciousness has motivated us to live the experience of inequality and abuse in every facet of our lives. It is by living the repetition of our immature soul lessons that we will finally learn truth and reveal our dual soul as a trinity of consciousness.

Recognition and acknowledgement of the Christ Consciousness within us is essential for the transition of our dual soul from the external, negative, and fearful perception of life to the internal, positive, and loving perception of life. When we fulfill this precise phase of our evolution, as our immature soul ascends into the wisdom, understanding, absolute truth, and unconditional love of ourself and other people, we will become the Second Coming of the Christ Consciousness upon earth. As we complete our transition and enter into the second half of the journey of our evolving soul consciousness, we can look at ourselves and clearly see the value of what we have learned. Because we are seeking to balance our matter, dual soul, and spirit, we must spend as much time in the mature side of our soul as we have spent in the immature side of our soul. The difference in our mature soul journey is that we will have given up living the "hell" that we have created in our immature soul journey, and we will happily create a "heaven" to replace it. Hell is our chaos. Heaven is our harmony.

Having reached the transitional level of our dual soul journey without having a conscious awareness of more than one life has created a convolution of the duality that we are living. The religious belief that we have in only one life is a dramatic wall of denial within our intellectual soul mind. Our denial triggers us to repeat and live multiple levels of fear in all facets of our life. The three primary levels of our fear are acted out in our language and behavior as judgement which creates control, manipulation, and seduction; anger, which creates conformity; and rage, which creates rebellion. It is only when we reach the level of rage and begin to rebel that we are willing to face changing our beliefs.

Judgement as our first level of fear is an insidious and destructive energy that sets the stage for change because the consistent judgement is usually delivered in a language of nagging that can only be tolerated for a limited period of time in any relationship. Judgement can take the form of control, manipulation, or seduction and therefore it is not always recognizable because of the illusion that it creates. Listen to the language, because judgement is frequently delivered in a constant, repetitious form of nagging that is the most insidious level of talking. Nagging is talking as a distraction for one's own mind and not as a form of communication to another person. Naggers will frequently have a habit of talking out loud to themselves because they find the sound of their voice reassures them that they remain in control.

Anger is our stasis level of denial. We will conform to our anger despite the external image of ourself that we want others to see. Those individuals in the stasis level of anger and conformity seek revenge for each and every feeling of anger in a subtle and hidden way. Revenge can be directed towards money, destruction of the person, destruction of relationships, destruc-

tion of life, or destruction of a career. It is our anger that has escalated the litigation in all manner of relationships purely to seek
revenge and punishment. This is especially true in divorces, med-ical care, and in any situation where wrongdoing is felt as rejection, abandonment, or inequality. Our anger seeks external
revenge with pain, suffering, and punishment as a form of personal redemption to justify internal shame, guilt, and sin.

The third level of our fear that has turned to rage will be
acted out in rebellion. In rebellion we seek our revenge as a
form of external destruction and external self-destruction as
physical abuse of our body. External destruction of other people
or things will be the first level of rebellious revenge. This means
that we will behave with a total disrespect for life, possessions,
honor, and value. Killing people will be commonplace. This
takes place externally because there is no love internally for self.
As we rebel and seek revenge externally, we have expectations
of abuse as support for our self-abuse as an internal punishment
or reward.

Our revenge that is directed towards ourself will take the
form of rebelling against beliefs, languages, behaviors, and
images that we hold as expectations of ourself. Suicide is a level
of rebellion against self that can bring about change for the
immature soul if the lesson is learned from the physical experience. Some souls will consistently commit suicide in many lifetimes before they learn the lesson of self-destructive rebellion.

All levels of fear are cumulative and therefore self-judgement,
self-anger, self-abuse, self-rage, and self-destruction are all knotted
together as the soul is working through its lessons in multiple
images. Each level of fear is internally self-directed first and mirrored externally to others through our thinking, language, and
behavior and completes its cycle by the evolution or devolution
of our soul.

True love of another person is not possible for our immature
soul until we learn to love ourself. Because we do not love ourself, our immature soul journey has been motivated by the sexual attraction of our physical nature, which has kept us in relationships, giving us an opportunity to see the image of our imma-

ture soul lesson in the other person. This has made it easy for us to see another's "faults," but it has been a challenge for us to look internally and see those "faults" as our own.

The illusion of love that our immature soul has experienced as sexual attraction keeps us focused on seeking the unconditional love of our spirit. Without our sense of "physical need" we would not grow and stay focused on the energy of love in our mature soul emotions that is magnetizing us to itself. The love and its emotions of happiness, enthusiasm, excitement, joy, bliss, passion, and ecstasy, that will be ours as we transition into the loving side of our mature soul mind and emotions, will far surpass all emotions that we have been conscious of in the immature journey of our soul. So far in the immature journey of our soul we have never experienced the truth of our mature soul and spirit love. Sexual love has become our illusion of life.

Gaining the knowledge to consciously understand the journey of our immature soul is vital to the growth of all humanity. Having reached this point of transition we must expand the collective consciousness of knowledge for all to change or some will change and others will devolve. The strongest force of consciousness will control the force of the collective motion of humanity. Change is the lesson of compassion for the soul and spirit, and internal compassion cannot be bought or given, it must be earned as knowledge by each soul. The knowledge gained must fulfill our understanding of the relationship of the knowledge to us as matter, dual soul, and spirit. Internal compassion is earned when our humility transitions the knowledge into wisdom. External compassion, as physical compassion, is the first image of the lesson on our journey in soul knowledge.

As we transition in the level of knowledge for our dual soul, we are completing half of our soul journey toward becoming integrated as a human being. Transitioning of our dual soul mind and emotions is an internal change that can only take place when we are ready to learn the internal lessons of our dual soul as a male and female consciousness with the freedom of choice in our thinking, emotions, and feelings. We alone must pull ourselves through the eye of the needle.

Understanding the knowledge of our invisible soul and spirit must be the first step to change. We can no longer deny that we are soul and spirit by externalizing our image of "God" as the

image of man. Externalizing the image of God from ourself is the first step of separation for our dual soul and spirit from our trinity of consciousness with our internal spirit reality. The trinity of "God" as the trinity of consciousness creation is reflected in each of us. Each of us is an immature soul of male physical nature consciousness and a mature soul of female Divine Consciousness. We are not separate. We are integrated as one. We are matter, dual soul, and spirit. We are one as a trinity of consciousness of male, female, and spirit.

Symbols, Myths, Superstitions and Rituals

ynesius (365 B.C.), Bishop of Ptolemais and a devout Christian of his time, once wrote: "A Spirit that loves wisdom and contemplates the Truth close at hand, is forced to disguise it, to induce the multitudes to accept it....Fictions are necessary to the people and the Truth becomes deadly to those who are not strong enough to contemplate it in all of its brilliance....The truth must be kept secret and the masses need a teaching proportioned to their imperfect reason." Synesius studied in Alexandria as a lifetime student of Hypatia, studying mathematics and philosophy. Hypatia remained his lifelong closest friend and he was devoted to her, calling her "the true exponent of the true philosophy."

This quote symbolizes the method in which all information has been handled from the beginning of creation, and including the present time. As we have been growing in the fear of our immature soul, we were simply not prepared to accept the reality of who we are and our purpose on earth, and therefore we created our approach to truth as relative to our beliefs and needs. Information has been given to certain individuals who have mastered the art of hearing since the beginning of our immature soul level of knowledge. But even for those who could hear, it was understood that most people would not be open to changing their beliefs and truth was altered to fit the times. Each and every sexual, religious, and scientific belief that we live as a karmic

101

belief today originated in our primitive lives from symbols, myths, superstitions, and rituals of our immature soul.

The biblical stories that we have treasured symbolize the cloaking of information until we are ready to understand the parable. In the same way that we believe God gave Adam and Eve clothing, we have had our knowledge of self cloaked in garments of symbols, superstitions, and rituals. The nakedness of Adam and Eve is the symbol of our mind being open at the time that we were created. Clothing Adam and Eve in the skin of animals symbolizes how our physical nature, as the animal part of us, clothed or hid our knowledge of creation from us by the cosmic shell of our belief system.

The missing information for us throughout our soul path is that we have not understood our dual soul and spirit. Without an understanding of both our dual soul and spirit as an integrated consciousness energy of our physical body, we are helpless to understand ourselves. When we can't understand ourselves, we focus on the myths, superstition, and rituals of our external physical nature. Our soul is the male and female consciousness of our dual mind and emotions that is being used to expand our consciousness of self. Our spirit is our indwelling "God" consciousness that provides us with the *"elan vital,"* or lifeforce energy, to live in our physical nature.

Man, in his attachment to myths, superstitions, rituals, and karmic beliefs, has made the image of God into his own image and worshipped the image of himself as his idol. In many ways our immature soul journey has been perfect, because as man has created the idol of himself to worship he is learning that he is the only person that can save himself. Our lesson of "salvation" has been cloaked in the garments of superstition and beliefs that have allowed man to live through the veils of each belief one step at a time.

As we have descended further and further into the depths of our emotional or female soul we have lost all memory of who we are and we have focused our beliefs about who we are on our physical image. The more intensely we direct our beliefs toward our physical image the more we cloak the consciousness of our spirit and mature soul and act out the sexual focus of our physical nature as our dramas of life. In the past two thousand years we have dramatically increased our focus on our physical image and have lived the reality of not being able to physically save ourselves from pain and suffering. Each generation is being patterned by our family, science, society, and religion into the negative beliefs and fears of our physical reality. Religion is the Antichrist Myths of the physical nature of our immature soul.

Our soul has learned in the same exact way that we learn, which is through the physical experiences of life. It is our need for physical experience to use as our tool of growth that required that our immature soul be designed in such a way that it could continue its journey through multiple lifetimes until it fulfilled its purpose of being human. Each lifetime has ascended our mind and descended our emotions in our immature soul. We have acted out our descending emotions by believing and living female inequality. The female symbolizes our emotions. By focusing only on our mind and suppressing our emotions, we have not lived the truth of our creation as a dual soul of male and female consciousness.

Because we hold our learned lessons subconsciously in our right brain and unconsciously in our cerebellum, our conscious intellect has not a clue of the miracle of life that the immature soul has been living. Our intellectual mind is a blank slate that must be repatterned in the first fourteen years of each physical life. Intellectually our ascending soul mind and descending soul emotions is about gathering knowledge for the soul mind of wisdom until we have enough knowledge to understand ourselves and enough self-love to sustain our emotional transition. Our immature mind descends as we absorb beliefs and behaviors that we are exposed to as children. We consciously work with the growth of our mind through education and knowledge, which we filter through our beliefs and behaviors subconsciously. If we are taught to be fearful, we will at the same time descend our female emotions as a suppression of love. Religion has created the foundation of our emotional suppression by physical suppression of the female, and it has also suppressed the mind by teaching blind faith as conformity to religious beliefs rather than expanding our knowledge. Blind faith controls the freedom of thought and emotions. As the symbol of the Antichrist, religion supports ignorance and creates religious beliefs as the most addictive habit of our physical nature.

Because of the organization of our fractal pattern, we have lived our eternal life and returned consistently into a new life without having a consciousness of the organization and discipline of our dual soul. Because of our belief systems we have not accepted our eternal life as a soul and spirit that requires a physical body and a continual physical experience as a necessity of evolution. Without conscious memory being passed from one life to another, we have believed that we live only one life. We have stored knowledge in our right brain and karmic beliefs in the ego of our left brain. In each life we block out our mature soul memory by our subconscious ego and we suppress our emotions that are limited by our religious beliefs.

Our left brain focus has kept us ignorant of how our dual soul and spirit functions as an integrated trinity of consciousness energy. Our immature soul mind believes the myths, superstitions, rituals, and karmic beliefs that it is attached to by ignorance. As we focus on scientific beliefs, we begin to ascend our mind beyond our religious beliefs by attempting to understand our myths, superstitions, and rituals. We create our entire world as the precise drama of life that we live from the focus of our immature soul mind and our descending emotions. When a large number of people have the same mental and emotional focus, we create a collective consciousness in society and within the world from that collective focus. Our collective consciousness of the "freedom of religion" has created our addiction to our religious beliefs. Freedom of religion is an illusion because as an immature soul we are kept dependent and in bondage by our controlling religious beliefs.

Because we have evolved with our karmic religious beliefs as immature souls, we are now revolving in that singular level of collective consciousness. We are fearful of any mention of change because we are fearful of the punishment of "God." Our old karmic beliefs in myths, superstitions, and rituals are the chains that bind our soul tightly within its descending emotional path and prevent our evolution into the ascending path. Our fears of death, hell, punishment, and the wrath of God create whole lifetimes of pain and suffering because of our attachment to myths that are illusions of our primitive ego mind.

Understanding the reality of ourselves and the importance of changing our perception of life as we continue on our journey as an immature soul has always been a major challenge for us mentally and emotionally because of our beliefs. As an intellect we develop beliefs and habits of thinking that we accept as the only way that we can think and live our life. Our intellect and ego is dedicated to its supremacy and sees new thought as a threat to its control. When the ego and intellect feels threatened by the internal soul growth, it does not understand and it will attach itself to addictions, beliefs, physical processes, distractions, hero or idol worship, and it will frequently pursue dependent intimate relationships. Our intellect will always be a part of us because it is part of our immature soul mind. Our ego faces change as we face change, but it does not face extinction. Our ego becomes our humility as we grow into our internal wisdom and love.

The ego has been created from the multiple fear beliefs that we have accumulated during our journey as a descending emotional soul. When we enter into the ascending emotional soul our ego is transformed into humility and it looks in total awe at the magnificence and wisdom of our mature soul. Supremacy and humility are opposite attitudes of our immature and mature soul, which represents our ego belief that our intellectual soul mind is supreme and our mature soul knowing that the ego isn't yet in the humility of the ascending emotional soul.

The book of Revelation is a perfect example of our myths, beliefs, and karma that we have clung to as truth throughout the entire journey of our immature soul. This biblical book symbolizes the journey of our immature soul and the transition that our soul is living as it awakens to the mature soul. The thinking and the beliefs of the day in which this book was written are symbolized within the text. Once the symbols are understood and the consciousness in which the text is written is acknowledged, the message becomes of utmost importance in helping us see how our soul mind and emotions are veiled within our belief system.

As Synesius said over three hundred years before the birth of Jesus, "The truth becomes deadly to those who are not strong enough to contemplate it in all of its brilliance." But today we no longer have the option of having our teachings proportioned to the "imperfect reason" of our intellect and ego mind. As a descending emotional soul that is persecuting ourself with judgement on the cross of our beliefs, we struggle to transition ourself and begin our ascending emotional soul journey. We are totally responsible for seeking the knowledge to transition. No one can absorb truth for our soul transition but us.

As a descending emotional soul we are trying to become internally aware of who we are, why we are on earth, and what our purpose is in being human as we struggle to reach our loving ascending soul. But our literal intellect and ego is holding the memory of our good soul and spirit separate behind its cosmic shell of beliefs. In its supremacy our intellect and ego thinks that it is absolutely right and it is fearful of personal responsibility for its freedom of choice. The fear of being wrong is intense within our intellect and ego because it fears punishment. The expectation of being wrong enhances the fear and the cosmic shell of beliefs becomes more dense to protect the intellect.

Because we came into our immature soul with a focus on our intellectual mind and fear emotions, we of necessity looked at everything around us in relationship to our thoughts and fears. Because of our primitive perception of life, we developed superstitions that we accepted as fact. Our belief in needing to be saved by Jesus, by medicine, or by a relationship strikes fear and damnation within our immature soul mind, causing us to expect our myths, superstitions, rituals, and karmic beliefs to protect us as our saviors.

Our ancient superstitions were the result of our myths and our beliefs are the result of our superstitions, which we developed from our perception of life as we were living it. Our rituals became our adaptive habitual behavior that we accepted as the way we "must" be in life to be accepted by God, our peers, and society. As immature souls we were learning and doing the best that we were capable of at the precise time that we were living the experience. Our generational times change every thirty years, and every ninety years our physical change is more pronounced within society. An individual will change very little within a ninety-year cycle. This allows attrition to bring about more subconscious change than we realize in a physical lifetime. We have consistently evolved in our consciousness and now we must review the beliefs of our past and understand ourself on a different level. Everything that we have learned and lived has been necessary to our growth. But the primitive beliefs that we remain attached to today no longer serve our growth as a dual soul mind and emotions that is entering into the ascending or loving consciousness of ourself.

It is important that we do not judge what we have experienced in life, but we must also not hang on to old primitive beliefs as supporting, motivating, or inspiring to an advancing soul. Our attachment to primitive and mythical physical processes has deadened or hypnotized our spiritual senses until our feelings no longer trigger our soul emotions. A supreme self-centered mind and ego focus allows us to kill, lie, cheat, and be sexually abusive without any emotional feelings being triggered in our heart. In effect, we become more animal than human in our reaction to life when our consciousness is limited to the concept that our physical needs are supreme.

The beauty that is eternal in the way that we have learned has been perfect for us. By learning what we don't want we have more clarity in choosing what we do want. Unfortunately we have not made much progress in the past two thousand years because we have been living the level of stasis as our soul mind and emotions have attempted to balance themselves. We have focused upon our intellectual mind and ego while suppressing our emotions, which has allowed us to destroy the harmony and rhythm, or the dance of life in the soul that allows it to transition.

In the past two thousand years we have fallen into a state of revolution. For two seven-thousand-year cycles we have been living in chaos without a clue as to what is going on internally in our soul consciousness. Each time that we are provided with information about our dual soul and spirit, we deny it immediately because it does not fit the belief system that we are revolving and stuck within. It was fourteen thousand years ago that we began our obsession with "God the Father" and the crucifixion of man on earth. During those years the male physical nature has seen itself as supreme, and the female Divine Nature has kept the internal memory of the good within us alive. Many of the most gifted philosophers of the past fourteen thousand years have been female. These female philosophers have heard the message of their spirit consciousness and have shared the knowledge with those who were ready to listen. As we became obsessed with "God the Father" we also began to hear only the male voices as philosophers and prophets, and it is the male voices that have been recorded in history. As we began our belief in "evil spirits" women were no longer spoken of by name. Women who were teachers or married "Gods" as teachers were called Goddesses. Married women without children were called Virgins. Older women were called Divine. Women of the age of marriage were called Nymphs. Women not yet of marriage age were called Sprites. These common titles protected them from possession by "evil spirits."

We evolve through every aspect of our dual soul consciousness and our physical life in an organizational pattern based primarily on the numbers one, three, and seven to infinity, which creates the fractal pattern of life and fulfills our Principle of Eternal Truth. We establish our pattern of equality based primarily on two, four, and eight to infinity, fulfilling the Principle of Equilibrium. Our dual soul persona pattern as male and female is based primarily on the numbers five, six, and nine as our eternal Principle of Unconditional Love. The female Divine Nature is always represented in this trinity of numbers as nine, which is divisible by all of its component parts. Together these numbers make a unity of one. The Universal Principles that organize our soul pattern are constantly guiding our physical lives. Myth and superstitions have been connected to these principles since the beginning of time. The yin and the yang symbolize the six and nine of the male and female soul relationship.

This dual pattern has been understood for millions of years and has been defined by philosophers such as Pythagoras over twenty-five hundred years ago. The pattern is dual or opposite as an invisible and visible energy, dual soul mind and emotions, and dual as soul and spirit. The soul itself is dual and opposite in every aspect, and this is the reason that each person on earth has a twin soul of the opposite sex. But the Divine Nature of us has our spirit consciousness as its inspiration for life. Our spirit consciousness remains the lifeforce energy of our physical matter. All of the so-called "mysteries" of life can be understood once we understand the pattern that we use as a soul and spirit to create our physical body, life, and our physical experiences.

In the beginning our consciousness was spirit with the inspiration to expand itself, which it did as it created our male and female consciousness as our dual soul mind and emotions. As we became a living soul and spirit consciousness, we created our physical design which became our physical structure. Our immature soul consciousness became more and more primitive as it attached itself to the belief that its physical nature and body was its total identity. As we have descended into the depths of our physical nature, we have lost the memory of our integrated dual soul and spirit. Our memory loss increased our belief that our male physical nature was supreme and the male became the focus of our reality, which denied the female soul and spirit within us. As we transition into our Divine Nature as an ascending emotional soul we will remember our soul and spirit consciousness. We are eternal as a living soul and spirit consciousness with universal memory. It is our body that has no life once the consciousness of the dual soul and spirit leaves our physical matter. This is why our physical body is finite and will continually face death as a way for our immature soul to begin again with a new soul agenda. The myth that our male physical nature is supreme over our Divine Nature set the stage for the last two thousand years of religious thought that has molded every aspect of our physical experience, our societies, cultures, and governments.

ness and separated it from the Divine Nature of our soul and our spirit consciousness, we began to think and feel that our physical image was the supreme "God" of us. When our internal mind focus became unaware of other consciousnesses within our mind, man created the image of God in his own likeness and the inequality of the female became religious law which remains today. Since we were negative and judgemental, we created our image of God as negative and judgemental in our belief systems and we have worshipped the illusion of God as our male physical nature since that time. Each myth of our primitive belief system had its start in our sexual core, and when the myths were judged in relationship to the male and female the inequality of the female became the primary persona of our male soul in its physical nature.

Our beliefs were formed from the perception of our mind that attached itself to the negative thinking and behavior, including the belief that we have only one life. Because we enter into each life without conscious memory of our creation, past lives, and soul purpose, we find ourselves clinging to the patterns that are introduced into our immature soul in each new lifetime by the family, society, science, and religion. A child lives what is repatterned into its intellect in the first fourteen years of life. When we understand the repatterning that occurs in each lifetime, we will consciously repattern knowledge and love, and fear and inequality will lose its control. Many of the so-called "facts" of our present educational system are obsolete, because they were never true facts but simply the beliefs of our primitive mind. Gradually we have changed some of these irrelevant "facts," but many changes are still to come if it is our intention to continue our growth as an immature soul.

The power of our "truths" that are relative only to our belief systems has been lived on earth from the beginning of our immature soul journey. Galileo, an astronomer, scientist, and philosopher who lived from 1564-1642, challenged the Catholic belief of the day that the sun rotates around the earth when he published his book, *Dialogue of the Two Principal Systems of the World* in 1632. To avoid being imprisoned for life he had to rebuke his own theory that the earth was not the center of the universe. He was excommunicated by the church and put on house arrest until his death. In 1992 the Catholic Church gave Galileo a dispensation from his excommunication because they now admit that he was right, the earth is not the center of the universe.

Today's beliefs are just as difficult for man to change, especially in relationship to our health and religion. Hippocrates (460-375 B.C.), a physician and philosopher, taught "We are what we eat," but his wisdom has been lost through time. It was Galen, a physician and philosopher who began psycho-somatic medicine, who said "the best physician is a philosopher." This has never been more true than it is today, when each of us must understand our invisible dual soul and spirit and its relationship to our physical body if we want to heal ourself.

During the immature journey of our soul the blank slate of our intellectual mind was unaware of other lives, accumulated knowledge, universal memory of creation, and depended solely upon the repatterning introduced into the memory bank of our intellect. As we traveled the immature journey of our soul, we also developed a cosmic shell of karmic beliefs that became the subconscious ego mind of the intellect. Many of our primitive beliefs were the result of the religious perception of ourselves that came from the negative and fearful focus of our ego and intellectual mind that was being influenced with myths that were accepted as truth out of our ignorance of ourselves and our purpose on earth.

As we attached ourselves to the negativity and fear we expanded our religious fears, which created the reality perception of our consciousness as the personality and character of our mind and emotions. The further we descended into our left brain soul mind and emotions the further we were from the consciousness of our loving soul and spirit. The superstitions and myths that our mind conjured up became the reality that we accepted as fact and created as our religious laws. These distorted facts became our karmic religious beliefs and controlled our mind and emotions in our male consciousness as they do even to this day

In his day Hermes was depicted to the masses as a shepherd carrying his lamb to safety. Hermes lived thousands of years before Moses. Later, lambs were sacrificed on the altar to symbolize man's sins being washed in the blood of the lamb to convince the various gods that were being worshipped to save man. Jesus was seen by the Roman Catholic Church as the sacrificial Lamb of God who died for the sins of man and was depicted on church relics as a shepherd carrying his lamb. Until A.D. 700 the official image of Jesus was not as a crucified man but a good shepherd who was gently holding a lamb. In A.D. 625 the Council of Constantinople proposed the adoption of an image of Jesus hanging on the cross. The Council of Trullo finally adopted this decree in A.D. 695 as the representation of Jesus Christ, the Messiah or Savior who takes away the sins of the world. Several years were required to remove the images of the lamb and to paint the image of Jesus Christ being crucified on the cross.

St. Agnes was a mythical saint whose creation was based on the story of the sacrificial lamb and who became very popular in Christianity. St. Agnes became a marketing tool used successfully by the papacy to sell wax cakes, known as "Agnus Dei." Each cake was stamped with a picture of the lamb and carried the papal blessing promising absolute protection against "acts of God" such as volcanos, fires, thunderstorms, destruction, drowning, and childbirth. The marketing of religious relics and symbols was a highly profitable activity for the papacy as the image of God and the church, which was rewarded by its fearful, frightened followers seeking redemption for their sins.

The lamb was associated with the resurrection long before the advent of Christianity. The resurrection of ancient times related to the lamb as the symbol of our innocently coming back into a new life without conscious memory within three days of our death. Once we experience death we enter life again as an innocent lamb of spirit consciousness. Life begins at the moment of conception and the body develops from the fractal pattern of creation that is stored in soul and spirit memory. The story of the resurrection that was created again around Jesus' life was a repetition of the same story. The superstitions and rituals that have been created around these ancient myths have had a profound effect upon our karmic beliefs of today and are holding us back from our personal evolution.

Christianity does not reveal that the purpose of Jesus' mission on earth was to help us enter into our ascending emotional soul by understanding the truth, love, and equality of ourself. Although this information has been given numerous times through the prophecy of spirit consciousness, the myths have been changed to superstitions and rituals that have controlled our beliefs and made us dependent on a fearful god.

The intellect gave the ego the task of holding on to all beliefs that were responsible for lessons that the soul was determined to learn. These karmic beliefs were then reinforced by our exposure to family, cultural, societal, scientific, and religious beliefs in our development into each new life. At the end of each life when death occurred, the consciousness of our immature soul would store those lessons that were learned in the mature soul mind. In this manner we have developed a powerhouse of wisdom that is simply waiting for our consciousness to tap into it as we begin the journey of our mature soul.

Our indwelling spirit consciousness holds the entire memory of our creation as humans, earth, nature, and the universe. The consciousness of our mature soul mind and emotions has all that we have learned in our immature soul journey as humans. Our immature soul mind and emotions is designed with each new life. We enter into our immature soul journey with no memory of our past experiences available to us with the exception of the old karmic ego beliefs that we are to work upon in this lifetime. Our soul designs our physical life in such a way that the old beliefs, myths, and superstitions of our soul lessons will be triggered by the physical family, culture, and physical experiences that we have chosen.

Our soul is never a victim of circumstances but it follows the form, structure, organization, discipline, and free choice, inten-

consciousness and our spirit consciousness
that is created as a fractal pattern of the image of the Spirit Consciousness. The true emotional essense of our mature soul consciousness of wisdom is love. The true emotional essense of our spirit consciousness is unconditional love. Fear is the emotion of our physical nature as we live in our immature soul.

We each have a dual soul mind and emotions and a spirit consciousness. As souls we were created from the fractal pattern of our Spirit consciousness and that same spirit consciousness lives within each of us as our indwelling spirit. Our male and female soul consciousness is the method of evolution for our dual soul consciousness but it remains the child of our eternal spirit consciousness. As the "child of spirit" we have an inherent purpose of expanding our spirit consciousness through the physical lives that we experience as a male and female soul consciousness as we learn the art of creation. Since our purpose on earth as a trinity of consciousness that is using our dual soul as our expanding consciousness is to learn the art of creation, we create every thought, emotion, and feeling in our physical reality as a way of learning our soul lessons.

When we were creating ourselves from the fractal pattern of our spirit consciousness, we designed our physical form from the elements of nature and we integrated into each cell of our body the fractal pattern of our cellular memory as our soul mind and emotions and our spirit consciousness. It is because we created our physical body and the function of our mind and emotional energy from the elements of nature that we must use the purity of the foods of nature to restore the cellular structure of our body. We have constantly used the air, water, foods of nature, and sex that were given to us as our biological needs to create ourselves as healthy beings, to continue our eternal life, and to create our physical reality.

There is no mystery to why we are now experiencing dramatic diseases that are "incurable." We have spent hundreds of years polluting the elements of nature that must sustain us physically, mentally, and emotionally. But we have been so busy looking externally to find cures that we have stayed in ignorance of the true relationship between ourselves and nature, earth, and the universe. All of life works together in a hierarchy and when one level of our hierarchy is destroyed the walls come tumbling down for the levels that remain. Our body was not created simply for the pleasure of sex, eating, and drinking. We have a higher purpose of sustainability or eternal creation on the physical level.

RELIGIOUS CULTS

Our creation and journey as an immature soul is defined in the book of Genesis, but the interpretation of these words has come from our immature soul mind and fear emotions. The entire Old Testament is a compilation of parables of our immature and mature soul consciousness that are interpreted in the vernacular of the descending soul consciousness so they would be understood by the culture for which they were given. We no longer live in the culture that existed at that moment in time, which was around 1650 B.C.

All of the biblical stories are parables, allegories, and embellishments of myths that have been handed down as beliefs, superstitions, and symbology from the beginning of our creation. Our beliefs were created by us from these superstitions and assumptions through our negative mind and emotions. When we look at the prophecies of ancient times the words are cloaked and veiled in the beliefs of the time. When we look at the same prophecies with the enlightenment of our mature soul, we read the truth of who we are, why we are here, and what our purpose is in being human.

We have allowed these ancient words to wear the same garments of interpretation since they were originally written. We have looked at these words and taken them literally, forgetting that the beliefs may have worked thousands of years ago, but with the knowledge of science our religious beliefs have no logic today. Jesus was born to teach us about the love in our mature soul. The teachings were given to us as parables because we were not open to hearing truth. Not many of us would want to wear the same garments for four thousand years, which was the approximate time of Moses' prophecy. The truth of our creation and soul evolution is hidden in the parables of scripture. Four thousand years ago we were totally externally focused, and as Moses heard the voice of "God" within his mind and revealed his teachings he was suspected of plagiarism, as the teachings of Hermes had revealed the same messages.

The superstitions of the ancient interpretation came from the word-of-mouth stories that were passed down through the previous time period as myths, or the traditional stories of ancient cultures. During the earliest period of mythology most of these cultures had not yet learned to read or write and history was kept alive by the stories that were shared verbally from one generation to another. This is equivalent to playing the "tell a person game" today, when the story that was told at the beginning of the circle has no relationship to the story that is told at the end of the circle. As a spirit and soul consciousness the story of our beginning cycle as an immature soul will be totally different from the ending cycle of our mature soul because we will have expanded the consciousness of ourself into understanding.

Since all of human life has been motivated by the enlightened soul consciousness and inspired by our spirit consciousness, we have subconsciously and unconsciously been on the journey to understanding ourselves, despite our lack of consciousness of what we are doing. This has allowed mythology to dwell on the stories of symbols, rituals, and supernatural beings, both in the evil beliefs of the "devil" as well as the "angel" or good beliefs. Our fascination with the energy that surrounds us and the "supernatural beings" and "events" has allowed us to bring the unknown into relationship with the known, which has created beliefs, superstitions, and mythical stories that served the purpose for our primitive mind. These beliefs gave us a reason for our physical focus of fear, war, and victimization in our life, and at the same time they gave us a form of hope and faith which we needed.

The parables began with our creation as a male and female consciousness. The Garden of Eden is the parable of learning how to live our biological needs as our fractal pattern of eternal life that is part of the hierarchy of earth. Each lesson is symbolized in the parable and was passed down through the generations of our soul as myth. It takes our soul seven generations times seven to infinity to learn a lesson and change our behavior. This is why the "sins of the father are passed down through the generations of the son."

The father is the symbol of our physical nature and all lessons are passed down as karmic lessons from one physical generation to the next. Physical, mental, emotional, and sexual abuse is a good example of how lessons are handed down from father to son in our physical experience. As our consciousness has expanded it has still taken seven generations of family abuse before there will be a change in the abusive behavior. If it is not changed at the end of seven generations within the family, the family will continue repeating the behavior in seven-generational cycles. A soul generation is 30 physical years. Seven generations is 210 years.

The mythical stories of our beliefs became the basis of many of our sciences, cultures, religions, and sexual behavior. When man became literate he began to accept these myths, superstitions, rituals, and beliefs as his only knowledge and they were recorded into books and believed as literal fact. We are our own ancestors, and when we can see the journey that we have lived as an evolving soul mind and emotions we can clearly see that our old karmic beliefs are no longer in harmony and rhythm with our transitioning soul mind and emotions. It does not matter if our old beliefs had their origin in our family cultures, religion, science, or sexuality: what matters is that we look at them realistically and be willing to change them to continue with the journey of our mature soul.

The old karmic beliefs that we are working with now as a human species are our beliefs in inequality, abuse, judgement, control, dishonesty, and fear. To learn the lesson of these beliefs our soul must learn to live in equality, truth, and love. We are the miracle of eternal life. If we resist learning in one lifetime, we will simply continue being born again into the same chaos until we complete the lesson within our immature soul.

When Jesus was born as an advanced soul, we were stuck in the revolutions and stasis of our fearful beliefs and behaviors. We had literally hung ourselves on the cross as we became stuck in our transition as a soul. It was important to Jesus that he live the same experience of physical life in the identical manner that humanity was living in the immature soul. Our Higher Spirit Consciousness was the collective consciousness of Jesus and he wanted to experience living in the identical level that we were living as humans to see if it was possible for us to survive the depravity and continue with our soul evolution into our ascending emotional soul without another period of rest.

As spirits we understood that we could live through the chaos but our collective immature soul minds created a woven fabric of external myth to conceal our internal knowing. Our later attachment to the concept that Jesus would save us became another superstition that was marketed and exploited by religion as a means of controlling the flock. Dependency and control are both lessons of inequality. Whether we depend upon our roles and identities as male and female, religious beliefs, or scientific beliefs, we enhance the lessons of dependency and control for our immature descending emotional soul.

As we have focused our beliefs on superstitions, we have resisted and denied our own personal responsibility for growth and change. In our denial we have accepted our beliefs as fact and closed our mind to new relationships between the information that we have gathered and our creation, health, and evolution. Our denial and resistance have led to an expanded dependency, control, and self-judgement, which in the physical reality expands our depression, disease, physical, mental, and emotional abuse, crime, dishonesty, war, competition, and our overall attachment to inequality. At this time in the evolution of our soul we are being motivated and inspired from within to find the relationship between what we believe, what we know, and who we are. If we are attached to ancient beliefs by dependency, control, fear, anxiety, depression, judgement, anger, addictions, and rage, we are creating an opportunity for our soul to devolve into primitive and abusive behavior. As our soul devolves, we focus on primitive memory nodes of our ancient past when our behavior was more primitive and no longer in harmony with our beliefs of today. As we relive our primitive behaviors, it puts us out of step with our present-day society.

Examples of our attachment to ancient beliefs would be as follows: When we focus on a memory node of total disrespect for human life, we will kill others, both children and adults, without any feelings of guilt or remorse. Or when we focus on a memory node of cannibalistic behavior, we will repeat that behavior as part of our present personality and we will have no control over our behavior. When we focus on a memory node of totally unconscious sexual behavior that responds only to biological need, we will have dramatic sexual abuse throughout society. When we focus on a memory node of a past life, we will try to relive the memory of that past life in beliefs, attitude, dress, and relationships. The mind and emotions of an individual who is focused on primitive memory nodes has only a vague sense of being out-of-sync with current beliefs and will proclaim total innocence and persecution by society as part of the intense belief in past memory. Large sub-cultures have developed as cults among people who are focused on primitive memories, such as religious and New Age groups, and those who have adapted sexual or physical body fetishes.

The consciousness of our dual soul mind and emotions follows the General Theory of Relativity that Albert Einstein discovered in 1915. Our consciousness moves through space, time, and gravitation with three primary movements: soul evolution, soul revolution, and soul devolution. Our physical laws are also Universal Laws. If we don't understand our dual soul and spirit consciousness and the soul journey that we have been living, we will not be conscious of the activity within our soul mind and emotions and the relationship of that activity to our health, society, or the world.

A few years ago I chose to watch a talk show of psychiatrists, psychologists, and physicians in a discussion of consciousness.

I was fascinated by the group's total ignorance of the soul and its relationship to the conscious mind, subconscious mind, and unconscious mind and their ignorance of what our consciousness truly is and the role it plays in our lives. These are basic truths that are found in metaphysics and yet are relatively unknown or misunderstood by the masses of intellectual people within our society, despite their educational background. The sad thing about this lack of knowledge is that we can never understand our physical body, mental and emotional health, or our belief systems until we clearly understand our dual soul and spirit and how our consciousness evolves. Once we understand ourself it becomes easy to understand our relationship to earth, nature, and the universe. Knowing the history of myths, superstitions, rituals, beliefs, and our behavior begins to map the precise historical path that we have lived as humans. History, science, and religion become our allies when we are serious about mapping our journey of consciousness.

There are a number of mythical beliefs that have led to our present devolution as a descending emotional soul. Holding on to these beliefs at this time in our evolution as a soul assures us that we will deny ourself evolution and choose devolution. It is our ancient primitive beliefs that have evolved from our myths that limit our soul today.

Our belief in only one life gives us a sense of powerlessness, inadequacy, and hopelessness. We cannot relate the experiences that we have to only one physical life because if we try nothing makes logical sense to us. At this time we are feeling the gravitational pull of the loving side of our soul, giving us a sense of duality between what our mind believes and what we feel emotionally within our heart. Our consciousness of this duality leads to depression because we feel unbalanced as we look at what we have been taught and what our soul memory is allowing us to feel. Looking at our life from the karmic beliefs of our immature soul allows nothing to make sense. In time, the feelings that we have internally to respect and honor our life will help the experiences that we have lived to fit into the empty spaces in the puzzle of our mind. In absorbing knowledge we can see the entire picture of what we are doing and why we are living our duality of thinking, emotions, and feelings.

Our belief that someone else is responsible for saving our physical body and our soul expands our helplessness, dependency, and feelings of being controlled. When we give our power away to religion to save our soul and medicine to save our body we have placed ourself into a role of being controlled and dependent on someone else for our life. Since our mature soul is waiting for our immature soul to learn the lessons of control, dependency, fear, and anger to give us the strength and courage to change our mental and emotional focus, it is important for us to take back our freedom, independence, joy, and love in our experience of life. Being dependent on someone else is the myth of our "need to be saved." Our soul has its own agenda and the concept of someone physically saving us is a belief that our ego has created, but it is not part of the mature soul journey and, except as a lesson of denying change and living in devolution, it has no influence on what happens to us internally. Our mythical and primitive beliefs in guilt, shame, sin, and persecution allow us to abuse ourself and others. We have been taught to abuse ourselves with our fear emotions, which are secondary to the beliefs that we have accumulated in our ego mind and that our intellect is controlled by and dependent upon. The beliefs that we are guilty, shameful, sinful, and victimized by life are all the result of our fear of separation from God, and his judgement and damnation, which are only mythical, superstitious beliefs of our immature soul mind. As the physical nature of our immature soul was learning about itself, we created every thought, emotion, and feeling as our physical reality. We needed a physical organization and discipline to follow in which we could learn the spiritual values that we kept in our core self. Our immature soul created its organization and discipline out of fear and ignorance of its eternal self and we were first exposed to the opposite of our ethical values and being of love. As we removed ourselves from the memory of our trinity of consciousness as the form, structure, organization, and discipline of our soul and spirit, we entered the world of chaos.

Living the duality of fear and love is providing the dual soul with a dual view of life. Our physical nature has lived in its fear but as we transition into our Divine Nature we will be living the love that is inherent within us. This gives the soul a clear picture of the fear it does not want to live and the love that it freely chooses to live. Our fear of God's separation and judgement reflects the internal separation of our soul mind and emotions through our self-judgement that we unknowingly indulge in as we measure ourselves as unequal in relationship to our beliefs. Our fear of separation can be seen in every aspect of our society as families become separated by judgement and anger, physicians separate the body into individual parts and no longer treat us as a whole living organism, the political parties seek to bring separation within the public as they judge each other, and religion separates God from us as an external image of man. The examples are endless as we look within ourselves, families, societies, and the world. Our fear beliefs are an electromagnetic energy that keeps our physical nature limited in the same way that a buried electric fence will keep an animal confined in a limited space.

Our belief that all food is good food and nourishes our body allows us to innocently abuse our body, dual soul, and spirit. Our focus on what we like allows excesses and deficiencies to predominate rather than maintaining the eternal Principle of Equilibrium of the chemicals in our cellular body. In allowing our body to become unbalanced, we invite disease and death which allows the soul to begin again with a new body. Imbalance mutates the soul pattern and can become part of the lesson for the soul as diseases are brought back into life as a lesson not yet completed. As we created ourselves we did so from the elements of nature that we chose as part of our fractal pattern. When we eat food that does not restore these natural elements, we begin a slow but persistent disintegration that will lead to disease and death. This condition of imbalance can take many lifetimes for the soul, giving us ample opportunity to change our balance by changing our perception of food and its effect upon our body.

Since medicine has lived with the beliefs that "all food is good food" and that "food has no effect on disease" we have not been taught the importance of food to our physical and mental health and well-being. Fortunately many physicians are changing their perception of the role of food in our health, but nutrition has not yet become an absolute requirement in medical schools. The responsibility for what we eat is personal and we must take the initiative to eat properly and prevent disease. Disease is an internal lesson for our soul. We are not only learning to balance our chemical physical body but we are learning to balance our internal chemical dual soul mind and emotions as we internalize the lesson of disease.

Our religious belief that faith is superior to knowledge has been a myth as a major form of denial for our immature soul. Our blind faith in the information that is fed to us allows us to innocently abuse ourself as we give away our power and become a follower without seeking additional knowledge. Knowledge is opposite to blind faith and knowledge is the current level of our soul evolution. Blind faith is the path to devolution at this point in our soul growth. In the beginning of our immature soul journey we needed some blind faith because we were learning in the darkness of our immature mind while suppressing our female emotions. We did not have memory of our creation and no library of stored wisdom that we could use. But at this point in our evolution, we have a mind full of knowledge and wisdom and we can hear the mature soul mind and our spirit mind guiding us if we are open to listening. This is commonly called "insight" and "intuition," which is acceptable terminology in our society.

Knowledge is the transitional level of our soul consciousness, which is the level in which we transition from our immature soul to our mature soul. We are changing from our physical nature to our Divine Nature as we make this transition of our thinking, emotions, and feelings. Knowledge is the only level of our soul that is divided between our Cycle of Awareness as a physical nature and our Cycle of Understanding as a Divine Nature. Now we are aware of huge amounts of knowledge, but when we transition into our mature soul we will understand all of the knowledge that we have gathered as a soul in relationship to ourselves. Understanding will be equivalent to our being aware that we have a tree growing in our yard but once we understand that trees are the lungs of earth we will love the tree and not cut it down.

Blind faith is the source of all beliefs where fear has controlled the soul mind intention, motivation, and inspiration to seek knowledge and instead has manipulated and seduced the mind into control and dependency upon beliefs of inequality and ignorance which removes our freedom of thinking. Our addictive beliefs deny the history of the soul and allow the fear to continue with the manipulation and seduction of the intellectual mind. Blind faith creates followers and has established the religious cults that control the soul journey of our physical nature. Blind faith breeds inequality because in blind faith control must be established by a supreme being, which establishes several levels of inequality within every society as the pyramid grows.

Many within society have been willing to play the role and identity of supreme beings, which denies the inherent equality of the human species. Negative beliefs are the illusion of our fearful soul mind and emotions, and it is our fear itself that attaches our soul to the addictive beliefs of worship as inequality. When there is an intense fear of the "hereafter," we fear death as the ultimate change and we have an intense "need to be saved." Our fear will control us until the mind seeks and finds the knowledge that allows it to see the illusion of the addictive beliefs, denial, and resistance of our immature soul mind and emotions. As the immature soul has revolved within the beliefs of fear, the fear itself has become the limitation that holds the mind and emotional soul in the darkness or ignorance of the intellectual mind and ego.

Our fear is ultimately our soul's denial of its freedom of choice. When we deny that we have freedom of choice then we must have blind faith as a follower to survive. In our fear we become dependent on someone else to save us and we ignore our internal power. Fear itself enhances the fear of not believing, which allows the soul to continue in the stasis of its controlling and judgemental fear beliefs. Fear beliefs create anger, but the anger responds by conformity which we live as an emotional seduction that is trying to avoid punishment. With time this will send the soul emotions into rage, which will bring on rebellion and the beliefs will begin to change as the soul chooses to seek knowledge. At this time in our society everyone is living some level of rebellion.

Our addictive religious belief in the identities and roles relating to male and female has created our sexual beliefs in the inequality of the male and female. The myths of identities and roles continue with a controlling influence within our religious cultures and society as our ego physical nature is resisting our soul transition into our Divine Nature. The religious beliefs in sexual inequality have been supported by government, science, medicine, education, and every other facet of our lives. The physical nature of man was taught that man was made in the image of God and that godliness within man gave him dominion or possession and rule over woman, child, and all of earth. These were convenient misinterpretations of prophecy that helped our physical nature create its beliefs as physical reality. Man was substituted for the word "human" and the stories of creation were misinterpreted to support the belief that man was superior to woman, which created the perfect physical environment for us to live our lesson of inequality. Our belief in inequality limited our consciousness to our identities and roles in every facet of our family life, culture, and society. As the female became submissive in her inequality, we created the suppression of our emotions as a soul.

KARMIC BELIEF IN FEMALE INEQUALITY

Our belief in inequality has been an example of how "the sins of the fathers are passed down through the generations to the sons." Our physical nature has repeated its beliefs throughout the journey of our soul because they were believed to be truth. Of course the truth in our physical nature is relative only to our conscious belief systems and not to our dual soul reality.

The rules and identities have been determined by religious beliefs, but these same beliefs were transferred from the myths of men into all other systems of our society because men controlled every other system of our society. In reality our female Divine Nature is superior to the male physical nature and this is why the change of consciousness is important for us. All males and females have been focused upon their physical nature in the immature journey of the soul. This is why some women feel that submission is an honor, because they are conscious of only their male beliefs within their soul mind and their emotions remain suppressed, which keeps them from being aware of the emotions in their Divine Nature or their present life in their physical nature.

Our belief in inequality between male and female, different age groups, the disabled, different races, different cultures, different lifestyles, different status images, different educational backgrounds, and all other aspects of inequality governs our physical world and creates our family and societal cultures. Inequality is the lesson our immature and childish soul is living now and that it has been living throughout the Cycle of Awareness of the immature soul in our physical nature. We must learn the lesson of inequality in our physical lives to facilitate the internal alchemical marriage of our male and female soul consciousness. Without a meeting of the minds internally, we will devolve rather than evolve in our dual soul consciousness. Our transition into our Divine Nature is the intention, will, and choice of our soul consciousness because our transition assures us of continued evolution in wisdom, understanding, and love.

If we didn't have a belief in inequality, we would not have a belief in blind faith. Inequality and blind faith go hand in hand in the ego creation of supremacy. When supremacy exists within our consciousness, judgement, fear, control, dependency, anger, and conformity are the rules that we live by because we feel unequal to others. As an immature soul we reflect our inequality into our beliefs, behaviors, persona, and lifestyle as we persecute ourself and others. If we didn't have a belief in inequality, we would not have a belief in dependency, control, fear, conformity, seduction, manipulation and all of the other negative beliefs that we live. Our belief in inequality allows us to reflect the unequal image of ourself in anger and judgement to those who are in external relationships with us. We reflect our fear and judgement to the other person because we are fearing and judging ourself. As we hang ourself on the cross of persecution, we want to control others because we are attempting to control our own fear and judgement. All of our negative thinking and emotions, as well as our blind faith and inequality, comes from living the myth that woman is unequal to man because man is made in the image of "God the Father." Man himself created this myth to support his ego fear and superiority.

Our belief that we must be a follower and worship false idols as superior to ourself is also a creation of religious myth and ritual. Idol or hero worship consistently influences our children and adults and is part of the belief in blind faith that allows us to see others as superior to self. Hero worship impacts the minds of our children and patterns them into primitive behavior. Hero or idol worship is the pattern of our male and female sexuality, science, and religion and has therefore influenced our many cultures from the very beginning of time as a lesson of inequality and blind faith. When we recognize the beauty and wisdom of ourself, we no longer want or need to live vicariously in someone else's shadow. When we worship love relationships we set ourselves up to live our inequality on a daily basis, and when the relationship ends we feel unlovable, inadequate, and worthless as a reflection of our belief in inequality.

Our belief that only the physical world is valid motivates us to make every thought, emotion, and belief physical. This belief allows us to deny the existence of the invisible world of our soul and spirit and to stay ignorant of the knowledge to understand the energy of our physical body, dual soul, and spirit. This belief is supported by many scientific disciplines. As science has denied the presence of an external God it has been reluctant to look within itself to find the internal and integrated spirit and soul consciousness that is our inspiration and motivation of life. Because our soul and spirit is unrecognized by our physical intellect and ego does not mean that we stay ignorant of our soul and spirit when we transition into our right brain. The lack of religious and scientific understanding of our dual soul mind and emotions and our spirit consciousness is creating extreme hardship for many people at this time as they find themselves transitioning into the right brain with no one to help them understand what is happening to them. The changes in the way that our soul mind and emotions transition is beyond the imagination of our intellect and can allow people to think they are losing control of their mind. Accepting a societal opinion that puts the blame on "mental illness" is supporting scientific and religious ignorance and is self-abusive. Our need to victimize others reflects a closed mind that sees the sexual and physical world as all that is.

Our belief that we know all there is to know keeps us from opening our mind to our Divine Nature. This belief exists on an individual, scientific, and religious level. It is a belief of consciousness distraction that keeps us in ignorance as we refuse to open our mind to new knowledge and to the relationship of old knowledge to understanding ourself. This is an intellect and ego belief that pulls us back into physical processes and creates the revolutions and stasis for our soul. It occurs as a reflective reaction to our limited consciousness as the ego goes into its denial mode. Although denial of knowledge begins as an individual distraction it soon becomes a collective consciousness within cultures, religions, science, and sexual groups. This distraction can be seen in cults that are not only religious cults but also sexual and scientific cults. When we believe that "we know all there is to know" we close our mind to any and all knowledge that doesn't fit into our belief patterns. We will use any method in our power to distract ourself and create an attachment to some physical process or primitive belief, such as our superiority over others. We can also accept some different perceptions of knowledge but evaluate what we learn by our primitive and ancient beliefs, which creates relative truth, not absolute truth.

Cults used to have only a focus of religious worship but now many people worship human or physical idols such as money, clothes, celebrities, lovers, people, science, aliens, and sexual fetishes. The key word to describe a cult is "worship." The act of worship makes us unequal to our object of worship. Our need to worship is our belief in inequality and our blind faith "knowing" that someone else is superior and knows it all.

Our beliefs are all karmic beliefs that have very ancient religious origins and can be found in the mythical biblical interpretations and rituals. Our cultures have been founded by our physical nature and the male is the symbol of our physical nature. As we are evolving into our mature soul, we are beginning to feel our Divine Nature of love and wisdom. If we fear the Divine or female nature within us, we will resist and deny our soul growth and let our fear overwhelm us. Karmic beliefs will continue to be current lessons for each soul life until they are released and the knowledge to understand them is related to the dual soul, spirit, and physical body as an integrated whole.

In examining our religious beliefs in creation we can see the beginning of idol worship and the male and female inequality. Many religions have taught us that woman was created from the rib of man. This belief defies what we have lived as the creation of new life throughout the immature journey of our soul. The Divine Nature, as symbolized in the female, gives birth to the physical nature of the infant. Whether the infant is in male or female form is of no importance, as both male and female are currently living in their physical nature as they have from the beginning of creation. The male is the symbol of our physical nature, and although the male plays a role in the conception he does not play an actively participative role in the development or birth of the infant. This allows us to understand the importance of transition into our creative, Divine Nature. The interaction that women experience with their Divine Nature allows women to feel better during pregnancy than at any other time in their lives.

For aeons of time the male has been thought to be superior to the female and to have the right to control the female and her life. Therefore it is through the male physical nature that the systems of earth have been designed. Now, as our soul is evolving more rapidly, the female Divine Nature is evident in both the male and female body. The physical nature is also evident in both the male and female body when the soul is in resistance and denial of its own growth. Both the male and female have experienced the journey of the immature soul with their mind and emotional focus living within the physical nature. This is the symbolism of the story of the "rib" in Genesis.

The third version of the Creation that is found in Genesis 2:21-22 AV (Masonic Edition) says: "And the Lord God caused a deep sleep to fall upon Adam, and he slept; and he took one of his ribs, and closed up the flesh instead thereof; and the rib, which the Lord God had taken from man, made he a woman, and brought her unto the man." This is the parable that explains the living soul being formed into a dual soul mind and emotions and the journey that we chose to follow as a male and female consciousness living equally in our physical nature as an evolving soul consciousness.

This parable symbolizes God as our indwelling spirit consciousness and the Lord as our dual soul of male and female consciousness. Our soul's choice was to focus both the male and female consciousness on the left brain as our male physical nature. The state of "sleep" or unawareness symbolizes the loss of memory in our intellect, which we would live within our physical nature. When this state began we entered "the land of Nod," and God and our male and female consciousness as the Lord saw the wisdom of physically separating the two lobes of the brain and allowing us to begin our soul evolution in our physical nature without the conscious memory of any of the previous events of our creation as spirit and our physical development as a living soul of male and female consciousness in a physical body. Our spirit consciousness in conjunction with our dual soul consciousness as male and female as our "Lord" became our trinity of consciousness. As "Lord" we have used the physical magnetism, which was symbolized by the rib of emotion from the heart of our female Divine Nature as Eve, to draw our male physical nature as Adam by the magnetism of our Divine Nature through the space and time required for our soul journey of evolution.

Physically it has been our female emotions that have magnetized the male to the female and the female to the male as both sought the love within self. Our love emotions were seen by our physical nature as the external "need" for sexual pleasure. Our emotional magnetism acted as a way of continuing the act of pro-creation as our sexual creation to fulfill the Law of Continuation or reincarnation for our soul, while animating the soul memory with the love of the Divine Nature for magnetism, and sensory stimulation as our pleasure.

As God separated the female Divine Nature from the male physical nature of our dual soul, both man and woman were committed to live life from their physical nature as an immature soul. The emotional magnetism of the rib gave woman the power to conceive as the soul memory of the pattern of creation. We were focused mentally and emotionally on our left brain as our male physical nature and we had no knowledge of how creation occurred or for what purpose. This brought equality into our immature soul journey, because both our male and female self would be using our male physical nature without any knowledge of our creation throughout the immature soul. As both the male and female were focused within the physical nature in their descending soul, it would give them total equality in the physi-cal nature and allow both to experience equality in their ascend-ing emotional nature as they used both their physical nature and their Divine Nature as an integrated soul mind and emotions. This placed our male physical nature and our female Divine Nature in a state of mutual hostility or competition through fear and negativity, which kept both sexes focused upon their male physical nature; and we have remained unaware of our female Divine Nature until now.

SYMBOLS AND THE BOOK OF REVELATION

Symbols were used by ancient cultures as a method of com-munication which included the laws of the culture and they were understood by everyone. The symbols and what they represent-ed were passed down from generation to generation as mythos or mythology. Mythology was communicated as stories which were acted out using the symbol as the meaning that it represented. With time the actual meaning of the symbol was lost and superstitions were built up around the symbol that may not even be close to the original meaning of the symbol. Symbols were created early in our soul journey before we were overwhelmed with fear. Our fear began during the level of knowledge in our soul journey. Our fear began as the cause and effect of religious moral law that believed in inequality, right or wrong, judgement, blame, inequality, dependency, and worship. Religious moral law was created from the interpretation of ancient prophecy that related to the duality of our soul. When the duality was interpreted as inequality it was natural to believe in good and evil, right and wrong, male and female, as we lived our inhibition and not our excitation. Our interpretations began our beliefs in our female Divine Nature as evil, and evolved into the image of man as the image of God or good. These symbols expanded our beliefs into the inequality that we live today.

The book of Revelation is the story of our creation, the journey of our immature soul, our transition, and the journey of our mature soul. When Jesus came to earth nearly two thousand years ago he came to see what was taking place in our physical nature that was holding our soul journey in revolution and stasis. He lived his life through his unconditional love, truth, and equality. None of Jesus' writings were left on earth because he knew they would not be understood. Jesus destroyed his writings himself before he began his ministry. Jesus denied his role of savior to the world. But the ego of man has held Jesus in the Savior belief, myth, and superstition which has begun the devolution of many souls. Jesus came to show us how to live our love but our fear beliefs could not accept his teachings of love as he lived them.

The book of Revelation defines our dual soul and its seven levels of change and growth as it lives its evolution as an immature soul. It uses the symbolism of candles to indicate the evolution of our soul through its seven levels, which allows us to see the true essense of love and light that lives within our soul. The Principle of Eternal Life is acknowledged in Revelation 1:18: "I am he that liveth and was dead; and behold I am alive for evermore, Amen, and have the keys of hell and death." This relates to the soul and its eternal life as it continues its cycle of expression of birth, life, and death eternally, and it clarifies that the keys are understanding and knowledge for our soul which explains the unknown concept or "mystery" of hell and death. Hell is the physical reality that we create in our immature soul when we do not understand ourselves. Death itself will be less frequent in our mature soul when we realize that we are a chemical consciousness and a chemical physical body that can be restored with the chemicals of nature. As we evolve into our mature soul with knowledge and understanding we will consciously create a heaven on earth.

The symbol of the lion's head has represented the sun-goddess as our Divine Nature for many ancient cultures. The image of the lion within the sun represents the fear that our intellect and ego mind are attached to when the memory of our Divine Nature is triggered in our immature soul consciousness. The lion is also the symbol of man living from his animal instincts while in his physical nature.

The stars symbolize the lessons that the soul has learned, as stars in our crown. Lessons of the evolving soul continue from one life to another as a karmic memory and when they are learned we have a star in our crown as we move one step further in our evolution. The lessons that we learn as a soul become our wisdom and pass from one life to the next as memory nodes in our mature soul. These memory nodes of wisdom are the stars in the crown of our soul.

The double-edged sword is the symbol of our dual soul mind and emotions, which represents the duality as opposites that will be found in every aspect of life as we live the journey of our immature dual soul. Our dual soul is dual in every aspect of itself as male and female, mind and emotions, fear and love, dark and light, negative and positive, external and internal, and inhibition and excitation.

The twin serpents are the mythological symbol of our female Divine Nature and our male physical nature which is symbolized physically within our body by the brain stem and spinal cord as the double-edged sword wrapped in twin serpents. This represents the knowledge we gain as we switch our physical gender from male to female and female to male in our eternal journey of life. The brain stem and the spinal cord create the cranial nerves and the nerves that control our body as our indwelling spirit consciousness. The twin serpents that live within our body are connected to our cerebellum which is the seat of our spirit consciousness. Our brain stem, spinal cord, cerebellum, and all of our nerves represent our spirit consciousness that is integrated into every cell of our physical body and that stimulates our senses which expands our soul and spirit consciousness. When any part of our body as a spirit consciousness is damaged, we are either dead or physically paralyzed depending on the point of trauma. The twin serpents symbolize the core of our dual soul consciousness as the power of our thinking, emotions, and spirit senses, and our body defines the expansion of our spirit consciousness as we live our physical experience as an evolving dual soul. The spirit is the universal memory that creates the relationship of all knowledge into understanding, and therefore the twin serpents also represent the "Lord" of knowledge as the dominion of our integrated mature soul and our universal spirit mind as the trinity of consciousness that is absolute truth.

The symbol of the beast with eyes before and behind shows how we will live the transition as we look backwards and re-live our primitive memories in our physical nature. Retrospectively our immature soul will understand the journey of our soul in our physical nature and recognize the beauty and wisdom of the design that we have lived. The symbol of the beast tells us to look at our past to relate our knowledge to our immature soul.

The symbol of the churches represents the seven levels of the immature soul and the many mansions of the mind consciousness that are found in those seven levels of our soul growth. This symbol shows us that all lessons learned through our physical experiences are good in the eyes of our soul. Each level of our soul has magnetized itself toward love to reach our next level of growth.

The Holy Grail is symbolized by a chalice and it represents the enlightenment of the dual soul mind and emotions by our Divine Nature as our cup that runneth over. The passion for life and the ecstasy of life that we will live from the moment of enlightenment as we enter into our mature soul of wisdom and loving emotions relates to the myth of the camel being pulled through the eye of the needle, as we take our full cup of knowledge into our soul of wisdom. As we understand and live a spiritual life our emotions of passion and ecstasy will expand the consciousness of our mature soul into the integration with our spirit. We are living in the vortex of negative energy as an immature soul and we must enter into a vortex of positive energy in our mature soul before we can expand into our comfort zone of loving emotions. It is the vortex of our negative immature soul that has closed our mind to the eye of the needle.

The crown symbolizes the truth and knowledge of all soul lessons that are learned within the spirit that envelops the body with love and equality, and it can be visibly seen as a golden halo of light by the enlightened soul mind. Our crown or spirit consciousness expands as we live and learn through the physical experiences of our immature soul consciousness of physical nature and our mature soul consciousness of our Divine Nature. The soul lessons that we learn become stars in the crown of our spirit and mature soul.

The crown of thorns symbolizes the cosmic shell of our religious belief systems that holds our intellect captive through the pain and suffering of the immature soul that we are persecuting on the transitional cross of our eternal life design. The crown of thorns represents each individual belief from which we torture and punish ourself in our need to be saved instead of accepting responsibility for saving ourselves by living our love, truth, and equality.

The frogs symbolize the resurrection or rebirth of the soul as it moves from one physical life to another. The frog symbolizes the soul's rebirth as a fractal pattern of our mature soul changes to the smaller fractal pattern of our immature soul as the soul is reborn once again into the purity and innocence of our spirit consciousness.

The Philosopher's stone, as a white sponge-like stone, symbolizes the female Divine Nature of our mature soul of wisdom and love that easily absorbs knowledge and emotions while seeking an understanding of ourself in relationship to the universe, earth, and nature. It has always been the female that creates new life and the philosopher's stone symbolizes the Divine Nature of the female as the energy of rebirth for the soul and the human species.

A black or ebony stone symbolizes the male mind of our physical nature that resists knowledge as water running over the surface of a solid rock. This stone is worshiped by some religious cults as a symbol of blind faith in the Gods. Ebony symbolizes the closed intellectual mind of our physical nature and its resistance and denial of change and rebirth as a soul.

The horned "goat" god symbolized the redeemer "god" who took human sins upon himself as the divine nature of Gad or Baal. The "goat god" symbolizes our physical nature and its victimization and illusions of sexual power. This is the societal role today of President Clinton as people persecute him and want to sacrifice him to redeem their physical nature from the guilt and shame of their sexual sins.

The lamb is the symbol of the total innocence and perfection of the spirit consciousness and represents the soul and spirit as it is reborn and lives the first seven-year cycle of life of each physical rebirth.

The white horse is the symbol of the purity of the human soul as it begins its journey as an immature soul. We began as pure spirit consciousness to create the design of our immature soul to live in physical form and to learn the lessons of our soul evolution with the strength, courage, and grace of a white horse. The white horse also represents the freedom, wisdom, and beauty of the human soul as it lives and evolves. The white horse also symbolizes the choice of our soul to keep the mind open during a lifetime as it was in the first two levels of consciousness for our immature soul.

The red horse symbolizes the level of our soul consciousness as we evolved in our sexual appetite and began to examine our consciousness of inequality. As we became conscious of the difference between the male and the female, blood played a significant role in the creation of our beliefs and our behavior. Blood continues to play a role in our male and female inequality and symbolizes the periods of our fascination with the meaning of blood. Our fascination led into baptism with blood, sacrifice of the first born, circumcision, and blood as our communion with God, plus other rituals such as war and human sacrifice.

The black horse is the symbol of our physical nature as we descended into our fear, judgement, and blame. The black horse symbolizes the limiting of our intellectual consciousness by the cosmic shell of our ego beliefs. During the black horse period we withdrew into the dark cave of our mind and we attempted to define ourselves and our lives by using the symbols of nature. We had no other knowledge to which we could relate, allowing us to make our nature symbols a form of communication with each other.

"Leukwarm" symbolizes the soul that is living in stasis and is apathetic about life and living. Leukwarm creates a climate that allows the soul free choice to evolve or devolve, and it represents the colorless life of one who lives without the spiritual passion of making its free choice. Boredom and apathy are the feelings of the leukwarm soul that feels no motivation from its mature soul or inspiration from its spirit.

Wrath symbolizes the cold and unfeeling fear emotions of an immature soul that is flirting with devolution as it lives in total rage and resists and denies change. Wrath is the temper tantrum of the ego, intellectual soul, which has not yet the strength of transition and change but is acting out its physical belief in the wrath of God as the image of itself.

Passion symbolizes the hot, passionate love emotions of a mature soul that is living through its creativity, motivation, and inspiration. This soul is actively evolving as it searches for more and more knowledge that allows it to relate itself to all that is. When we live with a passionate love of life we are living the magnetism of our Divine Nature. When we live our sexual passion we are living in our physical nature and our limiting beliefs.

The myths, superstitions, symbols, rituals, and karmic beliefs that we are attached to are the very things that are holding us back from moving our thoughts, emotions, and feelings into the mature soul consciousness of our Divine Nature. When we can look honestly at the miracle of our life, we will begin to be in awe at the cleverness of our soul. If we feel that we are stuck in not knowing how to change, then we must begin to look at our beliefs and behaviors and those that we are uncomfortable with, we must be willing to change. In changing our behaviors first, we will become aware of how our beliefs have been creating each behavior. We must live the changed beliefs and behaviors for at least three months to begin developing a new pattern within our thinking, emotions, and feelings. Have patience with yourself and say "I am love," which will give you the strength to help with any internal change.

The myth that our world is going to be destroyed and we will be destroyed with it is a symbol of our ego fear that the world is coming to an end. Our world is not coming to an end. Only the focus of our soul consciousness is going to change. It is the ego that feels its "world of control" coming to an end that lives in desperation. Don't accept this ego belief because it expands fear and strengthens our immature soul. We have the same amount of time to live as a mature soul as we have already lived as an immature soul. The difference will be in the pleasure we are going to have in our comfort zone. Once we begin to see ourself with love, life itself inspires us to seek peace, joy, and comfort while we enjoy understanding ourselves, our life, and the excitement of our family relationships.

Our ancient symbols, myths, superstitions, and rituals have created the foundation of our religious beliefs and behaviors. The religious beliefs have held us in bondage as an immature soul and are acting as the cause and effect of today's societal dramas.

THE CAUSE AND EFFECT OF OUR EVOLVING BELIEFS

Our beliefs limit our physical lives and therefore they limit our aware consciousness that soul evolution is occurring within our dual mind and emotions. Our beliefs are intellectual interpretations created by the judgement of our physical nature and its concept of inequality, which we accept as "fact." Our interpretation of our "factual" beliefs controls our perception of ourself, other people, and life. For example, our belief in inequality is reflected into religion, science, business, and our multiple relationships as our behavior. Our belief in inequality has created inequality for females in religion, science, politics, government, education, the judicial system, corporate business, and in relationships. Female inequality has been established as a form of lifestyle belief and behavior in all societies and religions on earth. As a soul of male and female consciousness, we are always equal. Inequality as a belief has allowed us to live our ignorance until we have the knowledge to release the belief.

All beliefs exist as the electromagnetic energy of our ego consciousness which controls our intellectual mind, suppresses our emotions, and limits our physical experience. As our beliefs suppress our emotions, we become self-centered in our focus on intellectual "facts," and we are totally devoid of any emotional response and growth. When we fail to grow in our emotional response we limit our ability to expand our consciousness from

139

our intellect as we imprison our mind in our fearful shell of beliefs. Our beliefs are all karmic and they live subconsciously as our ego cosmic shell

We become attached to the regurgitation and repetition of intellectual fact and our mind stops expanding because it has reached its destination of memory. We are literally afraid to go beyond the comfort of our intellectual memory. Our emotions are so consumed with fear that all of our physical experience is judged from our biased and limited view of reality, turning us all into intellectual robots imprisoned by our beliefs.

It is our restrictive ego beliefs that box us into our physical nature and allow us to see life negatively and fearfully as originating outside of ourself. In our box of beliefs we have lost the relationship connection between ourself and each other, society, nature, and God. Our ego is not into change, but rather it is determined to repeat the same tired refrain that it has used from the beginning of our evolution as physical beings in our immature soul. The ego collects beliefs that support its self-centeredness, separateness, and greed. Anything new is antithetic and immediately labeled as wrong because it threatens the ego and its power base of inequality and worship.

Our attachment to ancient, primitive, and outmoded myths, symbols, superstitions, and rituals can become the cause of our soul devolution. Devolution is not a belief for those who do not believe in evolution, and yet devolution is evident in the way our society repeats its pattern of beliefs and behavior out of fear as we slide backwards into our warring and murderous mentality, fear emotions, and abusive behavior. When we look at our intellectual mentality and our fear emotions, we can easily see that both are immature and childish as we judge every facet of our life as either right or wrong, good or bad. Judgement defines our ignorance not our knowledge.

When our mind and emotions are unsteady and constantly fluctuating between good or bad, right or wrong, fear or love, sin or virtue, we are living the duality of our beliefs and our fear is reflected into our relationship behavior. Our dual soul, as our dual mind and emotions of our male and female consciousness, is determined to make us look at the beliefs that no longer work in our lives. Our spirit then continues to get our ego's attention by challenging us in our beliefs by changing our relationships, career, health, and money, so we can experience our emotional loss and grief. By challenging ourself to feel we challenge ourself to think about our beliefs and to welcome change in the transition of our immature soul consciousness.

Only our physical nature lives through its judgement and fear. As we try to move forward into our Divine Nature, we experience devolution by sliding backwards into the beliefs of our physical nature. When we are faced with challenges and we immediately externalize blame and judgement to someone else, we expand our challenge by expanding our fear emotions, which allows us to become conscious of our beliefs if we are willing to look at our thinking.

Our fear will erupt into our beliefs and be acted out as revenge, retribution, and punishment towards the individual that we blame, which distracts our ego thinking and keeps us from dealing emotionally with the mental beliefs that we are living. Our ego reliance on physical distractions that protect us from our internal thoughts and emotions is the way that our physical nature chooses to resist looking at our beliefs.

Why do we have these negative and fearful beliefs which limit our consciousness of our consistent mental and emotional change? Are we so firmly attached to fear that we are literally afraid of the joy and excitement of life? Yes, we are, and within our fear lies the story of our evolution as a spirit and dual soul consciousness. All of our beliefs are karmic and have accumulated as our immature soul has evolved. Each belief has its foundation in our primitive art of creation of symbols, myths, superstitions, and rituals.

We have evolved through many physical beliefs, but our willingness to evolve through our emotions is limited by our belief in inequality. We act out our inequality in our dependency on sex, religion, and science, which we believe are sacred to the survival of our body and soul.

We have evolved unconsciously and subconsciously but we

are afraid to become conscious of the evolution that has been taking place inside of our mind and emotions. Our fear is intense because we do not understand our dual mind and emotions as our dual soul, and our physical nature fears the unknown and unfamiliar. Our beliefs are seen by our ego and intellectual physical nature as our karmic protection that provides our balance in life by saving us physically and eternally in death.

Our ancient, primitive beliefs are in reality our most expansive and dangerous addictions that imprison our immature soul consciousness. If we were conscious of how our beliefs limit our mental and emotional creativity and our physical potential we might choose to change our beliefs, but to consider changing our thinking is threatening to our ego with its fear of change which makes change an unthinkable concept. Our ego sees itself and its intellect as supreme and it wants nothing to do with our loving emotions which it fears. Fear then becomes the impenetrable emotional denial that protects and imprisons our intellect. Our overwhelming fear is reflected into every aspect of our life and becomes the basis of our negative beliefs, thinking, behaviors, addictions, relationships, self-judgement, and self-abuse.

Our ego knows that a superior mind and emotions exists beyond the wall of its restrictive beliefs. But our ego is threatened by change because it knows it must change from self-centeredness to humility as our soul consciousness transitions. This motivates our ego and our immature intellectual soul mind to continue the crises, distractions, challenges, and chaos of our life, until we can finally accept the wisdom of change. Our ego belief that change is negative and fearful simply intensifies our intellectual burden of pain and suffering that we eventually reflect into our physical body as disease, trauma, and death.

Our negative and fearful beliefs have served us in the immature journey of our soul but they are no longer in harmony with our soul mind and emotions that are evolving into their mature journey of growth. We are an eternal spirit consciousness that is learning to be human. Within the understanding of our spirit consciousness "human" means a higher universal consciousness of Mana or Spirit Consciousness. We are following the fractal pattern of the Cosmic Consciousness by being both invisible and visible energy, and by living our soul consciousness as males and females. We are spirit consciousness, dual soul mind and emotions as a male and female consciousness, and a physical body seeking internal unity and creative consciousness expansion. As we evolve beyond our restrictive beliefs we are changing our human consciousness and expanding the potential of our physical reality. Our beliefs are relative only to the level of aware consciousness that we have reached. As we evolve our beliefs must change from external, negative, and fearful to internal, positive, and loving.

Our sexual beliefs have evolved into the scientific and religious interpretations of our physical nature as we related the difference in our male and female sexuality to our judgements of right and wrong, inferior and superior. Because our male physical nature judged itself "right" as the image of God, anyone that did not appear in the same physical sexual form and color was judged as "wrong" and naturally inferior. The emotional and intellectual vibrations from the single belief in inequality continue to reverberate into our consciousness as human beings even today.

Our scientific and religious beliefs adopted the accepted moral law of the male head-of-household and influenced the habitual roles, identities, and behavioral patterns of our male and female relationships. Beliefs of sexual inequality that began aeons ago relative to our physical appearance set the mold of inequality within our intellectual mind and fear emotions for the scientific, religious, and family beliefs that have held us in bondage in the dark side of our immature soul journey as we have descended.

But the joke of our male and female differences is truly upon us and our belief systems because we are all male and female internally and we have frequently changed our external gender during physical lifetimes. What our male physical nature has done unto our female Divine Nature, it will have done unto itself internally and externally when the gender change occurs in another physical life. This is the way that we are learning to love ourself in the unity of our physical nature and Divine Nature. Without living the physical experience of both sexual genders our dual soul mind and emotions would never understand the unity of our physical and Divine Nature.

It is only through the active physical experience of living upon earth that our soul learns and grows. Despite our beliefs in guilt, sin, inequality, fear, identities, roles, and our belief in only one life, our soul is continuing to grow and change into our loving mind and emotions. In effect, our soul grows and changes despite our level of aware consciousness, and that is our "truth of salvation" as the miracle of our eternal life gifted to us by our spirit consciousness. Our belief in being saved by Jesus is a misinterpretation of how we save ourself by growing into a conscious awareness of the Christ Consciousness that exists within us as the integrated male and female consciousness of our dual soul and our spirit consciousness. Our physical nature externalized our belief in Jesus saving us because we did not understand our consciousness mind trinity and the consciousness intention of our internal Divine Nature to help us grow as a dual soul into our personal Christ Consciousness.

As an example, as we seek to love ourself we will all experience homosexual relationships where we seek to learn to love the soul image of the opposite of ourself within the same sexual form. Therefore, even in homosexual relationships one individual will be living from his/her male physical nature and the other will be living from his/her female Divine Nature. Homosexuality has been the clever design of our soul to teach us internal equality while allowing us to see the inhuman behavior of physical inequality. Our need to love the physical image of ourself has become so intense that our sexual experience has become our identity of separation, rather than the lesson of loving the unity of ourself as male and female.

The ego of our male physical nature grabbed all the credit for creation, ignoring the reality of our female Divine Nature as forever continuing the pattern of creation. Our physical nature was created as the antithesis of our Divine Nature. When Eve gave birth to Adam it was the intention of the spirit to create the exact opposite in both visible and invisible energy. This exact opposite is evident in the physical body as well as the dual soul mind and emotions of the male and female consciousness. The male and female bodies, mind, and emotions fit together perfectly to show us the beauty of ourself as a whole physical being and as a trinity of consciousness.

In the immature journey of the soul our physical nature has created chaos to help us become aware of what we do not want in the mature journey of the Divine Nature of our soul. We are at all times a spirit consciousness, male physical nature, and female Divine Nature. When we began our journey as a spirit consciousness we understood that our immature physical nature could not accept personal responsibility for the power of our Divine Nature. With this understanding Eve gave birth to Adam as a physical creation of her androgynous and equal Divine Nature. Inequality was born as a core belief of our physical nature, but it has never been a creation of our Divine Nature or our spirit consciousness.

When our physical nature allowed its ego to take credit for creation it was following the clever plan of our Divine Nature and helping our physical nature gradually awaken to the power of its Divine Nature. Our physical nature was spiritually destined to follow the fractal pattern of creation by learning to accept full responsibility for its change and growth as essential to evolving into its Divine Nature. We will have reached the Cycle of Understanding within our dual soul as it transitions from the immature intellectual mind and fear emotions of our physical nature into the mature soul mind and loving emotions of our Divine Nature. As we mentally and emotionally evolve into our Divine Nature the beliefs of our physical nature are no longer appropriate and we must evolve our beliefs into the ethical values of our Divine Nature. The moral values of our physical nature are opposite to the consciousness of the ethical values of our Divine Nature.

As our male physical nature interpreted its creation it failed to understand the creative power of our Divine Nature and judged itself as having been molded through the physical hand of a "God man" greater than itself. With this interpretation we began our core belief in the inequality of the sexes as the ruling force of our physical nature. Our belief was only relative to our ignorance as we have repeatedly lived the pattern of "creation" as we create new life as human beings within the female Divine Nature.

In our society our physical nature continues to see itself as the ruling force over our Divine Nature, family, society, and the world. The behavior in our sexual relationships, religion, science, government, and business continues predominantly as beliefs of our physical nature. Although some behavioral changes have become apparent in the last few years as the result of challenge and chaos, we have not yet learned to live our equality. Equality, truth, and love are the normal values of everyday living for a mature soul. When the majority of people are living in fear, judgement, and suppression, we are living a lie as a society. Judgement, inequality, and fear are the lies of our immature soul, which we conceal as we live our hypocrisy.

Our interpretation of creation was our external, negative mind and our fearful emotions attempting to define who we are and where we came from. As we judged ourself unequal to our Creator, our judgement created all of our beliefs by relying upon our physical nature and its perception of reality. In our negative, external, and fearful beliefs we set the stage for the dramas that we have lived in the journey of our immature soul. We have lived each belief by making it real as a way of making it "truth." We continue with this habitual repetitive practice of externalizing our beliefs because in our physical nature the belief becomes truth when it becomes physical. This is how our belief in inequality became "real" when we began to live our inequality. When we live our equality, that will become a physical reality.

As we began our descending soul journey we were patterned into our four biological needs, our memory was removed, and we were given personal responsibility for our evolution as a "naked" soul that had no knowledge to conceal itself with. This left us with no realization of the cause and effect of our belief systems as our beliefs are returned to another life. Soul family members frequently return to the same physical families and their minds are repatterned with the same beliefs. In our soul journey, we began to desperately search for something or someone to worship as we realized that we were personally responsible for our growth. Our fear was created from the nakedness of our mind and emotions as our sensory response.

Our spirit consciousness, in its wisdom, created us as a twin soul in male and female consciousness and in physical form to allow us to experience life to its fullest as we lived our dual nature. As our physical nature created the belief in the inequality of the sexes, we molded the focus of our scientific and religious beliefs from the "fact" of our sexual core belief. We created our belief in the external separation of our physical body, soul mind and emotions, and "God." We denied that we had a soul and spirit within us because our reality was created by our external focus. Because of our beliefs in separation from God, God had to be created as external to us. Because of our beliefs in inequality, God had to become an external man. Our belief in control, dependency, and worship set the stage for "God" to become our Savior. Our beliefs vibrate outward like the ripples in a pond, and each belief begins multiple other beliefs which have been lived as the "truth" of our physical reality. Our beliefs about our spirit consciousness were lost in our external reality and we lived our external reflection of the separation between our physical and Divine Natures as our physical separation from an external "God."

With the separation of our body into male and female physical form our physical nature believed it was externalized from our Divine Nature into physical form and it felt anger and fear as it was placed in a position of personal responsibility. Accepting personal responsibility for ourself and our survival was a new perception for our immature physical nature and it was not greeted with excitement and enthusiasm. This began our bondage of fear and cast the pattern for externalizing, negativity, and fear within the physical nature of our immature soul. Our physical nature felt like an abandoned child and quickly lost its vision of the loving soul and spirit consciousness that never stopped supporting it.

Life had been beautiful when our universal mind was consciously inspiring our journey. In our separation we descended into our immature soul mind and emotions, leaving us with a

sense of loss and grief as our immature mind and emotional consciousness was separated from its conscious memory of the
Divine soul and our spirit consciousness. Our overwhelming feelings of loss and grief left our physical nature absorbed in its
external negativity and fear as we began our descent into the
darkness of our immature mind and emotions. With our external
focus we set out to learn the art of creation and to create our
beliefs as our physical reality.

Our physical nature took its core feelings of fear and inequality and related them to every facet of its physical life. As our
external feelings expanded they were accepted as "fact," and the
beliefs of our immature mind and emotions began taking physical form and became the accepted religious and moral law as our
means of human survival. As our core belief in inequality
expanded, our ego expanded and inequality grew and flourished
as a way of life, formulating all beliefs after the pattern of its parent belief. As inequality became the accepted reality of the sexes,
the belief spread into science and religion, limiting the awareness
of our immature soul through its limited judgement of right and
wrong. Since men began science, religion, government, and the
judicial systems they were naturally created from the foundation
of our external, unequal, and fearful belief systems of ancient
primitive vintage.

Throughout the journey of our immature soul, inequality has
become the standard for our intellectual perception and it has
controlled science and religion as it has boxed us into the limited aware consciousness of our externalized physical nature. Our
physical nature began to learn as it fumbled its way through the
billions of years of our evolution, basking in its supremacy of
intellect, sexuality, and control. Our physical nature fought its
way through each soul level by warring, murder, and greed. In
total patience our Divine Nature supported this unequal thought
and external behavior, giving our physical nature all of the time
that it needed to become conscious of its art of creation from the
dual energy of our male and female consciousness.

At last we have subconsciously and unconsciously returned
to the original point of separation for our dual soul male and

148

female consciousness, and our physical and Divine Natures are being challenged with a return to unity. The chaos of our dual male soul mind and female emotions, as it is struggling with its core belief of inequality, is being reflected into our society with a vengeance as we live our transition. Changing the external identities and roles of the male and female will only be completed by attrition as the fear controls many people in their external image beliefs. As the souls that are stuck in their physical nature beliefs die and return to new physical lives in more advanced soul families, the pattern of beliefs will change and the soul will break free from its beliefs and evolve. Because we are living our transition the inequality of our belief system is surfacing throughout our society, with the emphasis continuing to be focused on the inequality between the sexes.

Abuse is a significant belief of our physical nature that exploits the difference between our physical nature and our Divine Nature. Abuse occurs mentally, emotionally, physically, economically, and sexually within our relationships, cultures, and society as we attempt as souls to find equality within ourself. In tolerating abuse of any type or within any gender, we are practicing self-abuse. Self-abuse is our lesson of learning to love, honor, and respect ourself equally in every way. Self-abuse and sexual abuse are simply the internal and external versions of fear that we are living as our strongest and most virulent belief in our own inequality.

The cause and effect of our beliefs is being lived by each of us personally, by society, and by nations. Our belief in inequality is the root of all of the supporting beliefs that control our lives as well as our minds and emotions. As our beliefs have evolved from our original interpretation of inequality, we are coming mid-cycle in our evolution as a dual soul. From the roots of our belief in inequality we harvest war in relationships, societies, and nations, crime, mental and physical disease, greed, dishonesty, discrimination, hatred, abuse, and most of all the inequality that is rampant within our self-abuse. In choosing to change our beliefs and behaviors of inequality, we begin to change our dual soul into one loving soul mind and emotions. When we have the strength and courage within our heart to change our primitive and ancient worship beliefs we will create a Universe that lives in love in peace, compassion, communication, cooperation, and creativity. As a human species this will allow us to bloom like a rose as we take all of our knowledge and relate it to who we are internally. Creating our physical reality from the miracle of our life will change us, earth, nature, and the universe.

THE BEHAVIOR OF OUR
PHYSICAL NATURE

We live the soul consciousness level that we have evolved to by reflecting each belief that we have in our cosmic shell into our physical behavior. Our beliefs are subconsciously reflected into our behavior from the cosmic shell of immature soul lessons we have not yet learned because our beliefs become our point of view about life. It is the reflection of our beliefs into our behavior that keeps us focused on what the soul consciousness has chosen to learn through the physical experiences of our perceptions of reality. Our beliefs create the energy field of our soul persona or energy reflection that we wear as our "coat of many colors." Each lesson is reflected into our thoughts, emotions, attitudes, personality, character traits, language, and behavior. As we learn each soul lesson our intellectual consciousness evolves and the soul image changes.

Our physical reality is at no time in our eternal life separate from the influence of our soul and spirit. Our dual soul and spirit consciousness uses the physical matter that it creates as our body as its tool to experience physical life. Because we are focused upon the precise level of consciousness that we have reached as an evolving soul, we continue to focus our conscious thought into our belief systems that we have accumulated during our descending emotional soul journey. Our consciousness attaches itself to a belief and we subconsciously and habitually

live the belief until we can recognize that it is only a belief and
release it from our intellectual mind. Since our beliefs have a
strong hold on our mind they limit the capabilities of expanding
our consciousness.

Our beliefs are being lived in the guise of what we don't want
as the Antichrist influence. The Antichrist energy is negative,
external, and fearful energy that has become the attitude and
beliefs of our ego and intellect during the journey of our immature soul. It is only when we have the knowledge to understand
ourself as a physical body and its true relationship to our dual
soul and spirit consciousness that we are willing to release our
old superstitious beliefs and change our present behaviors.

Spiritual healing occurs when we release the beliefs that control our immature soul of the left brain and allow the left and
right brain to experience the freedom of being one brain without
the restrictions and control of superstitious belief systems. Bringing our male and female mind together as one soul mind and loving emotions allows us to awaken to our own spiritual hierarchy
of values. For centuries this has been referred to as enlightenment, or entering the "Kingdom of God," which clearly tells us
that the kingdom of God is within us.

Every few centuries since we have been revolving in our
attempt to understand our internal self, we have believed that we
have reached the level of enlightenment with each tiny step of
progress. The belief in enlightenment began long before Paul.
When Paul started the Christian Church, Christianity considered
that it alone understood the truth of God. Paul was not truly an
apostle of Jesus; in fact, he never met Jesus. Paul taught and
wrote opposite to the teachings of Jesus. Paul's beliefs and
behaviors as well as his teachings clearly show us that he was
opposite to Jesus in his soul consciousness. Jesus taught love.
Paul taught fear. Love is the consciousness energy of our mature
soul. Fear is the consciousness energy of our immature soul.

During the days of the Inquisition (mid-1500s) the Church
considered itself and some people enlightened but it put those
who didn't believe as it did to the guillotine test and separated
them from their heads. This is an indication of the strength of our

religious beliefs and how we have acted out our lesson of inequality by judging, blaming, and punishing those who think differently than we think. Our belief in right or wrong, good or bad has motivated our behavior for the entire path of Christianity. As we have lived our consciousness energy of Christian beliefs we have become the essense of the living Antichrist and we have lived the opposite of what our Christ Consciousness and God Consciousness are teaching us.

The behavior of beheading, burning, hanging, or imprisoning a person who has different beliefs clearly shows the level of the immature soul and how we have lived the lesson of inequality as part of our physical experience during our childish descending physical nature. During the past six thousand years of recorded history multiple wars have been fought over the different beliefs that people have about God. Religious wars have always been an indication of the beliefs and behaviors of our physical nature, not our spirituality. All wars have been fought because of basic differences in our religious belief systems, which have encouraged fighting as a method of determining who was right by the physical strength and power of the winner. Our belief systems have been formed from our primitive religious beliefs, especially our beliefs regarding male and female relationships, sexuality, inequality, fear, and deceit.

When Christianity began before the birth of Jesus it was the result of the Romans conquering the Hebrews in 63 B.C. and it followed the Greek philosophy of Plato and Ptolemy. The Christianity that was taught as philosophy by the Greek philosophers was that our spirit was imprisoned in the matter of our physical body. Jesus was also a philosopher whose teachings followed the theme of the Greek philosophers. Paul changed the dictates of Christianity when he began teaching that Jesus was Christ, the savior of humanity, and God was external to us. Paul's version of Christianity began the present intense focus on separation and inequality which we have consistently acted out in our physical behavior.

Paul was born as Saul of Tarsus, a Jew who converted to Christianity in A.D. 43. Although Paul called himself an "apostle,"

the term was coined for those disciples who learned Jesus' teachings from Jesus himself. The apostles of Jesus went out to spread
his teachings to the masses. Paul was not truly an apostle of Jesus
and didn't take up the banner of Christianity until thirteen years
after Jesus left earth. Paul felt ostracized by the Jews and became
a follower of Mithra, a Persian pagan god, before converting to
Christianity.

Many religions were flourishing before the birth of Paul's
Christianity (A.D. 43), such as Hinduism, Buddhism, and Zoroasterism. Hinduism began in 600 B.C. as the continuation of the
Vedic religion from about 2,000 B.C. Veda developed from our
earlier forms of nature worship based on the worship of pagan
gods, and one of its many branches is Sikhism which is now
prevalent in the United States; Buddhism also began around 600
B.C. and was started by the prophet Siddhartha Gotama (Gauta-
ma); and Zoroasterism began in Iran around 6,000 B.C. as the followers of Zoroaster the prophet. Mithra was a pagan god of
Zoroasterism. Islam, or the Muslims, followed the Persian prophet
Muhammad (Mohammed, A.D. 570?-632) and lived by the dictates
of its religious law rather than Muhammad's philosophy. The
word Islam means "submission," and as an ideal it is the total
submission of self to Allah. Men are expected to be submissive
to Allah, and women are expected to be submissive to man as
the physical image of Allah. The Sufis were the mystics of Islam.
In creating his form of Christianity Paul borrowed laws, holy
days, rituals, superstitions, symbols, and methods of worship from
various forms of earlier religions, including Hinduism, Judaism,
Zoroasterism, and various other religions of the time. Paul's Christianity began an intense period of revolution for the human
species as our consciousness energy became habitual and obsessive in its revolving beliefs.

As we have lived life after life in our immature soul we have
brought our soul lessons of inequality, untruth, and fear back
with us in each lifetime as our belief system. We have chosen our
parents as a way of repatterning our intellectual mind into the
beliefs, which will be reflected as our physical experiences and
allow us to continue living the lessons that we must learn. The

soul consciousness is always on target and inwardly conscious of its goals and purpose of life. We have lived without an aware consciousness of our soul because our beliefs have denied this knowledge by focusing on an external, fearful God, preventing us from being conscious of our internal soul and spirit. Despite the denial of our internal spirit consciousness, all religions have been based on some form of prophecy which has been interpreted as the external voice of "God."

As we became a living soul and took on a physical body to use as our tool of growth through living the physical experience of our lessons, we first responded to our biological needs. It is our beliefs and behaviors that have forced us to expand our consciousness in our immature soul journey. In our physical nature we live from the beliefs and behaviors of our sexual core as one of our biological needs. For billions of years our immature soul has been judging, blaming, and fearing our sexual core as the evil within us because it triggered emotions of pleasure and love that were opposite to our beliefs. Because of our loss of memory with each new life we have forgotten that our biological needs are the way of maintaining health and upholding the Law of Continuation for our eternal soul and spirit.

Attaching ourselves to religious beliefs that are reflected into our physical behavior keeps our soul lessons constantly in our physical experience of life and helps us change our aware consciousness. Each time that we repetitiously live a physical experience we become more aware of what we are learning from the experience. As our awareness expands our consciousness expands and we begin to see what we don't want, which gives us the freedom to choose what we do want in our life.

As an example: If we spend thirty lives being an alcoholic we will eventually begin to understand that it is not comfortable for us to live in that state of self-abuse any longer. As we understand what we are doing to ourself we begin to recognize that we can change our behavior and begin to love ourself. It is frequently necessary for an alcoholic to reach the very depths of self-disgust before being willing to accept the need for change.

Changing a destructive behavior gives us back our freedom

and independence as we begin to recognize our internal personal power. Having the external power of alcohol controlling our
life makes us dependent on other abusive behaviors to provide
ourselves with alcohol and we become dependent on the illusions that alcohol creates as our reality within our mind and emotions.

As we become aware that a belief and its resulting behavior
is not getting us where we want to go in our life, we become
conscious of the beliefs and behaviors that we need to change.
Change then creates an opportunity for us to move forward in the
aware consciousness of our immature soul mind and emotions,
which moves us forward to the next level of our soul growth in
consciousness.

The level of our soul growth that we have reached is the
level of consciousness from which we live our lives. Whatever
beliefs we are attached to in our ego cosmic shell determine the
behavior that we act out. In addition to our behavior, our beliefs
determine our attitude, personality, and character traits that we
live moment by moment as a result of our thoughts, emotions,
and feelings.

We wear the energy of our beliefs and behaviors as our "coat
of many colors," which reflects our beliefs and behaviors out into
the open for us to become conscious of as part of our reality.
Nothing about us is truly hidden from others. It is the consciousness level of our soul energy that allows us to be judgemental,
blaming, fearful, and abusive or loving, accepting, sharing, and
peaceful. In the immature journey of our soul consciousness we
are negative, external, separate, and fearful and the mature journey of our soul consciousness is positive, internal, unified, and
loving. In our mature soul we are never dependent upon external possessions, money, relationships or physical processes for
our personal power.

In exploring our mind to find our negative beliefs, we begin
to uncover the old karmic beliefs that are lurking in the shadows
of our subconscious ego mind. Many times these beliefs remain
so cleverly hidden that we must use the awareness of our adaptive habitual behaviors to trigger the memory of our beliefs.

Abusing children and women will symbolize sexual anger and inequality as a karmic or hidden belief.

Because our beliefs began with the inequality between the male and female, we have structured the roles and identities that we live according to the beliefs that surround the sexual core as our physical nature. The inequality that has existed within male and female relationships became the very basis of our religious belief in inequality and our constant behavior of inequality. Inequality is the core belief of our ego that sees the male image of our physical nature as the image of God and therefore superior to the female image. As Paul's version of Christianity was spread throughout the world the primitive beliefs and behaviors of sexual inequality and anger took on a new meaning in the minds of the mass consciousness.

It is our physical nature that is sexually aggressive toward our Divine Nature within our own dual soul mind and emotions. We reflect our sexual beliefs and behaviors into our physical nature and physical lives. We have consistently created our physical beliefs as our physical behavior. On a soul level our physical nature has suppressed our divine nature throughout the level of our immature soul, as we have obsessed on our need to create every thought as our physical reality. On a physical level the male has suppressed the female throughout the level of our descending soul. Whatever is going on in our soul mind and emotions is reflected into our physical experience to expand our consciousness. Therefore, as our mind suppresses our emotions, the physical male suppresses the female with inequality.

In our physical nature our sexuality is at the core of our consciousness, making our physical sexual image the priority of our very existence and the way that we perceive other people. Because our beliefs began with the sexual inequality between the male and female, our beliefs about sexual inequality physically affect each and every relationship that we have. This begins with our parents and continues throughout our lives. The role and identity of our sexuality is the first focus of our thinking, behaving, and consciousness throughout our physical lifetime as we move from one cycle of our life to the next.

Many times we are unaware of the impact that our karmic
sexual beliefs have upon our daily self-judgement, fear, and
behavior. If we feel that we are not sexually attractive to other
people, we will judge ourself out of our fear of not being loved.
Sex and love are opposites. Sex is the biological "need" behavior
of our physical nature that we support with a fear of not being
loved. Love is the emotion of our Divine Nature. Our sexual
nature magnetizes us toward our loving nature. To uncover the
beliefs and the controlling behaviors that we live in our sexual
image, we must discover what our sexual beliefs are and how
they physically affect our behavior on a daily basis. Using the
belief that "sex is love" we can then look at how we behave
sexually.

Is our sexuality seen as a physical need or physical release?
Do you consciously practice control in your sexual behavior? Do
you consciously strive for sexual submission? Are abusive sexual
practices seen as pleasurable to you? Does control enhance your
sexual fulfillment? Are you interested only in your own sexual
pleasure? Do you try to fulfill a fantasy role in the sexual act?
What are your feelings toward your partner after sex? Do you
immediately go to sleep after sex? Do you use sex as a way to
relax? After sex are your feelings of love enhanced? Do you have
a need to hug, snuggle, talk, and share with your partner after
sex? Do you resent being touched after sex? Do you enjoy sex
more after a heated argument? Do you have a fixed sexual image
of your ideal partner in your mind that you obsess over? Do you
crave a precise sexual experience that leaves you feeling unfulfilled if it is not met? If you are a man do you think that all
women want you sexually? If you are a woman do you think that
all men want you sexually? Do you experience jealousy if you see
someone else with a person that you are sexually attracted to?
Are you jealous of your daughter's relationship with a man? Are
you jealous of your wife's relationship with her father? Are you
jealous of your husband's relationship with his mother? Are you
jealous of your son's relationship with his wife? Do you think that
you own your children and your spouse? Are you jealous of your
mate's friends? Are you jealous of the time your mate spends

working? Do you believe that sex is love? Do you have sexual fantasies about someone you don't know? Do you have sexual fantasies about people in power? Do you have sexual fantasies about children?

When sex is practiced only as a physical need the emotions of both partners are suppressed. The physical act of sex can require very little time but loving sex can be an exciting interlude that is a constant play of loving, touching, and communication. Gentle touching, fun activities, courting, dining, and the sharing of thoughts and experiences can enhance the loving relationship for both parties. Love cannot be present if we do not respect, value, and honor the other person that is in our life.

Most people think about sex as something that comes naturally, and indeed it does when it is simply a response to sexual attraction or when it is a loving and shared experience. When sex is experienced as love the soul mind and emotions are involved and the heart responds for the spirit consciousness. With the physical experience of mutual love we feel secure and confident in our desire for sex. Without love there will be a physical sense of emptiness with sex and our heart will feel deprived and uncomfortable. Sex without love can leave both parties feeling sinful, shameful, and guilty as well as unfulfilled.

As we have been living the revolutions of our soul, sex has become more extreme and abusive because the pleasure has dwindled from the repetitious focus of physical sex that is not understood. As we become bored with sex we begin to associate sex with the need for pain and suffering to experience an abusive sense of a physical thrill. Our need to experience sexual pleasure has led mankind into many bizarre sexual behaviors in the ultimate search for the peak sexual experience. As we use sex only as a physical exercise and we suppress our internal emotions, we are left unfulfilled because our emotions trigger our senses which allow us to feel fulfilled and loved.

Our need for the ultimate in orgasmic thrills has led to sadomasochistic behavior, promiscuity, group sex, exchanging of partners, public sex, abuse, rape, incest, torture, and death. These behaviors are old memories of our primitive behavior that we

return to in an effort to get our attention and bring change into
our lives.

Promiscuity moved to a higher level of social entertainment
with our sexual boredom. Homosexuality and bisexuality became
acceptable. Group sex came into vogue and became a commercial venture. Tattooing played a revived role of primitive adorn-
ment and is used as a means of attracting people with similar sexual tastes. Body piercing and genital ornaments added a level of
pain and suffering that has returned us to our primitive roots.
Abuse, torture, and death as part of sexual fulfillment is thought
of by some as their right to fulfill their primitive sexual needs.
Sadomasochism is a sexual way of acting out our need to control
with the infliction of pain and suffering and our need to be controlled with the same behavior from another.

All primitive forms of sexual behavior inflict pain and suffering during the sexual experience and support our primitive religious beliefs that we must experience pain and suffering for Jesus
to save us. The more pain and suffering is used as a means of
experiencing sexual fulfillment, the more intense the pain and
suffering must become to meet our increasing needs. Our need
for pain and suffering is the symbol that we use to remind us that
we are suppressing our emotions and paralysing our feelings. As
we suppress our emotions and sensory response, we are unconsciously denying our female divine nature and devolving into our
primitive nature. When we believe that we must live in pain and
suffering to be saved, we are searching for a physical behavior
that will expand our awareness of our female emotions and allow
us to "feel." Our soul is acknowledging that pain and suffering,
as negative and fearful emotions, are better than no emotions. As
we feel pain and suffering it triggers our hidden soul memory
that we have emotions and feelings even when we deny their
presence.

The relationship between our sexual experience and pain
and suffering as the only true way to experience the ecstasy of
orgasm has its core in the sexual beliefs of our early religious
period. The longer we revolve in our repetitious and superstitious religious beliefs the more bizarre and abusive our sexual

behavior becomes as our soul attempts to wake us up to our unacceptable behavior and beliefs.

To free ourselves of these old religious beliefs and truly enjoy our sexual relationships, we must release our attachment to our need for pain and suffering being synonymous with sex. Our need for pain and suffering is so intense as a form of denial within our cosmic shell that we make ourselves miserable with our sense of sexual rejection, abandonment, and loneliness. We consistently judge ourselves by our beliefs relating to our sexual image and create pain and suffering within our mind from our distorted illusions. As we see ourselves from the illusion of our veils, we become obsessed with our sexual image which we judge as inadequate and worthless. As we expand our consciousness by our male and female consciousness coming together, we can no longer identify with our physical sexual roles. Internally we see ourself as equal in our male and female consciousness when we are willing to use our trinity of consciousness as thinking, emotions, and feelings equally in our life. The old stereotypical physical roles of male and female are simply not appropriate in our belief system at this time.

The Sexual Core of Our Physical Nature

As we expand our consciousness we will feel different because our consciousness level is no longer in harmony and rhythm with the mass consciousness of our family or society. Our old primitive beliefs begin to create rebellion within us as we find ourself unable to live by the worship of our sexual identities and roles. Our feelings of being different are frequently lived at the sexual core of our physical nature as homosexuality, bisexuality, and cross-dressing. Homosexuality is the soul lesson of learning to love the physical image of ourself. Bisexuality is a lesson of duality for our soul as part of our lesson of freedom of choice. Cross-dressing is the physical way that we act out our consciousness of our female and male self and is an image of our lesson of integration as a soul. Our dress always reflects our level of soul consciousness, and dramatic changes for our soul can be seen in the past thirty years.

Until we can truthfully open our mind to facing our religious superstitions as part of our ancient and primitive beliefs, we will not accept that our obsession with sexual roles and identities is needlessly robbing us of our loving soul. It is through our self-abusive, violent, and senseless sexual behavior that we are attempting to transition into our mature soul of love. Until we can understand that sex is better with the emotion of love to support it, we will scatter our sexual activities around in total abandonment as we search externally for our internal sexual satisfaction of integrating our male and female consciousness.

If we are open to examining our beliefs, the logic of not believing as we do becomes very apparent and we find ourselves more willing to change. Looking at our old belief that sex is love can begin the process of opening our eyes. Sex is a physical behavior that our physical nature has used as its symbol of love.

When we first began as a living soul we were a dual soul mind and emotions living in our physical nature and we had no memory of our evolving trinity of consciousness. We were given a biological need to breathe air, drink water, and to nourish ourselves by eating the foods of nature. These three biological needs for air, water, and food were given to us as a means of keeping our body, mind, and emotions healthy so that we could sustain life. Our fourth biological need is sex, which completes the fractal pattern of our eternal life.

But with our gift of life came the gift of death, which allowed us to experience a new beginning when we became too stuck with our perception of the physical that we could no longer evolve as a mind and emotions. Death was given to us as our safety valve so that we could spend three physical days looking at ourselves and choosing a new image of the lesson we were trying to learn.

The cycle of expression that we were given as a living soul and spirit in physical form was birth, life, and death. One could not be without the other. This cycle of expression is the fractal pattern of growth for our soul. Because we were to use our fractal pattern of birth, life, and death as a way of growth, we also needed a biological way of returning as a living soul into a physical body. This was solved by another biological need which we were given as our sexuality. It is our magnetic and emotional sexual "self" that has allowed us to unconsciously evolve as a soul.

As our sexuality became a biological need we had sex with abandonment as the need occurred. This gave the soul and spirit an opportunity to continue with its eternal life by continuing its soul evolution in another physical body. Since we always have freedom of choice as a soul, the soul can choose birth, life, and death in any manner that it wants and it can choose to work with any lesson that it wants. Our immature soul was not limited by beliefs in the beginning of our evolution. It has only been the development of our cosmic shell of beliefs that has limited our immature descending soul in its physical perception of life. Our mature soul that lives subconsciously within us always uses its freedom of choice, without our immature soul being able to understand that freedom of choice is a reality.

As we have lived our cycle of expression countless times as a soul, we have continued to use our sexual appetite with abandonment until we begin to understand the wisdom and beauty of a singular loving sexual focus in life. It is only within the past several hundred years that some souls have evolved into heterosexual monogamy. Many souls that are captured in their physical nature still do not understand that the unity and equality of the internal male and female soul is what we are attempting to learn in our sexual relationships. Eventually we will consciously evolve once more into a union with our twin soul during our soul journey of integration of our dual soul with our spirit.

From the beginning of our biological need for sex we have practiced all manner of sexual copulation. We did not discriminate, but rather we took what we wanted as we wanted it. This sexual aggression could only be practiced by the male, as the design of the physical body prevented the sexual aggression of the female. The female, on the other hand, learned control as manipulation and seduction and would flaunt her sexuality in front of the male of choice. The aggressive sexual behavior of the male and female has changed very little from the beginning of our immature soul journey.

Even today our society continues to use sexuality as the core
of advertisements, movies, songs, TV, books, magazines, foods,
and comedy. Foods are eaten in a sexual manner, lotion is
rubbed on the body with sexual intention, cigarettes are smoked
with a sexual connotation. The seductiveness of our sexuality is
exploited, commercialized, flaunted, and abused all around us in
our everyday life. Our need for sexual arousal has become so
intense that it is acted out as sexual abuse by rape, incest, torture,
and death. Nevertheless, our sexual pain and suffering remains
misunderstood and exploited as we judge ourselves in relationship to our sexual beliefs.

Old sexual beliefs are: Sex is love; I am supposed to be strong
and do what I am told; I will embarrass myself if I speak in front
of others; Women should be seen and not heard; I must be submissive to men so they won't get mad and be abusive; I must be
sensitive to other people's feelings; It isn't polite to talk back; I'll
be a sissy if I show emotion; It is wrong to cry; I must not be
angry; There is women's work, and man's work; If I tell the truth
I will be punished; I have to act like I enjoy sex; If I submit my
body sex will be over sooner; Women are not supposed to enjoy
sex; Men are stronger than women; Men should control women;
Women and children are owned by the male; I can beat my child
or my wife and no one can stop me; A woman should always be
ready to sexually "serve" her husband; A woman's place is in the
home; Men need a mistress; A man's sexual drive is higher than
a woman's; Men should control the family; Women will do anything for money; Only men have a carnal appetite; Women are to
service men without enjoyment.

Our sexuality contains the internal designs of many of our
soul lessons which are also interactive as a way of expanding our
consciousness of self into an understanding of self. Without our
biological needs to keep us continuing with our evolution we
would abandon our lessons of equality, truth, and love. Nothing
about us is separate or unequal. We can only be physical when
we are mentally and emotionally focused in our living soul and
spirit consciousness. Without this trilocular integration our physical body returns to the dust from which it began.

Sexuality, as the core of our physical nature, is enhanced by our biological need for air, water, and food. Food in particular feeds into our sexual image and our self-image. Food is used as part of the sexual attraction as a socialization or courting tool. Food acts as a sensory stimulant to our entire cellular, central, and autonomic nervous systems as the physical symbol of our spirit consciousness. As such, the foods of nature restore our chemical consciousness and expand our aware consciousness. This is the physical reason that eating dinner together is a sensory stimulation that opens our mind to having sex. Our sexual emotions frequently bring forth our diseases of eating such as anorexia, bulimia, obsessive over-eating, emotional over-eating, desperation, depression, need for socialization leading to alcoholism and drug addiction, and a search for love through promiscuous sex. Love is the food of the soul and when it is absent from our consciousness we always seek to restore it to our consciousness through the social integration of eating and sexuality.

As we work on our physical lesson of male and female equality, we reflect our beliefs into our behavior. In a very subtle way we exercise an intense self-control, which we reflect into our behavior with other people. We may not have a consciousness of how we control either ourself or other people but we will be living it if we are willing to look at ourself. As a person lives the lesson of loving self they will seek worship and control as the male symbol of our physical nature. Our male persona is frequently found in a female body. Today we mix and match our physical genders as a relationship of our soul persona.

In looking at the way that we have controlled our biological needs we need only look at the dead food that we are encouraged to buy and eat, the chemically contaminated water, the air that is being polluted with chemicals of all types, and the trees that we are cutting down which destroys our pure air to breathe. The behavior that we have considered scientific and intellectual is abusive to us in every aspect if it is not balanced with emotion and feelings, and as a result we are making ourselves sick as a way to get our attention.

Our focus on sexual inequality allows us to use our physical nature as our control in every aspect of our life. Our sexuality as a biological need is there to fulfill the Universal Principle of Eternal Life by giving us a way to fulfill the Law of Continuation for the soul. As an eternal soul and spirit consciousness we must have a way of returning into physical form by using the exact pattern of evolution that our soul has reached and the fractal pattern of creation that is inherent within our soul and spirit.

The creation of new life by the divine energy of the female through the electrical stimulation of the pattern by the male sperm allows us to live the equality and experience the truth of sexual love between the male and female as a physical experience. Therefore, the biological need that we have for sex keeps creating new life for the soul as another cycle of expression of birth, life, and death.

Our biological need for sex has given us the perfect method of survival as a soul, as it provides our soul with an opportunity to return to a new physical body. When sexuality becomes abusive, the abuse brings pain, suffering, disease, and death into our physical experience to change our consciousness of who we are and the importance of living our lesson of equality, truth, and love. At this point in our soul evolution sexuality is playing a dramatic role in the same way that air, water, and foods are playing a dramatic role in our internal lesson of disease. The primary diseases of our society that consume our attention are the result of our biological needs for sex and food, water, and air being abused.

Contagious sexual diseases are prevalent within both the male and the female because of our attachment to our physical nature. When we are attached to our physical nature we can choose sexual disease as our internal soul lesson. Sexual diseases also include diseases of the sexual organs that change the sexual image that we have of our physical body. These include cancer of the breasts, uterus, ovaries, prostate, testicles, and penis. Other sexual changes that can be seen as "disease" are menopause, midlife crisis, decreasing sexual drive, and impotence. Any sexual changes change the physical sexual image that we have of ourselves because of our beliefs in our sexual roles and identities. If we have lived with a sexual addiction, any physical sexual change will not be understood.

If we see our sexual role being challenged we must begin to look within ourself to see that we are far more than simply our sexual image. Losing our sexual image is also interrelated with losing our physical image. Our physical and sexual image are both related to our biological need for air, water, food, and sex. When our sexual image is challenged by an unhappy relationship, we will frequently destroy our physical image by abusive eating habits or addictive behaviors.

When the sex drive is different in marriage partners the sexual image of the individual with a higher sex drive is at risk. Frequently this brings us into the promiscuity of sex as a sense of rejection and abandonment. In addition, the individual with a lower sex drive may feel an enormous sense of abuse when sex is being forced through a mate's biological need for sex rather than love. These are two images of the lessons of equality, truth, and love that we consistently act out as control rather than communication, and both are typical behaviors of our physical nature.

Our soul always has free choice in every lesson that it is learning. There is no defined way that a soul must live a lesson in our physical nature. The soul can choose to be as creative as it wants to be in designing a physical experience that will allow it the freedom to learn and evolve. Those souls who are designed into interrelated lives have chosen to learn together and will frequently play opposite roles in the relationship to give each other an opportunity to experience both sides of the lesson. There are no accidents in life. We may have no prior conscious awareness of any other events that we experience, but on a subconscious level we have chosen the physical experience to expand our soul evolution.

Our living dual soul is the child of our spirit consciousness. We have learned to focus only within the immature intellectual soul mind and fear emotions of our male physical nature, which has been unconscious of the role it is playing in our soul evolution. The consciousness that we live in our physical nature is lim-

ited to our re-patterned beliefs and behaviors and the intellectual knowledge that we gather, which creates our unique perception of life as our reality. In our physical nature we have no memory of our past lives. In our transitioning dual natures we will be
exposed to past lives but we will interpret them in relationship
to the subconscious memory of our ego. In our divine nature of
understanding we will be reborn with total recall of all that we
have learned and we will have no fear. We will not stop being
physical but our nature will be one of love and compassion
because our mind and emotions will be enlightened. As we begin
to understand the design of our living soul we can have a greater
appreciation for our physical nature and the role that others have
chosen to play in our life. Not all roles will appear as positive
physical roles within our mind and emotions, although for the
soul all roles are positive as they provide us with an opportunity to see what we don't want, which expands our conscious
awareness of the soul lesson and our freedom of choice to
choose what we do want. At this time in our evolution the roles
of our physical nature have become dramatic and are definitely
being lived "in our face" tensely and repetitively to help us awak-
en to the wisdom and beauty of our mature soul and spirit.

When the physical body is seen only as physical matter and
it is not understood as a soul and spirit energy integrated in matter, we miss the magnificence of the physical experiences that we
live and we react out of our external fear rather than our internal
love. Our ego reactions connect us to our external concepts of
physical pleasures such as sex, junk food, physical fitness, alcohol, drugs, money, possessions, and status as our addictive ego
control issues. Our ego has the power to lead us to believe that
our behavior of ancient addictive beliefs is spiritual, which allows
us to intellectually believe that we have reached our destination
of evolution.

Our belief closes our intellectual mind until we create an emotional crisis to open it again. Our emotional crisis may involve
becoming totally disgusted with our own destructive, abusive
behavior. Many ego emotional crises will be lived as the external
abuse of our physical-sexual image, reflecting our intention of

self-destruction. The behavior of over-eating, anorexia, bulimia, drugs, alcohol, and body piercing shows us how we externalize our ego emotional crisis. It is the destruction of our physical-sexual image that frequently leads to suicidal thinking as we shut down our spirit inspiration, leaving us with no sense of worth and no hope of change.

The ego has no respect for the soul and spirit because we never respect what we can control. As our ego closes our intellectual consciousness to the presence of our soul and spirit, it controls the mature soul and spirit by denying it access to the immature soul of our intellect. Control is an ego issue. When our ego can control another person we see ourself as superior to that person, which creates the sense of inequality and disrespect within the ego. Our ego is only in control of our intellectual soul, but because the ego is limited in its vision it is unaware that the mature soul and spirit exist as part of our trinity of mind. Our ego believes itself to be the supreme "god" of our intellect. We reflect our intellectual and ego beliefs into our physical nature to create our reality. The reflection of our intellect has created the ego belief that man is made in the image of God and is therefore superior to woman. This is our ego and intellect attempting to convince us that our physical nature of fear is superior to our divine nature of love. The intellect and ego reflects our fear beliefs of control and superiority into our physical nature and we have lived these beliefs by giving the male control over the female and creating a relationship of inequality for the female in all aspects of life.

The ego senses that something else is putting pressure on it, but the ego is a master of denial and dependency on its beliefs and habitual behavior. Therefore the ego controls the mature soul and spirit consciousness through its ignorance of the trinity of our consciousness. Control is the opposite of communication for the ego. When the ego has the sense that the intellect wants to explore its spiritual self, it creates the belief that the intellect is the spiritual self.

Our ego is in total control of our mature soul mind and spirit consciousness, then, by ignorance, which closes the intellect to

169

the knowledge of soul and spirit, which it denies as part of us. ~~By refusing to communicate with the mature soul mind and spirit consciousness our ego controls the inspiration of our spirit consciousness and the motivation of our mature soul consciousness~~ of love. Our soul and spirit are viewed as an unknown mystery, showing a total disrespect for the value of our trinity of consciousness. Mystery closes the immature mind to the soul and spirit presence out of ignorance. The ego controls our intellect because it holds it imprisoned by the cosmic shell of our beliefs. When we have the belief that our intellect is all there is to our mind, we slavishly follow the adaptive habitual behavior of our primitive beliefs as our truth. Our truth then becomes relative to our intellectual knowledge that is filtered and distorted by our primitive ego beliefs.

In closing the door of our ego mind and ignoring the mature soul and spirit minds, we destroy our motivation and inspiration to create. This works well for the ego because it denies its need to change and it loves the familiar repetition that allows it to be in control. With the intellect closed to our motivation and inspiration the ego relies totally on our sexuality to keep us moving forward by the subconscious magnetism that exists as part of the sexual attraction of our physical nature.

All of our beliefs and behaviors have their origin in our superstitions based upon our sexual core. As primitive beings we were, and are, obsessed with our sexuality because our survival as an eternal soul depends upon our return to physical life. It was during this primitive time that sexuality was practiced with abandonment. All forms of sexuality were experienced, from heterosexuality to homosexuality, bisexuality, pedophilia, pederasty, zoophilia, necrophilia, sadomasochism, sexual abuse, incest, rape, statutory rape, voyeurism, exhibitionism, prostitution, promiscuity, group sexual encounters, sexual fetishes, public sexuality, terminal sexual orgasm, sexual mutilation, sodomy (anal intercourse), fellatio (oral intercourse), celibacy, sexual abstinence, and "masturbation." At the present time we are re-living the accumulation of our primitive sexual behaviors.

As we evolve from the primitive journey of our immature

soul into the mature journey of our soul we find our sexual attraction changing to a loving soul attraction and the sexually deviant behavior changes. Each soul evolves at its own pace as it begins to understand knowledge and the relationship of knowledge to self. Evolution must occur for the entire human species, and therefore every human will change whether it means change through crisis or through a willing excitement. As we change we are changing from the sexual focus of our physical nature to the loving focus of our divine nature.

TEMPER TANTRUMS OF OUR EGO PHYSICAL NATURE

Our biological needs for air, water, and food were given to us for the survival of our body, dual soul mind and emotions, and spirit consciousness. Our biological need for sex was given to us as a means of reproducing ourselves into multiple lifetimes, our magnetic evolution, and our sensory stimulation. At this time in our evolution, both our eternal and physical survival needs for pure air, water, and food, plus our eternal and physical survival need for reproduction have been forgotten, and we treat all of our biological needs as self-centered pleasure needs. Because we do not understand our journey as a dual soul consciousness, we have commercialized and demoralized our biological needs out of ignorance. We have turned the temple of ourself into a market place and we feel guilty when we experience self-love.

Our obsession with food, drinking, and sex has gone beyond the limits of our soul endurance as we find ourselves sliding backward into our gross, obsessive food fetishes, drinking fetishes, and our primitive sexual behavior. Our food and drinking fetishes and our sexual fetishes support each other as we begin to devolve as a human being. As it becomes more and more challenging to reach sexual satisfaction, we allow the sexual act itself to reach new levels of abandonment and abuse that reflects our need for pain, suffering, punishment, and even death. In many instances we rebel against our own sexual desires in total rage, which we inflict upon the opposite sex with our external perception of blame, judgement, and abusive behavior.

For a soul that is searching to release itself from the descending emotional journey but that is still connected to and controlled by the ego, sex, drinking, drugs, and food become the ego's way of control and revenge. When sex is used as anger, rage, and abuse the soul is working on a physical basis to reflect the internal struggle between the male and female soul consciousness. Food is used and abused as part of our sexual rage and can devolve the soul into cannibalistic behavior. All murders have a sexual component for our ego. "Used" and "abused" are key words that do not include the emotions of love but are simply the sexual exploitation of the physical body on multiple levels.

Sexual deviation and female abuse is an indication of our suppressed emotional energy, which is the symbol of our female self, that is acted out externally towards the female by anyone living in their primitive physical nature. The mutual hostility that was created when the physical male and female were both placed in the immature soul of their physical nature must be healed for the internal male and female soul to come together as one in the divine nature. Our soul lessons always become our physical lessons as we act out our internal dramas by creating our thoughts, emotions, and beliefs into our external physical dramas of life. We reflect our internal self externally into every facet of our physical reality as our art of creation.

As humans we always reflect the level that our soul is working within into the physical reality that we create. That is the way that we learn the art of creating our reality. There is no mystery to life once we can understand the journey of our soul. At this time in our evolution, history is our ally when we can see it truthfully and focus on the progress that we have made rather than the wars, competition, and superstitions that we have lived and are constantly repeating.

Because of our belief in the inequality of the male and female, most of history has ignored the intense role that has been lived by the emotional female in guiding the linear mind of the male through his physical nature. The role of the female has frequently been discovered by science and ignored or not reported as part of history. This has occurred primarily because women were

172

revered more in ancient times than they have been since the onset of religions. To support religious beliefs the male had to play a superior role over the female. The focus on the inequality of the male and female tells us more about the ego belief in the superiority of the male as a sexual predator than what really happened.

Our biological needs for air, water, and food have become as distorted as our sexual needs as we approach both with abandonment rather than understanding. This becomes our reflection of the struggle that is going on internally which we experience externally as we try desperately as a soul to break free of our male physical nature's obsession with its sexual core. At the present time as humanity struggles with this challenge we find a dramatic return to Eastern philosophies that emphasize our sexual core and the male as superior to the female, who is expected to be submissive. Hinduism, as part of the foundation for Christianity, is being revived as our primitive memories bind our intellect to our sexually focused ego and we worship the "god" of our physical nature as our sexuality. The meditation and inertia of guru control is opposite to our spiritual self that lives with a passion for the miracle of life.

All religions have fed into the inequality lesson for our intellect and ego soul. As long as we connect our reality to the worship behavior of any religion we stay focused on the ignorance of the inequality of sexual beliefs in our intellectual mind. Our superstitions and ritual worship all evolved from the symbols of our primitive mind as it attempted to discover and understand the relationship between the male and female mind and emotions as well as the human and earth. As we have evolved, our worship has changed only to fit the beliefs of the present time. But the core of our inequality belief continues to be rooted in the symbology of our ancient mysteries of life, which all began with our attempt to understand the difference in the male and female sexuality.

Today we think about our sexuality with a sense of freedom, but we live the abandonment as our personal "cross of pain and suffering" inflicted through our primitive religious beliefs and behaviors. Without the knowledge of why we are obsessed with sex, we behave sexually from our old, primitive concepts of abandonment which are acted out in our relationships as female control. Our belief in the male control of the female affects each and every aspect of our intellectual and ego lives from the board room, courtroom, to the bedroom.

As we crucify ourselves with our primitive sexual beliefs and inequality behaviors we are living the biblical quote, "Father, forgive them for they know not what they do." Living through the sexual core of our physical nature has allowed us to experience the control, manipulation, seduction, fear, anger, rage, conformity, and rebellion as the accumulated focus of our physical lives throughout the journey of our intellectual and ego soul living in our physical nature.

Fundamental religions such as Baptist, Catholic, Presbyterian, Methodist, Judaism, and Islam work intensely to control the political, educational, and social order of humankind. All fundamentalists see "God" as the male image and the male as the true representative of "God" on Earth. Inequality is the root of all religious worship and the fundamentalists present the strongest collective consciousness in society today as they labor relentlessly against a change to equality. Religion is the Antichrist of the human species which is being lived by our ego to help us understand the equality of our male and female soul consciousness.

Fundamental religions are the true Antichrist movement in our world because they are preventing a change in the fundamental and addictive beliefs which hold people attached to their inequality, fear, and control issues. Inequality, fear, and control create dependency, failure to accept responsibility, and the habitual behaviors of following addictive beliefs through the illusion of faith rather than knowledge. Addictive worship beliefs hold all of society in inequality, abuse, destruction, and deceit. Because we are seeking to change into our personal Christ Consciousness by living our love, the inequality, fear, and control of our ego prevents us from living our soul choice to change. Our Christ Consciousness is the Divine Nature of our female soul. Religion as the Antichrist wants us to believe that our female divine nature is unequal to our male physical nature.

Each day of our life our beliefs reflect our attachment to old adaptive habitual behaviors that we do not consciously realize are controlling our intellect and ego revolution. These behaviors become so commonplace and accepted as part of us that we have not a clue that the behavior is destructive and preventing our fearful soul from evolving into our loving soul.

It is impossible to uncover old superstitious beliefs without first looking at our behavior and how we support the continuation of our controlling male ego beliefs. Since we have been living in our physical nature, which has sexuality at its very core, we must look first at our sexual behavior. Our primitive beliefs as superstitions and rituals become the source of our unequal behavior. We can effectively change both our beliefs and our behavior if we can truthfully accept the logic of science and history.

We have been mentally attached to our beliefs and behaviors for many billions of years that have created a pattern within our ego and intellectual mind. We react to our beliefs by our behavior without a consciousness of why or how the karmic memory affects the pattern of our daily lives. The sins of the fathers are passed on to the sons as adaptive habitual behaviors that have followed us through multiple soul lives and that are looked upon as normal and friendly by our ego. The ego does not like change. Our ego has been in its glory as we have spent the last fourteen thousand years in the physical repetition of our soul revolutions, intensifying our ego beliefs in inequality of the male and female as we have created the foundation of our physical reality from our male physical nature.

Our ego behaviors always reflect our thinking, emotions, and feelings about ourself into the external world, and throughout our immature soul all crimes have been committed by our male physical nature regardless of the sexual gender of the physical body. As we live in our negative mind and fear emotions, we can only see the negative side of life. The glass is half empty—never half full. From our negative, external, and fearful mind and emotional focus we create self-destruction and world destruction. Our language and behavior becomes abusive as a means of protecting ourself and our personal survival. As we reach the point of change for our soul evolution our ego returns to negative, primitive behavior such as sexual abuse of women and children, cannibalism, and killing for the "fun" of killing as a way of ego self-protection to avoid change. Our physical nature literally collapses into an ego temper tantrum as it experiences a total failure to love self. In our ego fear we resort to old religious beliefs once again to keep from losing our male power of control. The collapse of our immature soul into primitive behavior is the fractal pattern of the universal "black hole."

Our judgement, blame, criticism, and copying of inequality, abuse, anger, rage, and hate are all directed towards anyone in our path that can be used as a societal example. Our male physical nature fears not being loved. Because of our expanded technology, personal experiences are being used as societal lessons of control, manipulation, seductive behavior, language, lying, deceit, anger, conformity, copying, fad-following, rage, revenge, punishment, sexual abuse, pain and suffering, self-abuse, and self-mutilation, where large masses of people can passively learn what they do not want in their lives and choose to change their beliefs and behaviors. Some souls will choose to become examples of lessons that society is attempting to learn. Religion refers to these souls as "victim souls." Our soul is never a victim because it always lives from free choice.

These emotions and mental beliefs create our thinking, feeling, and behaviors which cannot be separated from each other because they have accumulated into a cohesive attitude, personality, character, language pattern, and behavioral patterns within our society. Our physical nature has allowed us to become followers of inequality as we have worshipped others as superior to ourself.

As a soul we choose our life and make decisions during our life to support our dual soul in its evolution by our physical experiences. We act out these controlling behaviors without a consciousness of how our behavior affects others or what the behaviors mean in terms of our evolving soul consciousness. Since we continuously wear our precise soul energy persona as our thoughts, emotions, attitude, personality, character, language, and behavior, there is no mystery concerning the soul level of consciousness that we are living. Our acting out of beliefs and behaviors is truly our soul "coat of many colors" that does not live in any mystery except the illusion of the "mystical" that is created by our ego as smoke and mirrors. When anything in life is a "mystery" it reflects our ignorance or lack of understanding of that particular reality. When people say, "I see your aura," they are seeing the level of consciousness that reflects as energy to surround our physical body. Each one of us lives in our own unique level of aura or physical consciousness.

Any type of control is always our ego behavior. Controlling language always has a sexual connotation of inequality and superiority despite the physical sex of the individual. Females who are in their physical sexual nature will be more aggressive with language control than many men who are striving to open their mind to their divine nature. Listening carefully to the words, tone, intent, and quality of language allows us to see the power of control that our ego subconsciously uses with other people.

EGO LANGUAGE

"In the beginning was the Word." This is the explanation of the power of language as we live it through the cycle of expression as thought, word, and action. The cycle of expression that we live reflects the truth of our immature soul level of consciousness. We can only change the truth of our soul consciousness by changing the outcome of the cycle of expression with knowledge as an expanded awareness of life. With knowledge we choose to think from our divine nature rather than our physical nature. Each thought that we have is reflected into our language, which is again reflected into our behavior to create our physical experience as life.

We use controlling language as an ego distraction, which prevents equal communication and freedom of choice for other people in our presence by talking all the time, silence or refusing to speak, and speaking but not hearing. Our language controls our behavior in multiple images when we: tell instead of ask; refuse to hear until we get our own way and hear what we want to hear; lie and embellish details to entertain and become the center of attention; lie as fear of being wrong—fear of punishment; lie to create an "I know it all" self image; gossip—spreading information (I-know-it-all belief); use vulgar words and speech patterns, which control by the shock value of disrespect, dishonor, and lack of value for others, limit communication because of the flaunting of the need for attention, flaunt the aggressive image of our physical sexual nature, and flaunt the ignorance of the thinking and beliefs; intentionally control through verbal demands; intentionally control through the fear of punishment by threatening language behavior; and when we use language that focuses on expectations of behavior from another person.

Language is used for manipulation and control as a natural reaction of the level of consciousness of our physical nature. Manipulation is a form of control that is used as a subtle form of illusion. Manipulation is more covert than outright control and generally includes sexual seduction as an obvious distraction. The sexual seduction will also be subtle as a way of using language to allow the listener to hear what they wish to hear. Manipulation of language for the purpose of subterfuge is abundant in our society, and it plays on the beliefs and fears that come from our old superstitions. Lying is a major component of manipulation and seduction, and it is motivated by our physical nature because of our fear of failure to achieve our self-centered goals and be sexually desirable.

Manipulative language is based on various forms of lies that are used as a means of controlling the behavior of another person. The lies weave a web of deceit that captures the fear of others and makes them more pliable to the molding of language as an illusion. These lies are passed on as superstitions, gossip, innuendo, and as fact, which in time become our beliefs.

Religion, education, politics, science, and the family culture have all used manipulative ego language and lies to obtain the wanted response of believers out of fear. The superstitious illusions that we have believed have held us captive of other people's control, manipulation, and seduction from the beginning of our physical nature. We have manipulated and lived all of our physical art of creation through inequality, untruth, and fear so that we can experience the physical lesson of our soul and gain the skill and knowledge to change our beliefs and behaviors.

Religion has been the master teacher of control and manipulation with "the word," as ancient interpretation of prophecy. Science has learned the technique well and followed suit. Family relationships have taken the verbiage of religious language and demanded inequality between the male and female. Societies have adapted erroneous religious beliefs in inequality as the foundation of their governments.

"New Thought" or "New Age" that began again soon after the beginning of this century used manipulative language as a way of enticing followers back into the primitive memories of the physical nature of our soul. In the same manner, the word "Metaphysics" is now being interchanged with New Age, Religion, and Spirituality as though they are the same beliefs, philosophy, and behavior. The manipulation of language comes not only in the control of the words but the implied definition of the words and the implied relationship of different words. With manipulation the delivery is wrought with lies, misconceptions, and misinterpretations. Lies are intentional untruths, where misconceptions are perceptions that are due to inaccurate beliefs, and misinterpretations occur because of ignorance. Manipulation of truth is the outcome of language within our descending immature soul. Lies are motivated by deceit and inequality within our ego. All other misconceptions and misinterpretations are not necessarily intentional forms of manipulation, but are innocently believed because the knowledge is not understood at the time the superstition is adopted as "fact."

Seduction is a sideways method of control in the same genre as manipulation. Seduction has an added sexual flavor and may frequently be used as an outright romantic intention or courting to allow the ego to succeed. There is a courting that will take place that does not always have a sexual outcome as the intention, but the sexual ploy or behavior can be used simply as one more means of seduction to meet a variety of self-centered goals.

Spirituality is now being used as a word that carries a powerful-
ly seductive force. Without an understanding of what the behavior of the spirit is, the concept of being spiritual can be accepted
intellectually as part of the seduction of our ego religious beliefs.
Religion is the opposite of spirituality. Religion is focused on the
inequality of the male and female and worship of an external
"man-like" God. Spirituality is when we physically live the trinity
of our male, female, and spirit consciousness as the unconditional love that dwells within us.

The manipulation and seduction of religion in the control that
it has exercised over humanity from the beginning of the past two
thousand years is overwhelming. The persona of the Antichrist
has been a total behavior of external judgement, blame, control,
manipulation, seduction, negative language, fear, anger, and rage
(wrath) that we have allowed to seduce us because of our intense
victim consciousness that we have superstitiously created in
our immature soul. We believe that we are powerless to "save"
ourselves.

Fear is the emotion of our immature soul that has led us into
our need to control, manipulate, and seduce in an effort to convince our physical nature that the religious belief in inequality is
truth. We are all equal as human beings. Our ego accepts our religious behavior as truth and clings to control as its power, despite
the inequality, deceitfulness, and fear that we generate in others
through our primitive beliefs.

We can never rid our belief system of control and fear in any
of its images until we accept that we are equal, truthful, and loving and we can totally live the image that we see within ourself.
In living the equality, truth, and love within us we can transition
into our divine nature and live spiritual lives. We are never spiritual when we are living in our physical nature because it is
opposite to our divine nature. When we think that we are living
in our divine nature but our language and our behavior reflect
our physical nature, we are seducing ourselves intellectually into
thinking we are spiritual. We have lived the illusion that religion
is spiritual in our lives because of our fear of survival. When we
seduce our intellectual mind into thinking we are already spiritu-

al, we control the image of spirituality in the minds of the masses and deny our need to change.

As religion controls the image-definition of spirituality in our minds it manipulates a seductive worship of the religious as superior to and more intelligent than others as we live our inequality. The human species was created in total equality as the trinity of our dual soul mind and emotions and spirit consciousness. What one person can do all people can do. Not everyone will reach the identical level of accomplishment at the same time, but our potential lives within the equality of our dual soul. There is no mystery in the equality, truth, and love that we will live once we bring our dual soul together as a male mind and female emotions. As one soul of male and female consciousness, the alchemical marriage of ourself will be complete as the integration of our dual soul.

Language is our verbal behavior. How many times in a day do we verbalize the words *no, can't, won't, afraid, can't afford, I hate,* or *I don't know?* How many times do we verbalize vulgar words? Each of these words closes our mind and controls our soul evolution. Negative words put us down mentally and emotionally. Our language is frequently used as a means of suppressing our emotions by our ego showing disrespect to our intellect with abusive words that do not honor and value our self-image. Abusive language is a method of control and manipulation of our ego towards our intellect to show the superiority of our physical nature.

When someone tells you "no" do you accept their wishes or do you attempt to control them by aggressive behavior? Do you use the word "no" to control yourself? "No" closes the mind down and focuses us totally on what we can't do. We use "no" to control ourselves, which allows us to control another's choice of behavior by not acknowledging their response. It is challenging for us to understand that our "needs" are not identical with another person's choice.

When we attempt to persuade another person to live by our rules, we are controlling, manipulating, and seducing the other person. This is a form of personal control as manipulative salesmanship that is annoying and destroys the integrity value of friends and family. This level of interference comes from the ego and has no relationship to our mature soul and spirit, but a clearly reflects our physical nature.

When we learn to speak so that we allow everyone free choice, we are learning to live our love. In organizing another person's life for them, we create dependency and control which destroys the other person's independence and freedom of choice. Religion has been based upon controlling our thoughts, emotions, beliefs, and lifestyle behaviors, which has kept the human species controlled, dependent on being saved and worshipping their fear beliefs for thousands of years. To share knowledge and then provide freedom of choice is the very foundation of communication. Control prevents the freedom of communication, which allows worship to flourish as ignorance prevails, and the masses tremble in their fear of punishment.

We have learned to depend upon our control to get what we want in life and we use our need to control in a subtle and insidious way without a clear consciousness of what our behavior represents. Anytime that we interfere in another person's freedom of choice, we are controlling that person. When we tell anyone what they should do, we take away their freedom of choice. The appropriate behavior is to ask the question, "What do you want to do?" Control represents our fear and inequality. Questions create an equal sharing of information so that a conclusion can be reached by free choice, which we use as a method of respect if we have no fear and we are open to sharing knowledge as communication. Jesus taught the masses to ask questions which he answered in parables showing how their behavior was controlling; unfortunately we are still living our control and continue to be resistant to changing our behavior.

Religion itself adopted the ultimate control of the masses by teaching and living inequality, which is the exact opposite of Jesus' teachings and his way of life. But because we are attached within our own soul to external concepts, control, negativity, fear, and competition, we accept these beliefs and behaviors as a rational and necessary lifestyle that reflects our own soul persona. Our lifestyle of pain, suffering, chaos, and fear fulfills our expectation of a religious life and validates our belief that pain and suffering is necessary for our salvation.

With the inequality belief uppermost within our intellect, we resist seeing that making changes in our life is evolution. The difference for us is that as long as we were focused in our intellect and ego mind we evolved without a consciousness of evolution. Now we must consciously choose evolution as we transition into our mind of wisdom. Becoming aware of our soul and spirit as the trinity of our consciousness challenges us to live our equality, truth, and love through our freedom of choice, will, and intention. We now have the wisdom to understand, accept, and acknowledge our dual soul mind and emotions and our spirit and their integration within our physical body.

The perception of male and female inequality is supported by religion, science, and sexual relationships, and we find ourselves living our sense of inadequacy, hopelessness, and worthlessness secondary to our belief in inequality. Inequality is the opposite of what Jesus taught. Our theory that we are living the teachings of Jesus brings us to another behavioral lesson of the soul, which is our truth.

Lying and deceitfulness all come from the sense of superiority that is the reflection of our belief in inequality. Only the ego wants to control, manipulate, and seduce another by refusing to face the truth of life. Our self-centeredness and our self-image are created by our sense of superiority, which is the seductive illusion of our ego mind. This does not keep the ego from protecting itself and its image at the cost of another's self-image.

Because our ego is controlling, unequal, and fearful it will stoop to the lowest level known to man to prevent its change. Because of the male ego belief in inequality our entire immature soul journey has been lived in externalized negativity and fear to avoid seeing who we truly are in our physical nature. Our societal disciplines that have guided us through our immature soul growth all reflect the unequal behavior of our physical nature and its ego. Nothing escapes the influence of our unequal behavior, whether it is religion, medicine, science, politics, govern-

ment, education, law, or socialization. The reality that we have
~~created from living our inequality, untruthfulness, and fear must
now change as we transition into our mature soul.~~

~~The fractal pattern of our~~ dual soul comes from the fractal
pattern of the earth, nature, and the universe. At times and in certain places the earth splits apart and folds into the center of itself.
The universe also folds into the center of itself in what is known
as a black hole. Now, as we reach the point of self-actualization
where we must live consciously in our equality, truth, and love,
we have the choice of evolving into our ascending consciousness
or resisting change, which will allow us as humans to fold into
the black hole of our immature soul mind and emotions as we
devolve back into our descending soul.

Accepting personal change is our challenge. If we are fearful
we will resist change by denying that our beliefs and behaviors
are the reflection of our personal soul level of consciousness. Evolution is the most exciting part of our lives as humans, and
acknowledging the ascending soul mind consciousness as the miracle of our life is a gigantic step forward. When we are willing to
change our descending emotions and allow the double helix of
our mind and emotions to become balanced, we will easily evolve
into our mature soul consciousness. We have been taught to be
followers, attached to our symbology as superstition, and living
our repetition of beliefs and behaviors as our only concept of reality. When we are searching to understand ourselves we must be
willing to look at the miracle that we call life and how we relate
to each other and the miracle of nature, earth, and the universe in
which we live. As we change into our mature soul mind and emotions we begin to recognize that we are on the journey home to
our spirit as an evolving mature soul consciousness.

Religion teaches us to be fearful, angry, unequal, and self-
centered. Religion molds our government, education, science,
family relationships, medicine, judicial system, and every other
aspect of our lives. The core issues in religion are inequality,
deceitfulness, judgement, and fear. By accepting religious teachings we live the religious beliefs of worship as our daily behavior. Religions are the Antichrist that is spoken of in the Bible,

because religions have always taught the opposite of what Jesus lived as the true energy of his Christ Consciousness.

Jesus came to teach us how to live our Christ Consciousness as the mature soul of our Divine Nature, but the perception and interpretation of his teachings came from the physical nature of our male intellectual and ego mind that was not yet willing to change. The important message of Jesus was how he lived and not the written perceptions that remain as religious interpretations and teachings. Religions have always been the reflection of our ego and intellectual mind of worship. The ego and intellect are into control, manipulation, seduction, anger, conformity, rage, and revenge. The last level of our fear is rage and rebellion. When we reach the stage of rebellion we demand to be different and we act out whatever rebellious behavior that we can conceive that will allow us to live our differences.

Today's youth and the youth of the last forty years have been living their rebellion. We have been wandering in the wilderness for the past forty years in the same way that our soul has been wandering in the wilderness for the past forty billion years. We are acting out the primitive biblical parables in our own life and we continue to resist seeing the relationship of our evolution to our beliefs and behaviors as we make our beliefs, emotions, and behaviors real as our physical creation of reality. Our resistance will allow us to be swallowed up by the black hole of devolution if we choose to follow the physical processes, religious beliefs, and controlling behaviors that we have lived thus far.

The subtle and insidious behaviors that we live are always reflected into our thoughts, emotions, attitude, personality, character traits, language, and behavior as the persona of our physical nature. We continue to live these behaviors as our physical reality without a consciousness of what they are. Since we use our relationships as the fiber of our soul growth, each and every lesson is at constant play in our daily lives, reflecting our level of soul consciousness as our daily lifestyle dramas. Each soul is personally responsible for its own growth and its survival. As we live our external judgement and blame we are simply acting out our soul reflection in the lives of others.

The word "survival" represents our survival as a soul during this period of change from the revolutions that we have been living to our evolution of consciousness as the integration of our dual soul mind and emotions. When we are actively working with our soul survival, we will reflect the survival lesson into our physical reality as our physical survival with a focus on either disease, insurance, money, poverty, or relationships as different images of the same lesson. Our physical survival is equated today in terms of money, possessions, career, and relationships to show us that none of these physical realities bring us internal happiness. Therefore, as we live the changes that will assure the survival of our soul, we will also be living the physical lessons of money, possessions, career, and sexual relationships, which will affect our biological needs for air, water, and food to balance our physical body and soul. In using money as our survival we must do so with equality, truth, and love to transition into our divine nature. Without equality, truth, and love being lived we cannot break through our ego beliefs and behaviors and integrate our male and female consciousness.

If we are attached to control, fear, anger, deceit, and inequality, our beliefs and behaviors will put our physical survival at risk. This will create an opportunity that will allow us to discover our personal power or we will find ourselves mired in physical paralysis and depression. The soul has an investment in our clearly understanding what we have learned as knowledge. Just when we feel that we have learned a lesson we can find ourselves in the midst of a drama that will challenge us to use our free choice as a way of understanding our own growth. Recognizing our need for change and coping with it equally, truthfully, and lovingly without attachment to the drama shows our awakening to the understanding of ourself.

Living in a relationship where control is absolute, we will feel disrespect, dishonor, and a lack of value for ourself. The control will remove the last vestige of value within ourself as we worship the relationship. As the relationship ceases to live in terms of the loving mind and emotions, it will soon dissolve on a physical level. When the ego and intellect are in control the person will be totally unaware of the damage they are inflicting into the heart of their mate. Since control, anger, and fear are signals of war for the ego, it excites the ego to stay in "fighting" condition by living its beliefs in inequality and superiority. This "fighting" condition allows the ego to constantly be plying its trade in all relationships as it seeks its next battle.

If both individuals in a relationship are living their need to control, war will break out in the relationship because the ego and intellect will be in active competition with each other. If one person refuses to fight, the other person will feel rejected by the refusal. The ego expects fighting and sees a good war as a necessary battle well fought, and this returns the relationship to normal for the ego. The loving self detests war, competition, even the illusion of battle, and would rather switch than fight, even when switching means finding a new relationship.

Control destroys our self-respect and inflicts mortal wounds into our emotional love. Control affects the loving mind as a prison affects an innocent person. Control imprisons our beliefs and behaviors and keeps us fearful of change. It is insulting to the loving mind when someone who is living their self-centered control tries to inflict control into the loving mind as inequality. Being acutely conscious of our controlling behavior can save our intimate relationships, as well as our family and friends.

Do you tell people what you want them to do? Or do you ask people what they would like to do? Telling a person what to do removes their freedom of choice and places them in a controlled, dependent relationship with you. Asking a person what they would like to do gives them the freedom of choice to defer to your plans or to freely communicate their own wishes. Telling is control, asking is freedom which encourages further communication and clarity. Control is a reflection of our belief in inequality that we live through our behavior and reflect into our relationships with other people.

Interference is control. If we offer advice that is not sought, we are interfering. Interference is the behavior of the "I-know-it-all" belief. Interference is a common behavior of the ego and intellect and is found in every aspect of life. Gossip is an insidious form of interference. Judgement is an overt form of interference. Lying is a covert form of interference.

Dependency is an avoidance of personal responsibility. Religion has taught us the belief that "Jesus will save us," which removes our personal responsibility to save ourselves by our own change and growth. Making another person dependent upon our advice, our laws, our relationship, or upon guru worship is the most blatant form of overt control and interference within our society and it creates the need to worship and to be worshipped. Dependency removes our personal responsibility, which destroys our creativity, motivation, and inspiration to change.

Our belief that death is a sin affects every aspect of our life as we live our physical nature. Believing that death is a sin allows us to live our life with the constant fear of death. It is our belief that death is a sin that allows the medical profession to constantly be in competition between life and death. We view our pain and suffering in disease as payment for our sins and struggle to keep from dying because we believe we have only one life.

Once we understand the cycle of expression of birth, life, and death as a grain of sand on the beach for our soul, we see that death is not a sin and we no longer fear our new beginning. As a soul we return to multiple physical lives in our cycle of eternal life. The belief that death is a sin has been established by religion secondary to multiple parables: Our belief that Adam and Eve were cast out of the Garden of Eden because of the sin of sex, was reinforced when the Ark of the Covenant was built and it became law that to touch the Ark was a sin and the person who touched it would be put to death. Since sex is a biological need and we must procreate we see our sexual urges as constantly sinful, which subjects us to our belief in the sin of death as punishment for our guilt and sin of sex.

Still later, Paul's sexual temptations solidified the belief that death is a sin which we must pay for with our life as the price of our sexual needs. As the personage of the Antichrist, Paul has played an enormous role in establishing the persona of the Antichrist personality within the masses. In creating the religion of Christianity for the Gentiles, Paul taught the masses to live as he lived through the energy of the Antichrist, which was the totally opposite energy that Jesus lived and taught as a philosopher.

Paul lived in sexual pain and suffering because he was a homosexual who had an innate hatred and distrust of women. Although he tried to resist his sexual needs he did not always succeed, and he put the blame and judgement for his sexual choices upon his mother. Paul was a Jew with the birth name of Saul of Tarsus and his sexual preference was not accepted by his culture. His feelings of being an outcast within his own family encouraged him to become a follower of the pagan Persian god Mithra, and to dabble in the ancient Hindu religions with their nature rituals and worship of female submission.

As Paul took upon himself the mission of the Antichrist, he brought his pagan beliefs into Christianity and taught them as the teachings of Jesus. His hatred of women became the church teachings of the "male as made in the image of God," which placed women in an unequal position in the family, religious life, and all societal disciplines.

Paul, in his Antichrist personage, created God in his own physical image and set the stage for Christian inequality, deceit, fear, and control as the normal relationship between the male and female. As the Antichrist it was perfectly normal for Paul to hate women, because the female has always been the symbol of our divine nature and he was living the intense role of the Antichrist physical nature. The inequality of the female in relationship to the male continues to be a major issue in all religions to this day.

In terms of our soul it was necessary nearly two thousand years ago to awaken the masses to the truth of their internal love. By teaching inequality, deceit, fear, sin, guilt, control, anger, war, and competition, religion, as our Antichrist beliefs and behavior, has taught us what we don't want to show us what we do want. As our immature soul comes to its consciousness of transition and we move forward into the evolution of our mature soul, we can be thankful that we have lived the opposite of our Christ Consciousness so that we can fully appreciate the beauty, magnificence, wisdom and harmony of ourselves in total love, truth, and equality.

Awakening to the enlightenment of the trinity of our minds and emotions as our evolving consciousness is the purpose and goal of evolution. Our immature soul gives us every opportunity that we need to complete our journey home and fulfill our purpose of evolving into our own Christ Consciousness. We always have the strength to live the dramas that our dual soul designs into our physical experience. Accepting change within our beliefs and behaviors only challenges the ego and intellect to look internally instead of externally, to think positively instead of negatively, and to live our love instead of our fear.

Our belief that disease is our punishment from God allows us to create disease within our body from the concept of our sin and guilt. When our obsession with sexuality or food is involved, we will reach a state of abandonment in our sexual and eating behaviors. Since our sexual and food needs are both part of our biological needs, we create all disease from these two focuses.

In effect, we punish ourselves with pain and suffering to awaken to the trinity of our soul and spirit consciousness. Disease is an internal lesson and shows us the purpose of our advanced soul in challenging us to open our eyes to our beliefs, behaviors, and lifestyles that we are living. Disease gives us time to contemplate our beliefs that death is a sin, that disease is a punishment from God, and that we have only one life to live. These are three major lessons for our immature soul to learn, and we learn best by actively living our lessons. If we are not into resistance and denial, we can learn passively by observing others.

As a dual soul, our memory of previous lives and previous deaths is reassuring us that our old Antichrist beliefs are not valid. Until we can understand that our religious teachings have no validity because they symbolize the separateness and inequality that we have bestowed upon our male and female soul consciousness, we are not willing to change them. Without a willingness to change our beliefs we continue with our behaviors as a physical nature and we refuse to accept the existence of our female divine nature. If we do not understand the role of food, air, and water as our physical survival, we will continue to contaminate and threaten ourself with death by the imbalance of our body, nature, earth, and the universe. Our beliefs must be lived until they are learned. Once they are learned we can then consciously change our beliefs and behavior as we begin to live the equality of our male and female consciousness, integrated as one within our divine nature of love, truth, and equality.

SEX AND LOVE AS A
SOUL RELATIONSHIP

As we have evolved in our beliefs the cause and effect has been reflected in our relationships as we change our physical nature from sex to love. Looking at our physical nature allows us to see how we have lived with our belief that sex is love. In reality sex is not love, but the connection between sex and love in our minds has been an essential belief to allow us to continue gravitating towards our mature soul love. Today we are challenged by our belief that sex is love as we explore and try to understand what sexual relationships mean to us.

Our belief that sex and love are one and the same thing must now be changed so we can at last understand our responsibility for sex and love as separate levels of our soul focus. Sex is the primary focus of our immature soul and love is the primary focus of our mature soul. Since we are living our soul transition from our immature to our mature soul, we must understand that the core of our physical nature is sex and the core of our Divine Nature is love. Sex was created as the illusion of love to provide the sexual attraction of the male and female as the magnetic arc of the soul, for procreation, and for sensory stimulation.

The true story of sex and love goes back to the very moment when we became a living soul and created our physical body in both male and female form. Until that moment when we created our physical bodies as male and female, both sexes were in one physical form. We became physical twin souls as the separation occurred in our physical body and we reflected our male and female dual soul mind and emotions as two consciousnesses focused within our physical nature.

As our dual soul mind was separated into a male physical nature and a female divine nature, we reflected our sexuality as the core of our physical nature and our love as the core of our divine nature. The key to understanding our separation as a male and female body is to understand the separation of the physical nature and divine nature by our ego belief system. In our physical nature the male symbolizes our mind and the female symbolizes our emotions. Our beliefs have held both our mind and emotions in bondage as our physical nature.

Our belief system was created by the ignorance of our intellect as we searched externally to understand ourselves. We had to reach our own conclusions about life over the long span of our immature soul. Because we were fearful we found external symbols which we used to explain our sexual reality. Our symbology became our superstitions, myths, rituals, and later our ego beliefs. Our beliefs created our ego cosmic shell that has held us in a captive focus within our physical nature. Our sexuality is the core of our physical nature, which allowed our obsession with sexual symbols to create the foundation of our belief system as our initial basis of information. For our immature soul, sex was our lesson of focus. That focus has been learned. Now we must learn how to change our focus.

As we began life in our physical form both the male and female were mentally and emotionally focused, by choice, into the left brain of our physical nature to teach us to live equality, which created a mutual hostility or enmity in our relationship because we had no explanation for or understanding of our physical differences. This mutual hostility has continued throughout the path of our immature soul in our sexual physical nature, and as we have lived the hostility of our sexual beliefs it has provided us with a constant lesson of inequality which we have lived as our physical art of creation.

The sexual attraction that we have all lived as male and female has allowed us to gravitate towards the unconditional love of our spirit self. This design could not have been more clever or more in harmony with the principles and laws of the universe. Our sexuality was bestowed upon us for the very legitimate purpose of procreation, which supported the Law of Continuation for the eternal life of our soul and spirit. Sex was given to us as a biological need for procreation, an emotional magnetism that held our soul in the magnetic arc of evolution, and as a source of pleasure and joy as an expression of our wholeness as the male and female united again to create a total sensory stimulation.

The only biological needs that supersede our need for sex are our need for pure air, water, and the foods of nature. Our first three biological needs maintain the credibility and integrity of the soul pattern of our DNA and assure us again of eternal life. We lived the four levels of our biological needs in the first two primary levels of our evolving immature soul consciousness. And although we thought that we had mastered these four biological needs, it is easy to see that we have not. We have reached the end of our journey as an immature soul without any memory of what we learned in the very beginning of creation as we began our eternal soul journey as a male and female soul consciousness.

We are now living at the depths of our descending emotional soul and we are in a state of inertia and repetition in our sexual obsession that we have returned to as the primitive memories of our immature soul. Even our biological needs for air, water, and the foods of nature have been circumvented by our attachment to our sexual image, commercialism, money, competition, war, and greed. Our inertia and superstitious beliefs about our sexuality are destroying our freedom of choice, freedom of will as motivation, and our freedom of intention as inspiration and we are captured in our fear of change.

We have distracted our minds with the perception that sex is a symbol of our physical freedom, and because we have sex attached to our lesson of freedom we are living our sexual freedom with abandonment, not responsibility. Our rebellious approach to sexuality allows sex to play a major role in getting our attention through the outcome of sexual abandonment. The intriguing web of our sexual beliefs leads us into an abusive consciousness of ourself and our inadequate sense of sexuality whether or not we are living in the lesson of abandonment through our sexual activities.

Part of our fear is attached to our scientific and religious beliefs that "we know it all." Logic tells us if we have a society that is refusing to respect our sexuality and we think that we know it all, then we expect to live in a world of war, death, and fear. Our sexuality is a primary factor in the continued evolution of our soul, but if our soul doesn't evolve into love our sexual behavior can destroy us. Our belief that life cannot be better than it is keeps us conforming to our old worship beliefs and abusive, sexual, and addictive behaviors. Our fear is convoluted into our fear of change as an immature soul, which leaves us with a fear of changing our sexuality. We have not even begun to scratch the surface of knowing our mind and emotions and our spirit consciousness. As we begin to discover the truth of the love within our mature soul it will be easier for us to comprehend that we have been living in ignorance of who we are and that we have created a world of pain and suffering. By changing our beliefs, we will change our behaviors and create a new world of peace and love.

All of our superstitious beliefs and behaviors had their original source in our sexuality as we struggled to understand the physical differences between men and women. This was the beginning of our worship of the heavens and nature as "God," our fear, inequality, self-centeredness, deceit, and our sexual focus as love. In our loss of memory of how we created ourself we looked externally for symbols to worship as an explanation of ourselves, and today we are still looking externally for someone or something to worship and we are still attached to the same primitive superstitions, rituals, and worship beliefs. The image of our beliefs and behaviors changes to fit the beliefs of the time, but our core worship beliefs remain the same in our immature soul mind.

Science and religion were created by the curiosity of primitive man which then gave their stamp of approval to the beliefs and fears that were already present. Although we adjusted our beliefs to fit the times, we continued in our superstition and ignorance and looked externally for our answers in our attempt to understand ourselves. We have lived our immature soul journey by living our primitive beliefs and behaviors of fear, control, inequality, abuse, competition, war, and sex, which we have accumulated as the foundation of our physical reality in our soul journey.

Our challenge as a human species is to be willing to ask "why" and question every belief that lives hidden in the cave of our dark mind. When we are afraid to look within ourself, to discover the source of old beliefs and how we live them, the truth of our daily behavior will flow from our inherent beliefs in sexual inequality and change will be resisted and denied. Many individuals accept equality intellectually but emotionally they do not live equality. To change and to understand ourselves requires immersion of our mind and emotions in the knowledge of love, wisdom, truth, and equality. We must acknowledge our changing beliefs and live the reflection of our changing beliefs in our daily behavior. Many aspects of our daily lives are focused on our primitive sexual beliefs. The daily relationship that we have with each other is the reflection of our sexual beliefs, even when we are totally unaware of our beliefs. Sexual inequality is the basic change that we must learn before we can live the equality of our male and female consciousness. Our change is about us, not someone else. As long as the belief lives that "man is made in the image of God," we will live the emotional reaction of superiority and inferiority.

We have used our sexuality and our belief in the "need" for love as our primary external distraction to avoid looking at ourself. This was the very beginning of our belief that sex is love. As we have evolved, our belief that sex is love has allowed us to search for love in unusual places, with unusual emotional baggage attached. In our search we have confused abuse, fear, control, manipulation, seduction, pain and suffering, and persecution with love. Because we live our physical lives as both male and female, we change the image of the soul lesson as we change our focus from our male to female persona of consciousness, which allows us to live our duality so that we remain unconscious of what we live as our reality.

Love cherishes ourself and others and therefore love is the opposite of all of our fear emotions. All of our negative and fearful behaviors are the direct result of our hidden karmic belief that sex is love, which is predominant in the male persona. Both males and females see their sexual role and identity as who they are because they have no other point of reference that they can understand. Because of our sexual identity, science has become obsessed with our "physical image" as our "picture of health," but at the same time it does not understand how we create a perfect physical image of our health.

Religion has been obsessed with the belief that "man is made in the image of God." This religious belief has supported sexual inequality from the beginning of worship rituals, despite the fact that it is an ego sexual belief of glaring inequality and fear. This religious belief led to the laws in many countries that give the male total possession of the female and children and the ability to treat them in an abusive, controlling manner, and in some societies the right to kill them. Inequality, deceit, and fear are behaviors that we consistently see in religion and science.

We create illusions of our perception of love in our religious beliefs through control, dependency, fear, and worship. We say we love Jesus and he is going to save us. There are many people in the world who worship dependency and deny their personal responsibility for saving themselves, and they live their sexual behavior as their God. If we are to live our love as Jesus lived his love then we cannot be dependent on sex as love or worship our relationships. Jesus was not controlled by the sexual urges of his physical nature because he was enlightened and living in his divine nature.

Being truthful with ourself and living equally and lovingly while keeping the reality of sex in its rightful place keeps us from feeling the "physical need" for sex as love. Sex can be a celebration of love as equality, which elevates sex to a higher level than our focus on sexual need or sexual attraction. Loving within the sexual act goes beyond our beliefs in inequality, control, abuse, self-centeredness, and fear as it allows us to experience true happiness and joy. When we have the "physical need" for sex we are being controlled by our biological urges and our ego, and love will play little if any part in our sexual behavior. Sex without love is mutually abusive as it becomes emotional suppression.

When we think and believe that sex and love are equal and identical as behavior we can never understand love. Our physical nature focuses on sex and our divine nature focuses on love. As long as we think the two are the same we will not be speaking the same language in our relationships. Not only will our relationships be absent of love but we will be unable to love ourself, and we will judge, blame, and control ourself and our relationships out of our fear of not being loved.

A major challenge in relationships today is that many people are living at a higher level of consciousness than others. If we have any relationships that put us in the direct space of another's beliefs, attitude, thinking, emotions, personality, character traits, and behaviors that are being lived from a different consciousness level than we are living in our soul's journey, we can interfere with each other's energy fields. We simply will not understand each other and we will not understand how to relate to each other because we are communicating at different levels of language that define words differently. An example could be a male who sincerely believes that sex is love and he will not sexually satisfy a woman who is searching for love. If a woman is searching for love, she will not satisfy a man who is searching for sex. If we are in opposite levels of growth in our sexual relationship the relationship will not be comfortable, conversations will not be understood, communication from the heart may be impossible, chaos will be the game of life, and eventually the relationship will end or it could become mentally, emotionally, and/or physically abusive.

Most men and many women are focused within their physical nature and truly believe that sex and love are the same thing. Because of the shared belief that sex is love, the behavior will be identical. Don't expect any nurturing in the sexual relationship, because when sex is seen as love we believe that the physical act itself is giving the love and we accept no responsibility for any other loving words or behaviors. The remaining twenty-three hours and fifty-five minutes of the day the woman may feel like a prisoner in her own home and be fearful of any emotional expression.

First of all, sex is a physical act. Love is an emotion. Love, as an emotion, is not love unless the balanced soul mind and emotions of our life are dancing in harmony with the mind and emotions of our partner as the true celebration of eternal life. Love is not simply the physical act of sex and the sexual attraction to a physical image, but it is the essense of our mature soul life as thinking love, speaking the language of love, and behaving in a loving way toward ourself and others. Love is our emotional response to the passion of life. Sex without love is abuse at this point in our soul evolution.

Many sexual relationships are based on the beliefs of possession, control, manipulation, and seduction. When the moment-by-moment interactions within our relationship behavior come from fear energy and sex occurs, it does not occur in love. Our consistent daily behavior always defines the level of fear or love that we are feeling internally and living externally. To have an expectation that we can treat our mate with any level of cruelty and then expect sex as a reward of love is contrary to the emotional response of love within our divine nature.

When fighting, abuse, pain, and suffering are used as an integrated part of the sexual act, the participants are using old religious beliefs as the belief in the "father as God" bestowing grace and forgiveness on the female for the male's pain and suffering. This belief is not necessarily conscious but is being karmically acted out in the sexual behavior. Many men and some women can only reach a sexual climax when pain and suffering is part of the sexual act. This is a primitive soul that is attempting to absolve itself through a primitive focus of ritual sexual worship. The sexual climax becomes the absolution of all sins for the primitive soul and it can feel the "love of God" once again.

200

Those men and women who are living in their physical nature will not realize that being cruel, angry, judgemental, critical, or controlling at any time in a relationship will have a dramatic effect on their sexual relationship because many men and women cannot perform sexually in the presence of fear. This is the only proof that anyone should need to understand that sex is not love. In our very basic animal instincts of fear, guilt, sin, submission, and punishment, sex is emotionally abusive both to ourself and our mate.

Throughout the journey of the immature soul the male has believed that when he gives his body to a woman, even when it is not the woman's choice, he gives his love. This is why men who rape women will believe that their victims enjoyed the sexual abuse as much as they did. In our intellectual and ego mind there is no differentiation between sex and love. To our loving soul there is only love, and sex is a celebration of the love that we want to share with our partner. Our immature soul has lived the image of sex as love, and changing the definition of sex as the opposite of love is a major step in our evolution.

Our mature soul defines love as touching, caring, gentleness, sharing of dreams and ideas in communication, nurturing, and, most of all, quality time spent together enjoying each other's presence equally and having fun. These are activities of our loving, wise soul mind. Love and sex is a celebration of togetherness, life, being, creation, the body, joy, and passion. Sex without love is a physical indulgence of using another body for self-masturbation. We create the belief in our physical urge for sex as an illusion of love. Love is living our truth equally, lovingly, and gently with our mate and our family. Sex without love, truth, and equality is not love but should be seen only as a sexual act.

Passion is the sixth level of our loving emotions that we experience in our right brain, not our left brain. Passion is the holy grail of our consciousness of love. Ecstasy is the seventh level of loving emotion in our right brain, and it brings us into the wholeness of the creation of absolute truth through the integration of our soul love as our divine nature and our physical nature. The integration of our immature and mature soul creates

201

a "peak experience" of total enlightenment of the purity of love. The coming together of our male and female consciousness is the beginning of living absolute truth as our physical experiences in life and it completes our journey home as a soul.

It is impossible for us to experience these two emotions of passion and ecstasy while we are living in our physical nature. Our physical nature has created the sexual illusion of passion and ecstasy to hold us within the cosmic shell of our left brain. When we complete the integration of our dual soul as our male physical nature with our female divine nature, we will be living the passion and ecstasy that we have only dreamed about intellectually.

The intriguing way that our left brain seeks to control and possess another allows the physical nature to create the illusion of passion and ecstasy during physical sex that is the result of our sense of superiority and control or our sense of inferiority and the need to be controlled. The belief in passion and ecstasy as part of sex, not love, increases the physical abuse as pain and suffering, which we have been taught is our method of being saved through punishment and persecution. The abuse does not always have to be physical, because sex can leave mental and emotional scars that will outlast our physical scars.

When sex is forced upon a woman who truly wants love, the physical act itself can be abusive but the emotional and mental trauma is even more intense for the internal soul. Women will find themselves dreading the act of sex for a lifetime, when there is no love that is being lived within the daily interactions. When there is no "love" in the physical sex act the pain and suffering of the female can remain for years as a soul lesson of self-love. Sexual abuse has created large numbers of women who "hate men" without realizing that the hate isn't truly toward the man but toward his ignorance of how to share his love and her ignorance of communication. The longer this condition continues the angrier a woman will become. As a soul this woman is learning to love herself without a dependency on external sex as the symbol of love in her life.

Once we can all understand that our soul moves forward one step at a time, allowing it to live many lifetimes at one level of consciousness, we can see how different people are living different consciousness levels of soul growth that fail to understand the pleasure of sex and the joy of communication. Sexual relationships will fall apart not only because of the abuse to the more advanced consciousness of the soul partner, but also because the immature sexual drive is not monogamous. When the sexual drive controls the left brain it will always be looking for that "ultimate" physical passion and ecstasy with another person. Only love is monogamous. Monogamy can be practiced because of a low sex drive or because of religious beliefs and continue to be abusive to the partner if it is coming from the "sex is love" intellect and ego thinking.

Our physical nature has moved forward in multiple levels of growth but since sexuality was given to us as a biological need and sex has been the focus of our physical nature, we have carried our sexual beliefs through the journey of our soul evolution. Since we do not have a conscious awareness of our sexual behavior as also needing to evolve, it is our sexual beliefs that are at the root of our resistance and denial of change. Our sexual beliefs are based on the soul lesson of inequality, which we have lived in our immature soul.

Sexuality was the beginning of our beliefs system as we struggled to understand the difference between the male and female through our external observation of the human body and its function. Sexuality can be traced back to the Garden of Eden in the Bible, which is the symbol of the beginning of our "living soul" on Earth. Every discipline of our lives began with our beliefs about sexuality, which has led us into our scientific and religious beliefs concerning the inequality between men and women.

Our beliefs about sexuality, whether they are scientific or religious, are all of a primitive nature that has been established by our negative intellect and ego mind from the basis of fear. When we first became aware of the difference between the male and female we didn't understand that difference. We have paid homage to our ignorance ever since and managed to live by multiple rituals that can be traced back to our sexual beliefs, such as communion, marriage, baptism, and circumcision. The journey of our immature soul is reaching its completion and we are challenged to begin thinking, feeling, expressing emotions, and behavior in a totally different way to move into our mature soul path. To change this soul reflection of ourselves, we must change our sexual beliefs and behaviors. Since we hold most of our sexual thoughts, emotions, and behaviors secretly within our intellect and ego, our first challenge is to be able to look within ourselves in absolute truth and communicate our hidden sexual beliefs and yearnings to ourself without embarrassment.

No one is alone with the hidden sexual beliefs that create the yearnings of the mind and emotions because it is the sexual beliefs of our immature soul that have been totally attached to its physical nature. Because we were initially taught by religion that we committed the "sin of sex" and got tossed out of the Garden of Eden by God, we live with sexual confusion. We have "sin" beliefs that make us feel guilty because we have lived these old beliefs as our habitual, compulsive behaviors for aeons as the daily reality of our immature soul.

The twin serpents in the Garden of Eden are the symbol of our internal male and female consciousness. The physical design of our nervous system symbolizes our internal spirit and the manner in which it guides us to expand our consciousness through knowledge as our male and female sensory stimulation. The dual serpents as our dual soul symbolize the accumulated knowledge within our male and female consciousness during our journey home. Our dual soul mind and emotions reflects its pattern into our body in many ways but the primary chemical pattern is our DNA. Our dual brain and limbic system is the chemical knowledge that enhances our sensing which expands our level of consciousness. The story of the serpents tells us that when we have the knowledge to understand ourselves as male and female, we will once again become androgynous as the serpent is and as we once were. As we begin our mature soul journey we will live equal time to our immature soul journey, but in our mature soul we will celebrate love as the perception of our physical nature and life.

As we began our lives as an immature soul with no memory of where we came from or who we were, we were always guided by spirit inspiration which always comes from the universal mind of our spirit consciousness. As we descended, our mind was not open to hearing the spirit communications and our beliefs became our reality. Because of our unwillingness to listen to anything but our ego, we came to our ego conclusions and built our beliefs from our fearful and limited perception of reality. Our life was based upon our fear as an immature soul and we interpreted our perceptions of reality from our sexual beliefs that were forming because of our consciousness of the differences between the male and female physical form.

At the time we did not call ourselves "male" and "female," nor did we understand sex. Because sex was a biological need it simply occurred as our body reacted to its needs. There was no sexual selection involved because we had not reached the level of attraction. In the beginning sexual "incest" was common because we were reacting to body urging not to a stimulated mind or emotions. The hidden goal was procreation not differentiation, and therefore all forms of sexual behavior were practiced with total abandonment. Today we are revisiting many of our primitive sexual behaviors in our society as past life memories.

In the past four thousand years of our evolution we have had more of our old, primitive sexual behaviors occurring in society as our soul urges us to look at and understand the primitive sexual behavior that we must release. Our primitive sexual behavior also results in the primitive behavior of abuse, murder, mutilation, and physical violence in our attempt to become conscious of the importance for us as a soul to release our sexual beliefs.

Many people in our society are now "backsliding" into this primitive behavior rather than releasing their attachment to the physical nature with its sexual core of beliefs. Others are becoming conscious of the love within themselves and the dramatic expansion of sexual satisfaction when sex is the physical celebration of love. If two individuals from these opposite levels of the soul come together in marriage or in an intimate relationship, the relationship will be a lesson of dramatic trauma that can be learned or ignored and repeated.

When we excite the mind and emotions we will reflect our excitement into our sexuality. If our mind and emotions are paralyzed in fear, sex will only be a reaction to the biological urge and it will be self-fulfilling, self-centered, and abusive. Some individuals are so anxious and tense in life that they consciously use their sexual biological urge to relax the physical body so they can sleep. This is a habitual sexual behavior that we have become addicted to for sleep. This is why many individuals will fall asleep practically before the sexual act is complete. This form of sex is not the celebration of love which we should live every moment of our life.

When our sexual relationships can be based upon the same level of soul consciousness for our mind and emotions, we will have a more compatible sex life. Being attracted to opposites within our physical nature will trigger us to grow as a soul by expanding our consciousness of what we don't want. As we learn our lessons we will usually move on into other sexual relationships where we feel a greater sense of comfort with our partner. If we don't learn the lesson of the sexual experience, we will repeat the experience in multiple images until the lesson is learned by our immature soul.

In our mature soul we will be living the loving emotions of our positive mind. The loving emotions of our positive mind are happiness, excitement, enthusiasm, joy, bliss, passion, and ecstasy. These are the primary loving emotions that will direct our life and attract us to our perfect sexual relationship. Having a relationship where both parties are positive, loving, and excited about being together gives us a different perception of our life, our sexuality, and our love. Being positive and loving to each other for 24 hours of the day, 7 days of the week, and 365 days of the year enhances our sexuality into passion and ecstasy at the intimate sharing of each other's lives.

In our immature soul we have been attempting to reach this state of excitement, passion, and ecstasy but we simply haven't known how to behave. In our belief that sex is love, we assumed we could be mean, judgemental, abusive, and unequal and our partners would love us anyway. It frequently comes as a shock to find out that our partner is not willing to be our partner anymore. But if we are willing to look internally we should be able to see that an abusive, angry, boring, controlling, and judgemental nature is not loving, and it is far from exciting to our soul mind and emotions when we are seeking change. From our immature soul level of behavior we create fear. Fear is the opposite emotion of love and fear does not create loving sex.

Touch is the very first sense that we developed as we were busily developing the pattern of our living soul in human form. Touching has a special significance in the world of love because it is a challenge to make love without touching. Some religions have taken this challenge and done their best to avoid touch during sex by covering the body with garments or sheets. Our sexuality is normal and it is essential for procreation which allows our soul and spirit to be eternal. But it is also the physical behavior that keeps reminding us that it is our intention to integrate our male and female soul mind and emotions in the same way that we integrate our male and female bodies.

To relegate sex to the level of "sin" simply shows us that our beliefs do not understand the wisdom of our soul and spirit. Only the egotistical, fearful physical nature of our immature soul would even think such convoluted thoughts. Because we entertain multiple sexual thoughts and karmic beliefs in our intellect we give ourselves an opportunity to see our own ignorance along the immature journey of our soul if we have a level of maturity that understands sex and love. Because of our personal responsibility for life, sexuality should be saved for those who are willing to celebrate procreation if and when it occurs and the sensory stimulation of loving touch, rather than using sex as a contact sport or a form of physical exercise for stress release.

As we evolve into our mature soul everything that is beautiful and loving is just beginning for our eternal soul and spirit. In understanding our sexuality, we will be actively learning how to celebrate our love. We will erase the illusion that we can be physically, mentally, and emotionally boorish, abusive, and controlling yet continue to expect people to truly love us sexually or in any other way. Change is our soul responsibility. No one else can do it for us. As we change ourself we change our sexual beliefs and behaviors and we begin to truly experience the celebration of love as our communion of life.

THE FRACTAL PATTERN OF OUR SOUL AS OUR PHYSICAL EXPERIENCES

We physically live the reflected fractal pattern of our soul energy every moment that we breathe and experience life. Our physical body is given to us as the miracle of life that provides the dual soul and spirit consciousness with a tool to experience life as a sensory consciousness. The level of our immature soul consciousness that we are living will be constantly, moment by moment, reflected into our physical life as our physical experiences to capture our immature soul's attention and expand our spiritual, mental, and emotional consciousness. Each level of consciousness within our trinity of spirit, soul, and matter creates a fractal pattern of life which we consistently live.

Our male and female consciousness is our dual living soul. Our senses all have their source in our indwelling spirit consciousness. Our physical matter was designed by the living soul and indwelling spirit consciousness and is at all times totally integrated and functioning as a whole being whether or not we have a consciousness of our unity. As a physical body we have never at any time been separated from our living soul and indwelling spirit consciousness. When our living soul and indwelling spirit consciousness separates from our physical body we experience physical death. In three days our living soul and spirit consciousness will begin the creation of a new physical body.

As we have been living through the immature journey of our soul, we have expanded our intellect and ego consciousness and fear emotions. We have created the belief that "God" is external to us and we have separated ourselves by our belief system from our own internal reality of consciousness. We have been taught various beliefs concerning what the soul is, which in reality are all superstition because they are based upon the mystery of life as our illusion of separation. Mystery as illusion is the foundation of science and religion.

As we separated the image of our intellectual consciousness from the image of our living soul and indwelling spirit consciousness, we also separated the memory of our power from our intellect and placed it externally on "others" to be responsible for us. This abdication of power reflects our loss of consciousness of our freedom of choice, intention, and will. Our loss of consciousness of ourself has allowed us to look for dependent relationships as a way of saving ourselves. Science and religion became the "Gods" of our dependent relationships.

As our intellect and ego immature soul mind and fear emotions began to change the physical image of ourself into one of dependency, we limited our immature soul mind into being controlled, manipulated, and seduced by the inequality beliefs of others whom we labeled as "superior" to us. This fractal pattern of fear became the design of our immature soul, and the further we evolved from our spirit core the less we felt the presence of our indwelling spirit and living soul. Time has expanded our fear and our dependency on the external image of salvation. As we reached the point of transition into our mature soul we couldn't transition into love while we were still attached to fear. Our failure to evolve created our path of revolution, and we began living an expanded fear with an obsessive singular focus. It is our fear of change that holds us in a state of paralysis today as we cling to our old karmic beliefs and behaviors that we have created from superstitions, rituals, and worship.

For the past fourteen thousand years we have been in revolution and those revolutions have become tighter and more intense as our beliefs have revolved without change. This is the image of a tornado that is furiously spinning toward the ground, and at the point of hitting the ground it creates destruction and chaos. We have been mentally and emotionally creating an increasing level of destruction and chaos to get our attention for the past two thousand years. The longer we deny change and continue with our primitive beliefs and behaviors the more primitive our external and internal destruction becomes.

We have increased the destruction of ourselves and our lives through fear, disease, our intimate relationships, families, careers, and every other aspect of our personal lives because of our focus on our primitive, self-centered pleasure, indulgence, and fear. Our fear of expanding our consciousness, by turning loose of our old superstitions, symbols, rituals, and myths as our present day beliefs, is what is holding us in our destructive revolutionary soul design of repeating our karmic beliefs and behaviors.

As we move into the mature journey of our soul we begin to love and understand our soul and what it has been teaching us by living one physical life after another. It is the total release of old karmic beliefs that allows our soul design to transition from its repetitive revolutions of destruction to the freedom, love, and independence of our mature soul. Where we are in the level of our soul growth is the precise focal point of our thoughts, words, and behavior in our everyday physical experience.

It is our mature soul mind and emotions that holds the pattern of what we have learned, which guides us to the creation of each and every physical experience to expand our knowledge. In each and every relationship we reflect the thoughts, words, emotions, and behavior of our unique level of soul growth. There is no mystery as to where we are in our evolution because we are constantly living it. Because we have not been taught to understand our soul energy, we are unaware of how we live our precise consciousness level in our daily lives and reflect the identical energy into our thinking, emotions, attitude, personality, character traits, language, and behavior.

Our intellectual consciousness level is limited by our ego karmic beliefs. We wear the energy of our soul as a cloak that is designed from what we believe, which determines what we think, say, sense, and feel emotionally, and it is this soul design that creates our behavior. In understanding the energy of the soul we can clearly see the level that we have reached in our evolution. Old ego karmic beliefs are like thorns in our daily lives, limiting our thinking, emotions, sensing, feeling, and our behavior. It is our belief in our separation from God that created our first and most powerful fear. Our fear belief was created during our immature soul journey as we began to live the cause and effect of being human.

Our fear has controlled us ever since we adopted the belief as our physical reality. Once our belief in the separation from "God" became a reality, we reflected our belief in separation into every other aspect of our lives. Medicine separated our body parts from our body and our body from our mind. Our journey of worship reflected and expanded our beliefs by the escalating images we gave to our multiple gods, separating our indwelling spirit further from our memory as an external image of "God." As we reached the level of worshipping all men as "God" we made the image of physical man into a "God" who had become wrathful, fearful, judgemental, and controlling. This separation expanded the inequality between the male and female and focused us on the belief in inequality, which we have continued to live until this day as a judgement of our sexuality making us unequal. Our belief in an external "God" followed our belief in "evil spirits." Our fear of "evil spirits" created "God" as a method of saving ourselves. Our image of "God" as our savior required that he be more fearful than the "evil spirits" that he would be at war with in the physical world.

If we are living in judgement we will see our physical experiences as crises and we will cope with them from the fear that is in our mind. If we are living in love we will cope with our physical experiences lovingly and we will be conscious that we are learning from the experience. In our immature soul journey we have lived the reflection of our fearful soul without a consciousness of what we are expressing through our attitude, personality, character traits, language, beliefs, and behavior. When we shut down our consciousness we live in a state of limbo where we walk through our physical reality in total automation, feeling bored with life and yet sensing an internal restlessness and fear that we feel helpless to appease. Our internal emotions were viewed as our possession by "evil spirits."

As we began our immature soul journey, we had spirit memory during the first primary soul level of our evolution. The further we descended into the soul the more memory we lost and we struggled to find the relationship that we knew existed between nature and ourselves. Our left brain gradually limited itself with the fears that it was interpreting into superstitions, rituals, symbols, and myths as beliefs, which has allowed us to live in a state of chaotic desperation.

As the perception of our left brain was passed down from generation to generation, we created the reality of "the sins of the fathers are passed to the generations of the sons," and our fear and apprehension grew out of proportion to all reality. This shows us how our beliefs are repatterned into our children and continue to perpetuate themselves as reality. Because we are our own ancestors, we have continued to live the "Ark of the Covenant" where fear is confined to the box of our beliefs and covered by our multiple veils of perception. It was with the physical creation of the story of the cosmic shell of our ego beliefs that we created the belief that "death is a sin." We have no fear in our mature soul and spirit consciousness.

Change has been so insidious, as it has occurred through the seven-generational cycle of our soul as well as our physical lives, that we have remained unaware of how we have adjusted our ancient beliefs to our current beliefs and behaviors. Behind our veils we conveniently adjust each and every belief to fit the times and we never uncover our consciousness enough to be aware that the old superstitions are no longer truth for us.

We began to worship our superstitions, symbols, and rituals that we had created as our reality during our immature soul journey. We believed that our superstitions and rituals would save our mind from its determined plunge into the abyss of our beliefs, and as we began to worship the beliefs we passed the beliefs down from generation to generation as the reality of life through our mythology or historical stories. In our sense of unworthiness, we have always assumed that the generations that came before us were more spiritual than we are today and probably even smarter. This is the reflection of the sense of unworthiness of our immature soul, which exists despite the evolution that we have experienced in our descending soul.

These beliefs accumulated and patterned our consciousness. As the beliefs became the focus of our living soul through the moment-by-moment physical experiences of living them, we accepted the beliefs we worshipped as truth. As our immature soul mind and emotions was trying to live its illusion of truth it was doing the best it could with the information at hand. The more beliefs we created the thicker the cosmic shell of our ego became. Our ego was saving and protecting our intellect, and the less memory we had during our next return to life the happier our ego was. Our left brain intellect is an equal partner in the dual soul, but it is our blank slate of memorization that we created and provided as a tool in each life to seek and gather knowledge as a method of stimulating our aware consciousness. Our left brain intellect has been encouraging memorization to remind us of our mature soul memory that we have been methodically using as our eternal memory since the beginning of our creation.

When we were created we began as a spirit consciousness. It was our spirit consciousness that created our living soul, as Lord, to participate in the design of our physical body. As we enter into each new physical life we return as spirit consciousness and our spirit is there to help our living soul, as Lord, to create the design of our new soul journey. Our soul and spirit repatterns our physical body and intellect into the form, structure, organization, and discipline that is essential to our dual soul as it enters into the physical experiences of life. Our soul and spirit also knows that we have free choice, will, and intention in the way that we live. There is no period of time that our soul sees itself as a victim within the soul journey of learning from our physical experiences.

Our sense of victimization comes from our ego and is especially prevalent at this time because our ego feels threatened by the change that it knows will be happening within us. The ego sees change as its separation from "God" because it sees its beliefs as its "God" and change as its death. The ego assumes that change is the beginning of its destruction because it does not understand that when the ego experiences change it transitions into humility, opening the intellect to the light of our spirit consciousness and mature soul love and wisdom.

If we are repatterned in a negative way as a child, we will live that negativity until we see the wisdom of choosing to change. Our repatterning has less to do with our parents than it does with our soul. The first seven years of a child's life are crucial to the child in terms of the repatterning of beliefs, emotions, attitude, personality, character traits, language, and behavior, which are all learned as form, structure, organization, discipline, and freedom of choice, will, and intention as the soul begins in a new life.

With each new entry of our living soul into physical life our consciousness is repatterned by our beliefs of superstition, ritual, worship, symbols, and behavior because these are the foundation of the immature soul's lessons and will be lived until all twenty-eight images of the lesson are fully understood by the intellect.

Our soul lessons are learned in twenty-eight images seven times seven to infinity as a fractal pattern of the twenty-eight levels of our eternal life cycle that are each lived seven times seven to infinity. In our eternal life cycle the twenty-eight levels are lived as fourteen spirit levels and fourteen levels of the living dual soul, with each level being lived seven times seven to infinity. This fractal pattern allows our soul to live as many years and lives that we need to complete our soul lessons.

Symbols include words as language and rituals as behavior. Our mind can be repatterned into habitual patterns of thinking, feeling, emotions, language, and behavior and neither the parents or the child will have a consciousness of what is occurring. To get to the source of our beliefs we must be willing to look within ourselves to discover the patterns of attitude, thinking, feeling, emotions, language, and behavior which we personally use in our everyday living. We must understand history from the symbols, superstitions, rituals, and worship of the day and not accept them as the reality of today. In knowing how, when, and why we lived our karmic beliefs, we can avoid innocently repeating them in this lifetime.

Our beliefs become so factual within our soul that we are blind to the reality of our personal self-expression, behavior, and the influence of our beliefs on who we are as a person. When our mind is repatterned into a specific focus of beliefs we have closed our mind to change. When our mind is kept open to new knowledge we have the ability to change our beliefs and transition as a soul. In each new life we face our freedom of choice, intention, and will to keep our mind open or to close our mind to new knowledge and change.

In each physical life we either evolve, revolve, or devolve and the movement of our soul is dependent upon how we live our life. For the past two thousand years we have primarily been in a state of revolution as a human species, although some individuals are not in harmony with the masses of people. Evolutionary movement for a soul that is living in a revolutionary society is challenging but fulfilling, as the soul will be consciously working with its lesson of growth through patience. Devolutionary movement for a soul living in an evolving or revolving society will create multiple dramas and chaos for all of society.

When our soul is in a state of revolution the reflection of that revolutionary energy will create multiple levels of war upon earth. As the soul begins to slide backwards the dramas of life will include self-abuse, abusive and violent behavior, and an obsessive and fanatical attachment to ego beliefs that will be seen by the soul as its path to salvation. The wars will begin within our own soul mind and will be reflected into our relationships, including intimacy, family, friends, career, society, and nations. Therefore, war is the behavior of the revolutionary movement for the soul that is flirting with devolution. We have been in a revolutionary soul movement for the past fourteen thousand years, which has waxed and waned in harmony with the short spurts of evolution that have occurred. For the past two thousand years our revolution has been reduced to a tight and chaotic repetition of energy that has left the human species leukwarm and captured in our adaptive habitual behaviors and beliefs.

When each soul is reborn it is born with an open mind and the opportunity to evolve. If the mind is closed by the behavior and beliefs it is exposed to, the child will begin to revolve and will act out the repatterning through inappropriate behavior that can be out of synergy with society. This behavior will continue as a lifelong pattern unless the mind can be reopened by its freedom of intention to seek knowledge and change. Knowledge has the ability to change us unconsciously into an evolutionary pattern. Knowledge removes old beliefs and behaviors that have become habitual and opens our mind to inspiration and motivation.

Our old superstitions, symbols, rituals, karmic beliefs, and abusive worship behaviors are left over from our primitive perception of who we are, and it is our karmic beliefs that have created the veils that box us into our external, negative, and fearful concepts of reality. Our primitive level of consciousness has served us in the descending path of our immature soul but it does not serve us in the ascending path of our mature soul. Evolution requires that we constantly learn new knowledge and change our perception of self and life by understanding the relationship of the knowledge to ourself.

In the descending path of our immature soul, we have gathered knowledge but we have not understood how to relate the knowledge to ourself. Therefore, we have viewed all of life separately, consciously believing ourself to be separate from God, nature, earth, our soul, and other people. Even our body has been conveniently divided into parts and looked at separately. Our physical sexual image has been the primary focus of our mind and we have ignored the credibility of our cellular structure as being essential to the health of our internal and external body. Our belief in separation makes us compulsive, obsessive fanatics in our search for someone to love us, which will let us feel worthy by being joined to and loved by someone else. Our external perception of the DNA being solely a pattern of genetics from our inherent family keeps us from discovering the importance of the DNA as our soul pattern. Each of us has the power to mutate our own DNA and work out the physical experience of the mutation as a disease lesson of our soul.

Our physical nature uses its sexual core as the primary focus for learning and growing. Because of our sexual focus we have been trying to become aware of who we are by symbolizing all of our beliefs through the basis of our sexual core. Since we are focused on our sexuality as male and female, we have been trying to understand life from our sexual perception and we have ignored our dual soul and spirit. The male saw himself as unequal to the female because the female had the ability to create new life. Therefore the difference between the male and female became an object of worship and was symbolized in all of the symbols, myths, superstitions, and rituals that we have lived. Many of our beliefs are still based on these old vacillating beliefs in inequality, jealousy, and control. The sexual symbols of our primitive lives are used today with changed interpretations. An example of a sexual symbol that is used today as a religious symbol is the fish and the spear. The original meaning of this symbol was sexual intercourse between the male and female.

In the beginning the female was worshipped as the goddess of creation and man tried to create himself in the image of the female. This was the beginning of baptism, circumcision, castration, genital shaving, and fear. Man made God in his image approximately fourteen thousand years ago as we once again visited our belief that we should worship the male as God. This began our present lesson of inequality perceived from the male image of self-centered superiority. The further our immature soul has descended into the abyss of itself, the more it clings to old beliefs and behaviors as all there is in life.

The immature soul is afraid to turn loose of the old superstitions, symbols, worship, rituals, and karmic beliefs that have been its reality for aeons of time. We become comfortable with that which is known and we fear that which is unknown. Each time that we change our perception even a little we adjust our superstitions, symbols, worship, rituals, and beliefs to fit the environment of the day. Therefore, our beliefs of today have been adjusted somewhat from our ancient beliefs, which keeps us from seeing the concealed sexual symbology of our current beliefs and behavior.

Two perfect examples of this are the ritual of circumcision and the ritual of baptism. The rituals of circumcision and baptism started many thousands of years ago with the intention of creating equality for the male with the female. Both began with the belief that the male could become more divine if he was washed in the blood, as a woman experiences blood with menstruation. When animals were sacrificed to the gods for redemption, the males would lie down in the wooden grates below the animals and let the blood wash over their bodies. This was the beginning of baptism with blood, which through the ages changed as we changed. At some periods the blood was drunk, and today's religious communion follows this pattern with wine or juice used as the symbol of blood. The focus later became dual and both men and women experienced baptism and communion, using water as a baptismal rite symbolizing being saved by Jesus. Jesus was first depicted as the innocent and pure shepherd caring for the lamb of "God." Later the symbol of the crucifixion of Jesus was used to symbolize the crucifixion of ourself by self-judgement and our need for pain and suffering as an inflicted punishment.

Blood was also consumed as a drink to internally experience the divine energy of the female. The sacrifices to "God" as a female deity continued through aeons of time and eventually led us into human sacrifice, when "God" was seen in the male image. During this time the sacrifice of the first son of the family to "God" allowed his blood to be spilled as an acknowledgement that man was honoring the divine presence of "God." Many years later we decided that the penile foreskin could be sacrificed for all males and this would eliminate the sacrifice of the first male born within a family. Circumcision was also used to give divinity to the son as his blood was spilled during the circumcision, showing that he was equal to the divine female. Blood was worshipped as the divine presence of the Creator and women were envied because they could naturally spill blood as a symbol of their divinity as the creators of new life. None of these beliefs and behaviors began at the beginning of Christianity. These old, primitive superstitions, worship, and rituals began aeons ago in our immature soul journey and have been continually repeated within the seven levels of our immature soul consciousness. As Christianity began our concentrated force of revolution as a transitioning soul, our ancient worship, rituals, and beliefs were carried over as the foundation of Christianity to get our attention. The story of Jesus was the same story attributed to many "God-like" men before him that were passed down through mythology.

These old superstitions and rituals have remained as part of our belief system, but as we have changed we have adjusted our belief in the superstition and ritual to fit our current thought and life experience. Science took up the call and endorsed circumcision for the sake of cleanliness and therefore the ritual continues. The ritual of baptism with water also continues as a way of saving the soul, and little if any understanding is truly shared about the soul's journey of evolution. Superstition occurred primarily because people could not understand what the soul and spirit was and how it related to them as physical beings. Religion has been responsible for perpetuating superstition because religion was created by man in his need to conform to his ancient beliefs while exercising control over the masses.

During the first cycle of our physical life from birth to age seven we return with an intellectual blank slate for gathering memory. In our innocence we are dependent upon our parents, family, friends and physical experiences of life to repattern our consciousness. When the family, culture, religion, or society repatterns the mind with old superstitions and beliefs, then each and every soul will continue to live those beliefs until it reaches the point where it is willing to change. Some souls, and especially children of today, are coming into life without the intention of being repatterned into old karmic beliefs. This advanced level of consciousness shows us that we are living the last revolutionary cycle and we are transitioning into our mature soul.

In the second physical cycle of our physical life, we are facing the crucial test to see if our mind is going to close because of its patterning or if it is capable of staying open. The closing of our mind usually occurs about the age of eleven, but it can happen at an earlier or later age. Closing the mind at an earlier age can happen when the influence of the parents, siblings, family, culture, and society are persistent about fear beliefs, abusive discipline, and behaviors as an example for the child to observe and to live.

If the mind begins to close in the second cycle of life it will usually be totally closed by the end of that cycle, at the age of fourteen. Once the mind is closed the lessons must of necessity take on a different image of intensity, negativity, externalization, and fear. When this happens lessons will be learned as a crisis, and in many children an addiction will be formed to the daily adrenal rush of creating a crisis as some form of war or revolution. If we are repatterned to persistent crisis, we will believe that crisis creates our only sense of worth and we will become addicted to chaos as a lifestyle.

Our soul mind and emotions work through electricity and magnetism, which interact with minerals, fatty acids, amino acids, enzymes, hormones, and other chemicals in our brain. The interaction of these chemical forces is then reflected into our physical body. Our body is doing all that it can to survive, and when an addiction is created the mind will supply through control, manipulation, and seduction any drama that will support its needs. Crisis can become an addiction of the mind, emotions, and body because the body creates a hormone to handle the crisis and we have a sense of feeling good when our body feels the hormone rush of crisis.

This need for crisis can be repatterned quickly into the first cycle of life if the personality of the mother is one of crisis during gestation. If crisis is a major family issue after birth it can become part of the baby's personality in the same way that peace can become part of the baby's personality. This repatterning is accomplished through the energy resonance either in utero or during the early days of the baby's life.

Constant negative energy will help the mind of a child to close itself to past memory in both the first and second cycle of life. If the mind can stay open through the entire second cycle of life then the chances are very good that it will stay at least partially open for the rest of the physical life. When the mind and emotions can stay balanced and partially open, the immature soul can evolve despite the physical experiences of life in a revolving society. With an open mind the soul will be a seeker of knowledge and enhance the evolution of the soul.

Evolution will occur because the open mind and emotions will seek the positive within the experience and seldom allow the negative to have a long-lasting influence. When the negative is felt it will recycle through the soul to the open area of the mind and emotions and will then have the power to change. Each revolution will have the power to change the pattern when it reaches the openness of the mind and emotions, causing the cycle to expand and evolve as it seeks knowledge.

Childhood disease is an internal lesson for the soul in the same way that it is for adults. With children and disease the parents share the soul lesson. Disease is chosen for the soul as a way to expand the consciousness. Each disease will have a primary lesson on all three dimensions of energy. Diseases of the brain are primarily lessons on a transitioning soul level of chemical balance. Diseases of the physical body are lessons of the immature soul and can be defined by the organ that is involved. As an example: Diseases of the lung show the lesson of the physical mind attempting to balance the unconditional love of the spirit. Lungs represent the "miracle of life" as "breath," which comes from the Greek word "spiros," meaning spirit. Diseases of the heart are symbolic of the immature soul that is starving for love within its life.

Childhood disease is frequently chosen by a soul who has tried in vain to learn the lesson of the disease in one or several adult past lives. When we choose to work with a disease as a child we have the wisdom of our mature soul and our spirit consciousness to help us understand the lesson. Because children return to physical life in the innocence and purity of their spirit consciousness, they will be consciously inspired by the spirit and motivated by the mature soul memory to learn the lesson in all of its levels of equality, love, and truth.

Our life is a miracle gift from our spirit consciousness that constantly inspires our living immature soul with awareness as we learn to balance within our physical matter. The soul may choose to return, work through the lesson of the disease as a child, learn the lesson, and begin again with the purpose of living a longer life without the lesson of disease to interrupt the new life intention. On a soul level the parents are chosen and agree to support the soul as it lives the disease. Parents understand their role on a soul level but may have no consciousness of the lessons they are seeking to learn on a physical level.

As we begin the third cycle of our physical life, we begin to consciously live the beliefs and behaviors that we have repatterned into our intellect. This repatterning is triggered by the influence of family, culture, religion, and society, but the trigger brings forth the old karmic beliefs that are hidden in our ego cosmic shell which our immature soul has designed as part of this life purpose. Our choice of birth is absolute for the soul. There are no accidents in terms of what the soul is choosing to learn, but the parents can choose to influence in a positive or negative way through their own words and behavior as well as choosing the influence of society that they allow to influence their children.

This is what is meant by the parable in the Bible which says "the sins of the fathers are passed down through the generations of the sons" (e.g., Exodus 20:5, 34:7, Numbers 14:18, Deuteronomy 5:9). This parable describes the way we hand beliefs down through the generations of our soul and of our family, with both requiring a minimum of seven generations before change will be accepted. The "father" is the symbol of our physical nature and has been worshipped as the "God" or leader of the family for millions of years. When abuse is being learned as a soul lesson, the physical personality will be abusive in every aspect of life—mentally, emotionally, and physically. As children are repatterned by this exposure to abuse they too will act it out in their adult lives. As the transition is taking place within our soul the ego will focus on triggering the sexual core as a way to distract the mind and emotions. Therefore, sexual abuse will be predominant in families and society. Aberrations of sexuality will also enter the mind from the primitive memory experience of our immature soul.

These sexual beliefs will begin to surface during the third cycle of our physical lives and many times during the second cycle. All of our primitive beliefs have sexuality as their core even when the sexual core is not apparent in the belief of today. This occurs because we initially began to discover self by becoming aware of the sexual difference between the male and female. This difference has captured our mind and emotions from the beginning of time and our superstitions and beliefs have grown from the worship of our issue of sex, creating the beliefs of religion, science, and even our moral values. Many of these primitive beliefs and behaviors are the very issues that are being triggered in people's minds today because our beliefs provide the primary denial and resistance to changing our soul focus of thinking and emotions.

We are conscious of the reflection of these primitive beliefs in the behavior of our families and societies as sexual crimes, religious wars, inequality, and random killings. Other reflections of the same primitive beliefs are less intense and therefore less noticeable. Sexual inequality as a behavior has always been apparent in the inequality of religion, science, government, education, and family relationships.

Sexual harassment is a reflection of the inequality beliefs that exist at our sexual core. As our primitive soul faces its intention of purging its ego belief systems, the behavior that is seen in society reflects into each generation at a younger age. The first reflection that will be seen in the young will be the copying of adult behavior such as lifestyle habits, vulgarity, smoking, drinking, drugs, and early sexual activity. When the lifestyle devolves, the rest of the behavior devolves into teenage wars, societal and sexual crimes, murder, rapes, and then political crimes. As we purge our human soul, we live through the soul of earth purging itself, and in each of these fractal patterns we find chaos as the energy seeks to balance itself in harmony. For most of our life sexual harassment was considered the normal flirting behavior between the male and female. The aggression of either sex was accepted and has always reflected the behavior of our physical nature.

As we evolve into the ascending soul of our divine nature, sexual harassment is felt to be totally disrespectful and uninviting. Because women are moving into their divine nature in larger percentages than the male, sexual aggressiveness is not being accepted as the normal behavior because it reflects the lesson of inequality to our female soul. When a woman is sexually aggressive she is in her physical nature or male soul. When a man is sexually aggressive he is in his physical nature. The challenge of sexually aggressive behavior comes to the attention of society when the two souls that are involved are coming from a different soul level and, therefore, they have different sexual beliefs and behaviors that are incompatible.

Many abhorrent sexual behaviors, especially toward children, are remnents of our primitive behavior when we did not understand our biological needs as a way of procreation but we were experimenting with the pleasure senses of our physical body. Only recently in our soul journey have we realized that pleasure is a legitimate reason for sex within ethical terms for both the male and female, because when there is genuine love all of our senses are stimulated and our consciousness of truth, love, and equality expands. In our very primitive path sexual activity was primarily abusive because it was not understood as an expression of love for our soul. When there is no love being expressed all sexual interaction is ethically abusive and becomes self-masturbation, which abuses another person's body.

As our soul lives the physical experiences of the fourth cycle of its growth from twenty-one to twenty-eight years, it lives the illusion of the primitive beliefs that have been triggered. The soul experiences an internal sense of confusion when those beliefs are being lived in duality. After the age of twenty-one many young adults begin to live their personal soul journey, which can be opposite to the beliefs and behaviors they lived in their parents' home. The changing of beliefs and behaviors always presents the duality of their teachings versus the freedom of choice of their soul. The level of consciousness of the young soul will determine whether the young adult lives conformity or rebellion as their lifestyle.

As we have evolved and become stuck in the revolution of beliefs, we have also opened to a limited consciousness of our ascending emotional soul. Experiencing the beliefs of the descending mental soul at the same time that we are experiencing the love of the ascending emotional soul allows us to live our duality in the physical experience of our lives. We can also have an ascending mind and descending emotions, which creates another form of duality in our soul persona.

During each physical life in the fourth cycle of our immature soul journey our sexual core comes to life to add to our confusion and to expose us to abuse that is generally unrecognized. Our sexuality brings us back to our illusion of love and triggers the memory potential within us of the true love that is hidden in our ascending emotional soul. The third and fourth cycles of our life are cycles of experimentation with intellect, emotions, physical experience, and sharing ourself with others.

If we are repatterned by old beliefs, we will trigger those beliefs, which has the potential to confuse us even more as a love illusion is created in relationships. Old beliefs are based on old fears and superstitions, which will affect the thinking and behavior during this cycle of life. The soul will frequently challenge us during this cycle of life, and without a loving family the immature soul can choose alternative paths of living as an illusion of love in its desperation to be loved.

From the age of fifteen through twenty-one we have less guidance and more confusion than at any other time of our life and we find ourselves relying on our perception of what we think that we have learned in the first two cycles of our life. We can react to old karmic beliefs without an awareness of why we behaved in the manner that we are acting out. This can expose us to unconditional love or it can expose us to a feeling of abandonment and abuse, and we will reflect our feelings into our behavior as we search for love in all of the "wrong" places.

In this period our beliefs become more real as we subconsciously act them out image by image in our behavior as we relearn the art of creation as our physical reality. There is an advantage for the soul in acting out our beliefs through our behavior because it shows us in an "up front and personal" way what we don't want and what we do want. This helps us know ourselves in multiple ways, but most important of all it changes our level of consciousness when we become aware of what we don't want. In becoming aware of what we don't want we can make a choice to change. Change is good and it helps our immature soul grow through our mind and emotional consciousness in the same way that it helps us grow physically.

The dual soul is constantly moving us forward within each physical life cycle and it is constantly moving forward to a new life cycle as an eternal soul. As we begin our fourth life cycle we begin to reflect all of the beliefs and behaviors that we have been dealing with since the beginning of life. At twenty-eight we will have learned some lessons, and this gives us the freedom to move forward into knowledge with an expanded consciousness. Other lessons we will not have learned and these beliefs may capture us in adaptive habitual behaviors as lifetime addictions. If our consciousness of ourself and life is paralyzed and we live on "automatic pilot," we will continue to repeat our beliefs and behavior without an awareness of their influence on how we feel.

Addictions are not simply the physical addictions of alcohol, drugs, sex, possessions, money, relationships, and food, but we also habitually repeat our addictive beliefs as our thoughts and emotions, making them the behavior of our daily life. In fact, sometimes we may feel like we are revolving around a maypole, day by day, as we find ourselves living the same habits and behaviors in our lifestyle, thinking the same thing, speaking the same words, and feeling the same fears about life. We will avoid knowledge and change at all costs because of our self-judgement and fear.

The more intense our fear becomes the more loneliness we feel from our sense of being unworthy to receive love. The cycle continues with a centrifugal force fragmenting us physically, mentally, and emotionally into separate parts in our desperation. The less integrated our life becomes the more anxiety and depression we feel. As we find ourselves in the center of this fragmentation we are, in a roundabout way, searching for our personal self-realization by our very act of immersing ourself in what we don't want to get our attention.

Our attachment to beliefs as thought, emotions, and behavior can capture us in the same revolutionary cycles until we will feel our fear and boredom sucking the life from us. During this period we will begin to find crisis as a way of change and in turn become addicted to lifestyle chaos. What we realize as we "struggle" with our lives is that we feel lonely and anxious for love. Because we don't understand that our love is our internal spirit, we distract ourselves into the external world and attempt to substitute a physical person or process for what we think is love.

Our distraction sets the stage for us as our pattern of life to go from one crisis to another, because a crisis gives us attention from many people, which allows us to feel loved. As we follow this revolutionary cycle life after life as a soul, our crisis must get more bizarre with each life for us to feel fulfilled. This negative creation of energy will attract us to external negative energy and we will become followers of the negative in life, rather than the positive in life. Worship will become our obsession and we will worship multiple addictions.

The negative and positive energies of life are both always present in life, but the number of followers of the bizarre influences can tilt the balance of society into the negative influences as easily as it can tilt the majority of society into the positive influences. If we tilt society into the negative, inequality will bring about war, fear, and hate. If we tilt society into the positive we will bring about love, peace, and cooperation. Society becomes the reflection of the fractal pattern of the masses. Therefore, each individual that truly reaches self-realization is tilting society into the positive balance. This societal shift follows the Universal Law of Motion identical to Newton's physical law of motion.

We reach self-realization by realizing what we don't want in life and focusing our lives into thinking, speaking, and behaving in the focus of love, truth, and equality so that we live in communication, peace, and cooperation. It is only when we can live the love, peace, and cooperation of life that we are truly choosing to transition into our positive energy. Being a leader is living through your own independence and freedom. It is not leading other people because that becomes controlling. Leading is stepping up and living your own internal truth. Being a leader is being true to the internal Spirit Consciousness. Leaders do not conform. Leaders seek knowledge but they are not controlled by other people's thoughts, words, or behavior. Leaders seek knowledge only to open the mind to new thoughts and to see how life relates to self. Self-realization gives us freedom of choice, will, and intention.

Each time the soul attempts to open the intellectual mind the ego will have a temper tantrum. It will create distractions, crises, doubts, intellectual dissent, addictions, and it will especially focus us on the all-important search for love through a new relationship. This is the ego's intention of bringing us back to the sexual core of our physical nature. Because our soul has been eternally searching for the soul love within us, as its true essense of life, our ego uses our "need" for love as a tool to control us and distract us. As we transition our soul is learning to love itself as a male and female consciousness.

If we resist wanting to return to our sexual core, our ego will begin to tell us how unworthy we are, that no one loves us, how inadequate we are to be alive, how sick we are making ourself, and all of this information will bring our fear to the point of anxiety attacks, phobias, suicide ideation, fear of death, and mild to severe depression. Our ego has the power, through its control, manipulation, seduction, fear, judgement, anger, and rage, to bring us to our knees, so that we begin to worship and obey our ego one more time in life. The ego always tells us that our intellect is supreme.

Knowing our precise journey in life is not as important as realizing that we have the freedom of choosing our journey. We have no obligation to follow someone else's soul journey. In fact, we can never truly follow the journey of another soul because the experience of the soul always creates a uniqueness to the individual journey of the soul. We must make the best possible choice we can make in following the journey of positive consciousness energy in every moment of every day. If we wait to

figure out how someone else has chosen to handle a similar situation, we have missed an opportunity of choice and of growth.
Working within the framework of positive thinking allows us
to create our behavior in a positive way. If we need to make an
important decision in life and we are in a quandary it is important
to breathe deeply three times, calm ourself, and drink a full glass
of pure water before we think again. Breathing pulls inspiring spirit energy into our body and drinking a pure glass of water refresh-
es our soul. Water is our universal medicine and can help the body
and mind balance itself, because it is the symbol of the soul.
Breathe deeply again three times after drinking the water and you
will feel the peace and calm flow through your body. Now you
can think in a positive and logical manner to make your free
choice. Allowing anger is allowing your ego to control you in fear.

This is the cycle of self-realization and it is our personal
responsibility to seek knowledge, search for truth, and to live
from the positive energy of ourself in a conscious and mentally
open lifestyle. It is in our fourth cycle of life that we begin to
open our intellect to the awareness of self and how self relates
to all that is in our reality. No one else can change us but us, and
the journey we take will be the journey we follow in the next
cycle of our life.

During the fifth cycle of our physical lives, from ages twen-
ty-nine to thirty-five, we begin to understand the form in our life.
If we have reached a state of self-realization, or the knowledge
of ourself, in our fourth cycle of life we will use positive beliefs
and behaviors to create the form of energy that we choose to
live. If we became a follower and feel controlled, we will put the
negative form of energy into our daily living. This is the exercise
of choice for our soul, and of course our soul will be influenced
by the beliefs that we have absorbed and lived in the earlier
cycles of our life.

The beliefs that we have released become very important
actors on our stage of life because we will not conform to a belief
that has been released. If we refuse to conform to accepted
beliefs and behaviors, families and society will judge our changing beliefs and behavior, which they are attached to as expecta-

tions of us. As we choose to live in a different way, we help all of society challenge the old primitive beliefs within themselves. As mental and emotional "holdouts" to change experience the acceptance of changed belief and behavior, the active rebellion and the passive participation of viewing the rebellion give them the courage to change as a part of the majority. This allows the "holdouts" to change their beliefs and behaviors gradually as the societal beliefs and behaviors change, but they will be able to hold on to their need to conform, which is the behavior of anger at a level of fear.

Without the choice to rebel and to change we would not evolve as a soul. Instead we would consistently live our revolutions of thoughts, beliefs, and behaviors life after life until we are in a total state of inertia and decay begins. This would be the way to destroy the human species. Because we have been tightly revolving in the same belief systems for two thousand years and have been revolving nearly fourteen thousand years in the belief in inequality, we have been living our lessons of inequality throughout the past two thousand years as a conscious choice of beginning our evolution once again in another life.

Since 2,030 is the end of our immature soul journey, we must begin to evolve into our mature soul at a different speed to keep inertia and decay from overwhelming us and creating devolution. It is in the fifth cycle of our physical life that the majority of people face the choice of rebellion internally and externally, while others will be born rebellious. As part of nature, earth, and the universe, the human being as a fractal pattern of the immature soul energy of consciousness is also subject to the principles and laws of the universe. Our time of revolving and inertia is coming to an end, and we must accelerate or decelerate as a soul. Movement of the soul is the lesson of our freedom of choice. We live our freedom of choice in the fifth cycle of our physical life, and in the fifth level as a soul we revel in our freedom of choice as we begin to understand ourselves.

In each moment of our physical life, we face the same identical fractal pattern that we face as a soul. The physical pattern of life that we live gives us insight into the movement of our

231

soul and the level of consciousness that our soul is living as its physical experience. If we can experience self-realization as knowledge and understanding on a physical level, we will have proven to ourself that our soul can also move forward to balance the ascending emotional and mental soul. Once we begin to seek truth as knowledge, we will become passionate about the miracle of our life.

Knowledge is the level of the soul that we are living. The beginning of the level of knowledge for our immature soul is the self-realization or awareness of ourself as a trinity of consciousness energy which expands through knowledge. The ending level of knowledge for the soul is our movement into the mature soul journey through an understanding of ourself as we relate all of creation into the self-actualization of our wisdom as a civilized human being. If we can learn to change during the fourth and fifth level of our physical cycles of life, we will open our mind to understanding our soul journey and our physical self-actualization as a collective consciousness of beautiful power and wisdom. The soul evolution that is an opportunity for us now has never been possible for us before as an immature soul.

Because of our attachment to the same beliefs and behaviors, we have never before reached the level of knowledge where we could begin to understand ourselves as a soul and spirit. At this time our knowledge is greater than it has ever been and our mind is more open than it has ever been. This is the opportune time for the soul to transition into the love that is its true essense of life. In being open to changing our physical knowledge and understanding ourself, we invite our soul to transition into its true essense of love and understanding.

We become so engrossed with the dramas of life that we ignore the value of living. Keep an open mind and be consciously aware of what you are learning each moment of each day. Being consciously aware of how we are acting and reacting to life will allow us to see the mirror image of our thoughts and behavior in those around us. We teach primarily by example. We must never underestimate the effect that our language and behavior has on those around us.

Our children and our close friends can become carbon copies of us, because of the impact of energy attraction. If we are negative we will attract friends of like mind. If we are positive we will attract friends of like mind. If we are negative our children will be negative. If we are positive our children will be positive. The ethical values that we live will be the ethical values that our children live. Many parents have opposite personalities and values and this provides the children with the dual vision and exposure to the negative and positive energy, giving them the opportunity to be attracted to the energy they choose.

If all of our friends are negative, controlling, and judgemental it is important to look at ourself and ask ourself, "Why am I attracting this energy?" Never associate with friends that you don't want to be like. Energy is contagious. If others are excited, we get excited. If others are angry, we become angry. If others are judgemental, we become judgemental. It is important to choose our friends well. Our families are chosen by our dual soul and we are in life to teach and learn from each other. In choosing to be a positive example, we will influence the family and bring about change in each and every soul.

It is in the fifth cycle of our physical life that we must realize that there are no external answers for our soul. Our personality, character, attitude, beliefs, and behavior are coming from our immature soul energy internally. If we don't like who we are, we do have the power to change. Our internal energy spouts from within us as a volcano spouts its molten lava. Volcanos change with time and become dormant, tempering the chaos at its core. If a volcano is smart enough to change, then why aren't we? The volcano constantly shows us the pattern of chaos coming out from within and its ability to find peace.

The sixth cycle of our physical life is from the year thirty-six to forty-two, and if we have not yet begun to consciously awaken to ourself this is the time we will find our confusion increasing and our search for awakening will lead us on a straight and linear path to the plethora of physical processes of our primitive memories. The ego becomes stronger with each cycle of life and it has learned how to direct the intellect into an arena that it can

233

comfortably accept. This cycle begins the struggle between the externally focused fearful ego and the internally focused mature soul emotion of love

This internal struggle creates an internal sense of imbalance that makes us feel that something vital is missing from our lives. What we are missing is clearly undefined, but we are conscious of the void. We begin our search for balance when we are a newly born infant living in the innocence and purity of our spirit consciousness. In seeking to balance with the physical world we must repattern our memory of physical balance. As we get older we begin to remember the internal self and feel the need to stop focusing on the physical world and balance our mind and emotions. As children our intention to balance is so intense that we over-balance toward the physical, allowing our earthly attachments to become dominant. When we live with a physical dominance until the sixth or seventh cycle of our life, it will be a challenge for us to change.

When we are focused in an intellectual, linear fashion on the physical world, we very innocently think that we are removed from the laws of nature, which are there to support our balance. As we become repatterned to our beliefs as addictions, in addition to our physical addictions, we literally chain our mind and emotions to the physical beliefs and processes that have helped to create our imbalance.

In our sixth cycle the ego reaches for its greatest heights or depths, feeling that it is the supreme entity of life, or it can go in the opposite direction and believe that it has no worth. Arrogance or depression will be the primary personality and the mind can move back and forth between the two, giving the illusion of a mental roller coaster. When this occurs the attachment to money and possessions will be intense. The mind will use its physical attachments as distractions from the emotions that it is suppressing.

When the soul is attempting to trigger us into our mind and emotional balance the ego creates the illusion of money and possessions as being our balance. This shows that the emotions are suppressed and the ego is using money and possessions as the illusion of intellectual and physical power. Our true soul power is found in the magnetism of our emotions, which have been magnetizing our soul through its immature soul journey of evolution. As we suppress our emotions we are suppressing our growth into the mature soul and creating our revolving consciousness energy focus on the material as a distraction. In time this material focus creates the inertia or paralysis of our emotions, which resists any forward movement for the immature soul.

When the soul truly is intent on forward movement it can create disease as an internal lesson or family loss as an emotional shock. Disease and death remind us of the vulnerability of our finite physical life and show us that we are not really in absolute control of our life, even though we may have created that illusion through our money and material possessions.

If we have exposed ourself to these lessons of balance and learned them earlier in our life cycles, we will be open to the change and growth of our immature soul. Understanding knowledge and its relationship to us helps us to live with humility. Ignorance helps us live with arrogance. If we have not yet accumulated the knowledge and understanding of ourself that is essential, we will find ourselves desperately searching, and in our desperation and ignorance our ego pulls us backwards into the primitive memory of worship.

Because of our material focus, we will begin our search through physical processes because we firmly believe that the physical is all there is. Our search can cause an intellectual crisis and disillusionment if our emotions and the knowledge of who we are are being suppressed. When we find ourselves in a growth crisis we will deny that we are responsible for what we create and resort to blaming and judging the areas in which we have searched for help. This external blame is the result of the fear of the ego because it feels threatened and it is acting out its fear in anger and rage. The ego will not accept responsibility for its decisions or its creations if it is working with the lesson of personal responsibility, which is a major issue for the ego cosmic shell of our immature soul.

Because of our beliefs in being saved, inequality, dependency, and control, we have avoided the personal responsibility for our own behavior throughout the journey of our immature soul. If we have only one of these beliefs we will try desperately to avoid personal responsibility. Personal responsibility must always be lived as part of our normal and constant behavior if we want to transition into the mature soul. Living our personal responsibility is how we learn the positive soul lesson and release our addictions to inequality, dependency, and control.

Accepting personal responsibility for who we are, how we think, what we do with our lives, and how we feel about life is our challenge to break the spell of inertia that we are living. Inertia is recognized as a lack of excitement about life and we live our boredom by being threatened by personal responsibility, feeling bored with life, thinking that money is our security, and most of all our desperate, external searching for someone else to love us.

As these lessons loom expansively within our internal soul we are being triggered to awaken to our hidden potential of animation, creativity, knowledge, understanding, and love. Throughout the years of our sixth cycle of life our soul will be determined to help us awaken to our hidden potential. It will trigger us with crises, dramas, loss, grief, career changes, relationship changes, and disease.

It is appropriate for our immature soul to pay attention and not allow the ego to rule supreme. The ego will continue its temper tantrum as long as we reward its bad behavior. When we learn to communicate with our dual soul mind and emotions through the truth of who we want to be, and to communicate with love, our world will begin to change for us. We will begin to awaken to our inner beauty, wisdom, love, and our excitement about life.

As we face our forty-third birthday we are facing the reality of change. We can face it gracefully or we can let our ego live its tirade of anger and vulnerability. During the seven years between forty-three and fifty we will choose change or it will be cast upon us unwillingly and unwittingly. The dramas will surprise us in our lethargy and illusion of comfort. Every belief that we have clung to as though our life depended upon it can be challenged from the most obscure sources imaginable.

At this point in our life our soul has the intention of teaching us about changing our consciousness by making certain that we live change. When the balance of the soul is in the left brain, our beginning dramas will be external, physical crisis. If our soul is more balanced in the right brain, our challenges will be internal disease crisis. Either way our soul is determined to help us change and become conscious of ourself and life, one way or the other. Our soul will work with our belief systems if we have a physical focus and challenge us with every belief that we accept as fact. If our mind is tightly closed our crisis will be hard to handle and accept. If our mind and emotions are open our acceptance and response to the crisis will be easier.

Change is important for the soul during this cycle because this period of time in our physical life symbolizes the transition from the physical descending soul to the divine ascending soul. In our physical reality we are transitioning from the physical dimension of our energy to the soul dimension of our energy, which happens at the age of fifty. As we live this symbol of our soul transition in our physical life cycle it is important for the soul to expand our consciousness of the change in energy that takes place within us and external to us. Until we become conscious of our soul and spirit energy we will not allow ourselves to transition because of our ego beliefs and behaviors.

We have a soul intention of growing beyond these beliefs and behaviors and learning to understand ourselves through knowledge rather than superstition, rituals, and symbols. If the soul fails to get our attention it will give the intellect some time to work it through, but normally two more cycles of life will be the average life span if change is totally denied. The soul reaches the point where it understands that the immature soul intellect and ego are too stuck to change and then death becomes the ultimate change for the soul, which allows the soul to begin again with a new opportunity to learn.

In our physical nature we see our sexual core as the essense of ourself. In our divine nature we recognize our spirit consciousness as the essence of ourself. Our beliefs and behaviors will consistently be seen in the way we relate to ourself and others. The physical nature that we are living allows us to recognize within ourself the level that we have reached in our soul evolution. We wear the unique level of soul consciousness energy that we have reached like a shroud over our body. It is reflected into our beliefs, thinking, emotions, personality, attitude, character traits, language, and our behaviors. It is no mystery. We are wearing our consciousness as our "coat of many colors."

We have no mystery about us because we are constantly reflecting our level of consciousness into all of society. Anger, hate, blame, judgement, control, manipulation, worship, seduction, dishonesty, war, immorality, rage, violence, abuse, competition, deceit, inequality, dependency, and fear reflect the exact image of who we are when we are in our immature soul. If we are loving, communicative, equal, honest, independent, free, open, cooperative, and compassionate, we show a different level of consciousness growth. Some souls will vacillate from one image to another, which says the soul is actively attempting to transition. If we find ourself in this image we must immerse ourself in knowledge to help complete the transition.

It is when we are living the dual consciousness images of our immature soul and our mature soul that we will find ourselves experiencing panic attacks, phobias, anxiety, fear of death, disease, and depression. Millions of people are living this duality now. Living our soul duality gives us the sense that our world is coming to an end and we are going to die. The thought of death brings about an overwhelming emotional fear of death, which is our fear of change. We have an old karmic belief that "death is a sin" and that when we die we will be judged by "God" and refused entry to heaven. When we are attached to this old karmic belief system about death, we see death and disease as punishment from a wrathful "God." We feel that God has judged us as sinful and our punishment will be dying and living eternally in hell. The karmic image of our fear is enough to cause depression and anxiety in anyone.

The old karmic belief that death is a sin also allows people to see disease as a sin. Believing that we are being punished with the pain and suffering of disease because of our sins allows us to worship medicine, if we feel medicine has saved us from the sin of death. These beliefs are of very ancient origin and have no validity. "God" is not judgemental or wrathful or angry or any of the other negative versions of his personality. "God" is a trinity of consciousness energy and we are a seed of "God" as the same trinity of consciousness as male, female, and spirit. "God" is unconditional love and as a seed of "God" we are unconditional love at our core of spirit consciousness.

"God" is in everything within the universe. We have only to look at the pattern of nature to see that death is normal and we will live again. Flowers die during the cold season of their life but they begin again in the spring. We begin a new life three days after death. This is the parable of the resurrection, and several other biblical parables carry the same message, such as the story of Jonah and the whale. We die more frequently during the cold season of our lives and in the hot season we will live longer. In our cold season we are bored with life. In our hot season we are passionate about life.

In this seventh cycle of our physical life the most important exercise for our mind and emotions is to examine our belief systems and be willing to change our thinking and emotions. As we change our beliefs our consciousness change will be reflected into our changing behavior. We will stop living in fear and begin to live in our loving consciousness as the true essense of our mature soul.

Many times we are challenged to change our beliefs because we fear being wrong and the consequences of punishment by "God" if we are wrong. Looking at our beliefs and seeing the roots of these beliefs as they were created in antiquity will help us with changing them. Allowing old karmic beliefs to control us with all of the knowledge that is available to show us where they came from simply shows that our soul continues to be attached to its fear. Our present religious beliefs are the ancient superstitions, symbols, worship, and rituals that we began to learn aeons ago in our immature soul journey. Christianity and all other reli-

gions have repeated these beliefs with some adjustments to fit the
beliefs into the current time cycle and within the individual cult.
It is the fractal pattern of our habitual and primitive beliefs
that holds us back from changing the fractal pattern of our physical experiences, and these same beliefs hold the fractal pattern
of our immature soul back from changing into the mature soul.
No one can get to the root of our beliefs but us. If we will consciously spend time looking at ourself and at the list of beliefs at
the end of this chapter in relationship to ourself, we will begin to
discover our own level of soul consciousness.

The fractal pattern of our physical life is a direct reflection of
the fractal pattern of our soul. We never hide who we are from
others because who we are is seen in our beliefs, thoughts, language, and behavior as a fractal pattern of our primitive immature soul. Look carefully at yourself and welcome change into
your life. The persona that we wear every day of our life speaks
its own language from our soul consciousness.

When we begin the soul dimension of our life at the age of
fifty we face our own mortality and the beliefs that we hold about
life. With knowledge and understanding this can be the most satisfying and exciting time of our life. It is never too early or too
late to learn. In our transitional soul dimension of our physical
life we will live the duality of our two dimensions of energy,
which has the power to pull us in opposite directions. Knowledge brings us peace from the duality of the soul mind and emotions and gives us the freedom to be equal, truthful, and loving
with ourself and others.

Some beliefs that are important to look at in relationship to
your own thinking and behavior are: Death is a sin; Disease is
punishment from God; Jesus will save me; I can only get to heav-
en through pain and suffering; I have only one life; I am guilty,
sinful, shameful and must be persecuted as punishment for my
unworthiness; Faith is superior to knowledge; I am my physical
identity; I must play the role of my gender; The male is superior
to the female; Inequality exists between the sexes, races, ages,
cultures, and lifestyles; I need someone to worship and obey; I
must follow someone superior to me; Only the physical world is

real; I know all of that; All food is good food; I own my children; My friends are obligated to me; I am not capable of taking care of myself; I need someone to love me; Man is made in the image of God (Fearful, angry, judgemental and controlling behavior is in reality the image of man which man has reflected as his belief into the image of God. This allows man to worship his own self-image as God in defiance to "Thou shalt have no false Gods before me."); I won't go to heaven if I am not religious; Heaven exists in an unknown place; I will go to hell if I don't believe in God; I am unworthy in the eyes of God; God will punish me if I don't believe; It is not worth anything if it doesn't cost a lot of money; If I am good I will go to heaven and if I am bad I will go to hell; Why stop smoking, I am going to die anyway; I am stupid; I am bad; I am inferior; I can't help who I am.

Looking at these old beliefs will help you begin your change. Now begin to review who you are. Despite the fact that you may feel that many of these beliefs do not apply to you, you may surprise yourself and find a few truly do, if you are not afraid to look at your internal self. Pick up your journal and begin to ask yourself these questions. Write the answers that you hear in your mind.

Who am I? What is the condition of my physical body? Do I nurture my body with good food, water, and air? Do I take care of my physical body with exercise? Do I rely on medicine to keep me healthy? Do I rest and play for a period each day? Do I spend at least an hour in silence? Do I willingly give time and love to others? Do I judge and blame other people for events in my life? Do I willingly share the truth of myself with others? Do I think others are taking advantage of me? Do I give and receive freely? Do I cherish my friends? Do I feel that others should always agree with me? Do I try to control others in my life? Do I want others to be dependent on me? Do I feel incapable of taking care of myself? Do I feel lonely when I am alone? Do I appreciate the good things in my life? Do I focus on what I don't like in my life? Do I find it easy to make choices? Do I laugh every day? Do I sleep peacefully? Do I awake refreshed? What is my first thought upon awakening? Am I happy? Is my personality loving? Do I feel joyful about life? Can I look at my fears? Do I always speak my truth? Do I communicate my feelings in a loving way? Is my behavior consistent with my thoughts and words? Do I live with fear? Do I love myself and my life?

Reviewing these questions internally and truthfully in relationship to our physical experiences of life allows us to change our consciousness of ourself and helps us to change our physical experiences. Make this internal review at least once a week for three hours and continue for three months and you will change your level of aware consciousness of yourself. Use a journal and write an answer for each question each time. Date your journaling and at the end of three months review your journaling and note the change in your answers.

UNDERSTANDING THE
LANGUAGE OF THE SOUL

L anguage is the verbal behavior of our soul that reflects our
level of consciousness in our thinking, emotions, and feelings.
Language becomes a physical expression of our consciousness
but it begins as "the word" of inspiration before it becomes intellectual thought. Language can create truth, perceived reality, illusion, and total deceit. Our language is at all times dependent
upon our perception of reality that is governed by the level of
consciousness of our dual soul and it is reflected into words as
intellectual thought. Intellectual thought is at all times limited and
distorted by our ego when we are speaking from our immature
soul mind.

Language is a method of creating our consciousness level
into our physical world. We use our language for many purposes and the intention of the language can be read through the
energy tone, the vocabulary, the etiquette of the words, the rigidity, the stiffness, the depth, the height, the dialect, and the pre-
sentation. Language can be judgemental, controlling, manipulative, seductive, angry, rageful, and accusatory when it is coming
from the intellect and ego of our immature soul consciousness.
Language always reflects the image that we have of ourself.

As soon as we begin our first breath in a physical life, our soul
mind is focused upon stimulating the repatterning of language,
which is inherent in our cellular memory. Language is patterned

first of all from the family in which we live, our friends, the media, and other relationship exposures that we have to verbal expression. If our language is patterned within a negative mind, it will reflect our thoughts, behavior, fear, and our conscious and karmic beliefs. Language is the relative truth of our ego and intellectual mind. It is relative to the speech patterns that we have created within our mind from the patterns of language that we have been subjected to in our development stage of life, and it reflects our level of aware consciousness.

As adults we begin to repattern our language from a variety of external exposures to life, but we will maintain the patterning that relates to our strongest karmic belief systems that were repatterned in childhood. As our belief systems change from negative to positive, we will again experience a dramatic change in our language, which will benefit us in all of our life experiences. The purpose of our immature soul at this time in our growth is to transition our ascending mind and descending emotional immature soul from negative thoughts and languages to positive thoughts and languages. Because of our soul evolution the most important aspect of our life that consciously affects our language is knowledge.

When we choose our parents to return to life as infants, we choose them to help us set the stage for the lessons our immature soul is continuing to act out in our physical reality. Therefore, we bring back into each new physical life old karmic lessons from past soul lives which we want to learn in this lifetime, and the stimulus for those lessons is frequently an unconscious language expression. When we choose parents to teach us what we don't want, we are challenging ourself to accept the personal responsibility of learning independently as an adult. When we choose parents to teach us what we do want, we are reinforcing what we have already learned and want to re-live in this lifetime. Sometimes we choose parents who have opposite minds and emotions so that we can see what we don't want in our language as well as what we do want and freely choose what we want to make our own. Our choice in language patterns will reflect into our personality as we live each day of our physical lives. Sometimes we will choose both parents to show us what we don't want to remind us of what we may have lived in a past life. We can be determined that we do not want to experience it again, or we can copy the exact language behavior and create it as our physical experience for an entire lifetime.

As we use language in our everyday life, we are reflecting the level of our soul very clearly to those who are around us. If we communicate through controlling, dictatorial directives, constant nagging, judgement, criticism, abusive language, manipulation, seduction, and harassment, we are primitive in our soul level of consciousness. A controlling manner of speech is showing our addiction as an immature soul to the primitive lives that we have lived, which had a fearful and self-centered intention. The self-centered soul level of language will reflect the same intention as our beliefs and thoughts and it will be the intention of our physical behavior. Control will suppress any and all love emotions and we will live from our fear emotions that will control our primitive language.

When we look at the different cultures of the world and the accepted language patterns within these cultures, we see the reflection of the beliefs and behavior of the collective consciousness of the people. When the language in a country is cooperative, positive, loving, openly communicative, and happy, the culture is advanced. If the language is warlike, negative, judgemental, restrictive, and abusive, the country is struggling to understand its own negative, fearful, and primitive consciousness.

Obsolete or primitive thoughts and language cannot be used productively in our quickly changing world. Non-communication or primitive grunts do not pass for language communications. If we open our conscious mind to new positive language concepts, we can change gracefully with the changing world consciousness and we will feel the effects of our change in every aspect of our life. There are creative ways to think and speak without feeling depression, pain, and suffering as a major factor in our lives. We can be successful and happy if we are not afraid to change our thoughts, our language, and our behavior to make it happen. Living the joy and happiness of our mature soul mind and heart magnetizes wonderful friends and relationships into our life. Expanding the knowledge of ourself gives us an expanded language as our key to change and success at this time in our life.

Language is our method of communication and it is the first manner in which we share ourselves with other people. If we cannot communicate in personal relationships, we will reflect our inability to communicate in everything that we do within our lives. If we communicate negativity within our language, our fear emotions will affect our tone of voice and reflect our anxiety about life. If we are addicted as a soul to our primitive beliefs and behaviors, our roles and identities, and our dependency on ego control, our addiction will clearly reflect in the verbal language that we use as well as our body language.

The common behavior for an immature soul consciousness that is addicted to its primitive behavior is foul language, abusive behavior and language, lying, cheating, lifestyle addictions, and self-centeredness. These are warring souls that war against themselves and reflect their warring self into the family unit, society, business, classrooms, judges' chambers, political roles, the medical arena, and every other role and identity of life. Many of these individuals are subconsciously old and advanced souls that are consciously addicted to the primitive behavior as a necessary self-image that keeps them from exposing the feelings they have of being different on the inside from their friends. An old and advanced soul consciousness that keeps negative friends within its life will find the diversity of the consciousness energy pulling it backwards into primitive beliefs and behaviors. Soul devolution will be reflected first in our language patterns.

Our intellect and ego consciousness views change as tantamount to death. The subconscious ego does not have a consciousness of the beauty of change either in our language, beliefs, behaviors, or any other facet of our lives. We will hold on to the external self-image that we want to reflect in our language because we sense change with mortal terror of rejection, abandonment, and punishment.

It is important to change our language because it is the most obvious physical image of ourself that we constantly reflect to everyone around us. As an immature soul, changing our language shows that we are growing. As a spirit, changing our language is acknowledging our wisdom and truth. There are multiple effects that changing our language has upon us and those around us. Our language changes are the first changes that are noticed by another person, and this creates a perfect example for others to follow.

Changing our language changes the image that we have of ourself and the people that we attract into our lives. Our language is an energy force and will attract others with a like energy force. If our language is vile and vulgar we are revealing to those around us what our personality is and the personality that we attract will be the same. Changing our language reflects who we are, how we think, and how we behave in relationships. If we are confused, fragmented, constantly talking as a distraction, totally externalized in our perception of life, feeling inadequate, worthless, hating life, bored, discriminating, bigoted, religious, feeling sorry for ourself, or a host of other self-images, we will reveal them all in our language.

Changing our language helps to repattern the minds of those around us. When we have the insight within ourself to become conscious of how our language sounds and what it reveals about us, we can choose to consciously repattern our language to support our true personality. When we repattern our language those who are constantly around us will begin to conform to our changes and repattern their language.

Changing our language reflects the level of our intellectual soul consciousness. Many individuals can be highly intellectual and feel that their intellectual capabilities make them different from their friends. Our fear of being different will allow us to pattern our language in a manner that will hide or conceal our intellect. Some people will hesitate in speaking because they fear their language will reveal their intellectual focus and they might be judging themselves by being embarrassed about being smarter than the average person. To live our love, truth, and equality, we must be open and communicate who we are.

Changing our language clearly shows the intention of our

mind. Our language acts like the Indian scouts that track ahead to reveal any problems in our journey. Our language reveals our intention even when we are not consciously aware of our intention. If we are thinking one way but our language is revealing our hidden thoughts, it is important to listen to our own language to see the duality that is taking place in our minds. If we choose to consciously change our language, we will reveal the intention of our mind rather than duality or fragmentation. This can only be accomplished when we have a clear intention of hearing and changing our language. The change begins to have an effect on our thinking, emotions, and feelings. One perfect way to hear ourself is to tape ourself when we are with our children, a friend, or a spouse, and forget that the tape is running. Later, when we listen to the tape, listen to our language, the words that we speak, the tone of our voice, the intention of our words.

Our language mirrors our approach to life, i.e., a negative, external approach versus a positive, internal approach. If our language always reveals a negative, external perception of who we are, we will also hear the fear that is reflected into our words. Our dependency, control, manipulation, seduction, and anger will all be reflected in our language as the reflection of our thoughts. It may not be our intention to reveal everything that we are thinking or feeling emotionally, but if we listen to our language pattern we will find our thoughts, emotions, and feelings all concealed within the language that we speak.

Our language mirrors how we feel about ourself, i.e., judgement, blame, inadequacy or worthlessness versus love and happiness. Our negative, external, fearful immature soul consciousness has a language of its own that is more revealing of us than we usually realize. When we gossip, talk constantly, interrupt others, and do all of this with language that is judgemental and blaming, our language is telling us what our mind-set is and how much we are judging and blaming ourselves. We never judge and blame another person unless we are judging and blaming ourselves first. All language of judgement and blame reveals our sense of inadequacy and worthlessness. When we cannot love ourselves and be happy, our unhappiness and fear will be mirrored in our judgement and blame of others.

Changing our language acts as our most important learning and growth tool of awareness and understanding as it raises our level of soul consciousness. When we can listen to our language and become conscious of our negative and fearful emotions and how we externalize our internal emotions to other people, we can choose to change our language pattern. Having the conscious intention of acknowledging our language patterns and choosing to change to a loving emotion will dramatically support our immature soul growth. We have habitually used language that is self-depreciating in our immature soul consciousness. When it is our intention to transition our soul, changing our language patterns is a good intention to nurture.

Changing our language includes both speaking words and hearing words. Our language not only reveals our thinking, emotions, and feelings but it also reveals our behavior. We speak and hear from our individual level of immature soul awareness. If we constantly speak, we never give our mind time to hear. This is an ego maneuver that is calculated to keep us from changing our thinking. When we are speaking we are relaying information as language, which creates multiple levels of cause and effect in others. When we take the time to listen and to hear, we have the opportunity to learn. If we indulge in run-on talking, we are using language and our ability to speak as an ego distraction that is calculated to keep us from hearing and learning. When we are learning the lesson of inequality as an immature soul, our speaking and hearing must be equal to support our learning the lesson.

Many times we cannot hear when others are speaking to us because of ego trivia chatter that has captured our linear intellect. When we are consumed with ego chatter, the chatter will gossip at us, giving us the belief that we know it all because we heard it in our head. There is a tremendous difference between ego chatter and our mature soul or spirit communication. We can never hear our mature soul and spirit if our ego is into run-on talking. When we reflect run-on talking into our language pattern, it tells us that our ego is chattering at us and our mature soul and spirit cannot be heard. As we evolve we will have silence within our head, which allows us to be very conscious of our mature soul and spirit communication and the rhythm and tone of a lilting, passionate language of wisdom.

Changing our language represents us in our relationships by putting our loving thoughts into words. Our language has an absolute power to enhance or destroy relationships. If our language is always negative, fearful, or judgemental how much joy are we bringing into our relationship? Negative language is never supportive and loving, and it never motivates our partner to feel sexy.

Language is also dependent upon the definition of words. In relationships there can be two different levels of consciousness that are being lived. Words are defined differently by different levels of consciousness. The immature soul level of consciousness will think that sex is love. The mature soul level of consciousness will not equate sex with love. The mature soul will choose consistent beautiful, positive, and loving language as an expression of love. Loving language can inspire the physical act of sex as a celebration of feelings. When the emotions of love are present on a consistent basis, the sexual relationship will be consistent because the mature soul always seeks the sensory stimulation of sex to expand the sensory feelings and to stimulate a higher level of love emotions.

If language is negative, fearful, controlling, critical, vulgar, dependent, and a host of other negative perceptions, sex will not be inspired because the mature soul will pull away from the negative energy in an attempt to prevent suppression of the loving emotions that the mature level of consciousness prefers to live within. Language is a higher level of our power of creation when it is a reflection of the pure love within one's heart. If the love is not truth, language will always reveal the illusion that is being lived as our art of creation. A consciousness of how to define and interpret language is a valuable skill to possess in all relationships.

Changing our language changes our thoughts and structures our behavior in all intimate relationships, family relationships, friendships, and with co-workers. Language is a reflection of our self-image. If we love ourselves and we express our happiness in our language, we will have a profound effect on every level of our relationships. If we are in an intimate relationship, our positive language will create a beautiful experience of sharing and teamwork. In our family relationships our loving language is an expression of our loving emotions. Our family will show respect for us when we respect them with positive and loving language, and they will follow the example that we create. If a child grows up with a negative, vulgar, critical, judgemental language being spoken in the home, the child will pattern their language after ours because they accept us as their chosen teacher. Nagging is a terrible language to inflict upon children and it is always a reflection of the nagger's own fear and insecurity as they are living in the immature soul.

Our friendships will be more intimate and supportive when we express our loving emotions for friends in our positive, supportive, and loving language. No one needs a critical "friend." Our language defines our truth of being a friend or not being a friend. As we speak to our friends in loving words and tones we become an example for them to watch, hear, and learn in the relationship.

When our language is loving and supportive it changes our relationships into satisfying communication. Communication is a two-way exchange of speaking and hearing. When we share our personal experiences through loving communication we offer the opportunity for others to learn passively from our experience. We can avoid many crises by good communication. Not having to actively live an experience because we were able to learn the lesson from our communication with a friend is a gift of love. We must always look at our own language and not judge the other person. If the language that is spoken by someone we know does not support the loving environment that we choose, we can choose not to be in the person's presence until their language changes.

Changing our language changes our behavior and helps our mind and emotions transition from the negative to the positive and from fear to love. When we are thinking loving thoughts, living our loving emotions, and opening our senses to acutely feel the love around us, we will not want to behave in a negative way. We will also not want to expose ourself to negative language or behavior in others. As a mature soul we will sometimes find our friends dropping away if they remain living in an immature soul level of consciousness. This is appropriate, and when we love ourselves we will understand that each soul must grow at its own pace and that is the soul's perfection.

Changing our language improves our communication and provides us with an opportunity for sharing knowledge. As we grow we will find multiple opportunities to share knowledge by sharing ourself and our learning experience. When we begin to love ourself we want to be free of heart. We want to come out of our cave of mental and emotional concealment and share or reveal who we are to our friends, family, and lover. We must never be embarrassed about who we are, our life experiences, or our family. If we had not lived exactly as we have lived with each and every experience being important, we would not be who we are. We only grow through the passive or active physical experiences of life as a soul. If we had not thought as we have thought, lived the emotions as they appeared, and experienced the sensory stimulation of food, knowledge, family, sex, drama, and crises, we could not have reached the level of soul consciousness that we are now living. We learn to accept our power of creation by creating ourself, our life, and our world as physical creations. Our life, ourself, and our world are the open university for our soul.

Changing our language helps us to attract like energy to support us. As we change our internal energy, we create our persona or electromagnetic field of energy surrounding our body. Our persona defines our beliefs, thinking, emotions, attitude, personality, language, and character traits, which are reflected into our behavior. As our persona changes, our friends will also change. We attract other people of like energy from our own persona or energy field of consciousness. When we attract another person that we feel is negative into our life, we must look at ourself to find the thread of the lesson that remains within our life. Once we learn the lesson, we will no longer attract the energy of that lesson within another. We will choose to be around the energy that supports who we are, which expands our growth.

As we grow we will change our language from the negative and/or the dual intention to help us transition into our mature soul consciousness. Our immature soul consciousness is negative, external, and fearful. Our mature soul consciousness is positive, internal, and loving. As we transition we will move back and forth between these two personas and live our dual consciousness as our physical experience. Our duality can first be identified in our language. We will find ourself being negative and fearful one day and positive and loving in our language the following day. When we become conscious of our dual language, we can also become conscious of our freedom of choice. Until we reach the level of duality within our soul consciousness, we will have no idea that we always have the freedom of choice to use the language that will support us. Our mature soul has allowed our immature soul to grow through the experiences of life without knowing that freedom of choice, will, and intention are part of the soul's power. Once we understand that our freedom of choice is within our constant and consistent power as a soul, we will use our freedom more intensely.

When we first begin to feel the sense of our freedom of choice we will externalize that choice and feel the need to choose a different partner, geographical area, job, friends, family, possessions, house, car, clothes, etc. It is our habitual behavior to externalize in our art of creation. Our freedom of choice is the same exposure to freedom that launched our sense of sexual freedom, freedom as females, freedom of equality as males and females, freedom to work, freedom of education, freedom to have children outside of marriage, freedom to live without religious control, and the freedom to settle a new country in the name of freedom. Our sense of mental and emotional freedom is a heady elixir for the soul as it begins to mature. Language comes from the thinking in our left versus our right brain as we transition within our dual soul mind and emotions. Many old and advanced souls are on earth today and the left brain thinking is losing popularity as the right brain thinking verbalizes truth, equality, integrity in behavior, and protection of ourselves and our environment. Self-centered and self-serving behavior is being replaced by humanitarian behavior that is concerned with ourself, other people, and the earth on which we live. Without a change in our language, our behavior will not change. Without an internal language change, we are not capable of protecting ourself and allowing ourself to evolve into our mature soul consciousness.

Our soul wants to transition from the negative approach to life to the positive approach to life. To transition we must change the focus of our thoughts from the negative to the positive soul mind and emotions. We must perceive life from the love of our right brain and not focus on the fear in our left brain as our ego trivia language that we allow to control us. Our language and behavior must have personal integrity, protecting ourself, others, and earth. When our language is fearful and abusive, we reinforce our left brain and our primitive ego. When our language is negative and fearful, we create invisible walls of resistance and denial within ourselves that we remain unaware of for multiple lifetimes. When our language is positive and loving, we reinforce the evolution of our soul consciousness into our mature right brain.

We will not return to the ethical values of our spirit until we learn to think logically, speak with a positive language and tone of voice, and live the loving behavior of our mature soul consciousness. As immature souls we have the true knowledge of our spiritual values coded within our universal memory and our mature soul memory. Our ethical values have a language and a consciousness of spiritual integrity. It is important that we live from the spiritual values that are an inherent part of us. The family values that are considered essential in our left brain have a language all of their own that has not taught mankind loving behavior, compassionate language, equality of the male and female, absolute truth, or unconditional love.

Language is a lesson for the immature soul of learning the language of respecting, honoring, and valuing ourself and other people as equal. When women began to be accepted into different disciplines of science they patterned themselves and their language after the males within the discipline. Language that supports the male physical nature does not support the female Divine Nature. Language reflects our precise level of consciousness that we are choosing to live, but not the level that we are capable of living.

Language is a lesson for the soul and as such it is an image of the balance we are seeking in communication as thinking, speaking, and hearing. It is through language that we learn to balance our soul mind, our matter, and our relationships. Abusive, vulgar, and negative language does not honor, respect, and value who we are as human beings and it is a language of our primitive and constantly changing soul. Language must be consistent with our own personality and not be borrowed from another person just to be accepted.

As we find ourselves well into our soul transition of language, it becomes even more important to use the appropriate language if we wish to be understood and not misunderstood or ignored. When we are using our loving language with other people, our behavior must always be consistent with our words and intentions. Vulgar and seductive language will be interpreted by those who have the belief that "sex is love" as an open invitation for sex. Seduction, which is a primitive body and verbal language pattern, can be used and thought to be a loving language if we are living in our immature soul consciousness. The intention of the language pattern of seduction is not always the same, but deception can occur until we become conscious of the difference.

The internal energy of love is not comprehensible to those who are living in the energy of the negative, external, and fearful physical experience and seeking a sexual conquest. There will be multiple language challenges for society because of the confusion that will erupt over the difference in the descending emotions of language and in the dual meaning of the words in language. This confusion is the same as the male and female experience of inequality as they interpret language from their different levels of soul consciousness. A female can speak one language with the intention of love, while the male interpretation of the language can be one of implied seduction and sexual attraction.

In changing the way that we view words we will be learning to change the way that we speak and listen. Here is an example from a newsletter I received in the mail: "we...offer nutritional information only to help you to cooperate with your doctor in your mutual problem of building health." Look at the word "problem." If we think of our health as a problem, we are going to be facing a challenge in "building health." If we substitute the word "purpose" or "opportunity" for the word "problem," we see "building health" as a positive team experience between us and our physician and we are motivated to do what has to be done to bring about change within ourself. With a positive approach of language we can more easily accept the opportunity or purpose of becoming healthy.

"We must judge what is best according to circumstances." Look at the word "judge" and substitute "choose." If we "choose" what is best according to the circumstances the entire circumstances change and expand into another level of consciousness. "Choose" gives us the power and wisdom to follow our own mind and changes our perception of behavior. We do not have to judge to make a free choice. We must look only at our multiple choices and choose what "feels" best for us. When we allow ourselves to choose and to sense the energy of our choice we are actively using our thinking, emotions, and feelings.

Our soul motivates our growth and change by creating choices within our lives. The experiences of our lives will bring to our attention old karmic beliefs that we are learning as soul lessons. Repetition of our physical experiences will help us discover the soul lessons that we are learning so that we can discover what we are unconsciously living. Our immature soul creates repetition over and over in each of our lives and over and over as multiple lives. We create and recreate the physical circumstances that are essential for our immature soul learning through our perception of reality and the language that we use to define our perception. Our spoken language is the reflection of our thoughts, emotions, and feelings as verbal expression. We also use our body, our mannerisms, and our sexuality as forms of behavioral language communication.

Disease motivates our soul to internalize its lessons instead of externalizing them. Our language of disease has expanded to expectation, fear, and obsessiveness. Our language is focused primarily on the expectation of disease rather than health. Health is the normal state of our physical body. When our language is defining our expectation and fear of disease, we will create our expectations and fears as our physical experience. We are learning the art and the multiple forms of our ability to create our physical lives. If we fail to see how we create from our thoughts, emotions, and feelings, we will continue to act out our lives as the dramas of a staged play.

Disease is an important internal lesson of how we use the internal language of our thoughts, emotions, and feelings to create disease before we verbalize the language. Our disease language is our ego at its best. When we listen to the expectations of disease, the fear of disease, the genetic factors of disease, we have this ego trivia running around in a tight spiral of negative energy and fear within our intellectual mind. Our thoughts create what we think about and what we fear the most.

Soul memory will return at times when we meet old souls from other lifetimes. Having the spontaneous experience of past lives opens the mind to the reality of our living more than one life. Past life memory also opens the mind to language in multiple forms. We can hear the language, but we can also be conscious of a total sensory experience using all three dimensions of our senses. A past life experience might be defined as a "craziness of the mind" or "insanity" by the medical authorities, but it is not. If those people who experience past life memory had the support to understand the experience they would deal with the experience normally through knowledge.

Our language of bipolar disease shows us how our mind is using both sides of our soul consciousness. Schizophrenia is defined as hearing voices, having visions, and knowing things that aren't true, or the presence of a "split personality." These are the identical physical experiences that each and every one of us will experience as we begin the cross-fertilization of our dual soul consciousness. The language of manic depression is another definition of "mental illness" that defines expansive waves of consciousness which move from our immature inhibited levels of our soul consciousness to the "manic" or excitable levels of our mature soul consciousness. All mental imbalance is a combination of the brain chemicals and our knowledge becoming very unbalanced and unequal. The internal and external language that we use in our physical experiences creates how we live the experience.

Near-death experiences bring us face to face with more than one life when we are in absolute denial of our eternal soul and spirit. When people see the tunnel of light they can be doing something as simple as watching the cross-fertilization take place within their dual soul mind. Our language of experiences tends to conform to the things we may have read or heard others speak about. We may not have experienced any form of life-threatening event.

As we learn a major lesson, we can sense the opening of our mind, which creates a spiral of light. Our mind, emotions, and feelings all function by spiral energy forms. Our mind is electricity, our emotions are magnetism, and our feelings are all chemical. Our spirit consciousness is chemical and the electromagnetic energy of our dual soul is a result of the chemical reactions that take place within the multiple levels of our cellular structure, including our total system of nerves.

The internal language that we use to think about our physical body defines our perceptions of experiences. Our soul and spirit can leave our body and choose to return. This can happen whether or not we are medically resuscitated. Our soul always has the freedom of choice. Many people should die if the definition of death were strictly adhered to in all cases.

Our soul is not concerned with death. It is concerned with life. When we are living a stuck quality of life, whether from disease or boredom, our soul can choose to begin again. Our language for beginning again is death. The soul language for beginning again is life. Our beliefs about death can bring forth many hidden lessons for our soul. If we understand the language of our soul lessons we can become conscious of the lessons and learn. We will frequently live our anger by constant physical forms of distraction such as talking, traveling, drinking, smoking, crises, fear, and multiple other addictions. Because we do not understand the language of distraction as the language of our ego, we will not recognize our anger. Control is a language of anger. If we feel that we must control every aspect of our life plus everyone else that we know, chances are we will not understand the language of anger that we are living.

Living through the experiences of family deaths helps us to realize that life is eternal as our soul memory is triggered into loving language. One of the phenomena that occurs at death is that everyone forgets what they didn't like about us and they focus on what they did like. If we could focus on what we like about ourself and others while we are living, the soul could live longer and learn more. We have an ancient belief that "it is a sin to speak truth about the dead." Our belief means that if we speak only the language of praise the "evil spirits" will leave the soul alone and "God" can welcome the soul into "Heaven." Our belief that we must only praise the dead allows us to suppress our anger. The language of death confuses the soul of many individuals who are learning the lesson of truth, because we will feel the internal duality of our thoughts and emotions. Death is a language of our ego beliefs.

Disease is a language of our dual soul that is used as an internal lesson at the time of our transitional change. The disintegration of the cellular structure of our body into multiple diseases is motivating us to balance our soul mind and emotions as well as our body by changing our language from disease to health. Disease speaks many languages of the soul. Disease as an internal lesson is urging our immature soul to look internally, not externally, for the cause of disease.

We are a chemical consciousness. If we are chemically out of balance our soul will speak its soul language of disease to us to get our attention. Our chemical imbalance is the source of all diseases. The part of our body that represents the lesson will be the most vulnerable to a disease. Our excesses and deficiencies of chemicals within our cells can create havoc through the chain reaction of the chemical imbalance. Chemicals that are not normal to our simple cellular structure can cause major body and mind crises as they shut down the cell's ability to reproduce itself.

Experiencing the challenge of "cures" for physical disease is awakening the soul mind to our personal responsibility for maintaining the viability of our cellular structure, which begins in our thinking and language. Only the soul can heal itself. External healing cannot occur for an internal soul. Physical changes can be created within the physical body by external healing processes of disease treatment, but the body will create another disease. Our soul is seeking eternal healing from the stress of our journey home.

Rampant disease in society is triggering our soul to the memory of longevity. Negative thinking leads to negative language and negative behavior. Our internal language that says we will only live for a certain period of time can bring about an early death for the soul. Statistics are a physical language that create an ego echo within our mind and can bring about an early death. If our ego hears that the average life expectancy for the male and female are a certain age, it will essentially set its time clock to invite death in on schedule. Our ego language will tell us that our time is up and it is time to die. When retirement occurs our ego language can begin the nagging trivial pursuit that we have no value left to life and we will choose death as a new beginning.

The fighting of continual wars as a way of life is reminding our soul that war and competition are focuses of our left intellectual and ego mind and that this negative language is not appropriate in our soul time of transition. War is a judgement behavior of right and wrong. War is a major lesson of learning to be civilized, which we are continuing to live as human beings. The level of consciousness that we are living as a soul is clearly the language of war. War is uncivilized. Our mature soul lives from compassion, cooperation, and communication. Our immature soul lives from judgement, fear, and war. The immature soul lives from a belief that we should "fight first and ask questions later." This belief is a motivational belief for many "supremist" cults. It is accepted as a way of life by many men and a few women who are living the persona of their physical nature. War is a terrorist language.

Our soul is using disease, depression, and war as a signal for our need to change our thoughts, words, and our behavior. If our soul cannot motivate us to change within life it will motivate us to change through a new beginning. There is wisdom in longevity which allows us to spend our time consciously aware of our transition. The longer we live, the more we learn, and the more knowledge our soul can take with it into its new beginning. Only our knowledge survives the changing of the body for the soul. Our body is a protective source for our soul and spirit to live within. When we change in death and begin again, we change the guard or protective physical barrier of our body. In understanding the many uses of "the guard," we can understand that the language of the soul is spoken from a different dimension or perception of reality.

All language exists in three primary dimensions of thinking, emotions, and feelings. We have been living in the first dimension of our consciousness as an immature soul. We are now moving into the second dimension of our consciousness as a mature soul. As we change the dimension of soul from the immature to the mature, we are changing the dimension of our physical self from the dimension of our physical nature to the second dimension of our Divine Nature. Changing the dimension of our soul consciousness means that we must change our dimension of thinking, emotions, feelings, and language. We are expanding our perception of reality and our art of creation as physical beings. We are evolving as a soul consciousness in the language of internal communication.

Five major beliefs have controlled our language for the past two thousand years. When our language is controlled by beliefs, we are controlled by those same beliefs. This has been our period of revolution where we have habitually repeated and repeated our beliefs, behaviors, and language as one terminally reinforced the other while we have fought our wars to maintain our beliefs. Revolutions are deadly to those who fight in them, to those who live them, and to those who speak the language of revolution. Revolution is war. We have been living the war between our ego and our spirit.

Beliefs always control our thoughts and are reflected into our language. The major belief of our thoughts and language is "Jesus will save me," and it has its source in religion. This "need to be saved" belief is the very fiber of our lesson of personal responsibility. The language of this belief makes us dependent as we give our power to Jesus to control our life. We each become the king who has abdicated the throne of power. Jesus never at any time said that he would save anyone. We have been taught to live an illusion. Jesus of Nazareth said "I am not the Messiah." "Then he charged his disciples that they should tell no man that he was Jesus the Christ." (Matthew 16:20) The word "Messiah" means Christos or Christ. Jesus was never the Christ until Paul created Jesus in that language image. But the language of "Jesus Christ" has become our belief and we worship the image of someone saving us. The word "Christ" was added to Jesus by Paul, who was selling the belief to the masses that Jesus was the Messiah.

Man has not been open-minded to the true message of Jesus. The true language of Jesus gave us the responsibility of understanding ourself when he said, "I am not the Messiah. I cannot save you. You must learn to save yourself." It was Jesus' language that motivated the plot for the illusion of his crucifixion, yet his message is not fully accepted to this day, partly because the biblical language of Jesus was created by other people.

When we do not want to accept responsibility our language will reflect only that part of a message which we are open to accepting and our mind will be closed to the rest of the communication. Language includes the art of speaking as well as the art of hearing, which together is the art of communication. What Jesus truly spoke no one wanted to hear, and therefore the language of the communication became distorted by our intellect and ego.

Beliefs limit our thoughts and focus our mind into negative perceptions and fear emotions, resulting in controlled and dependent language. Negative and fearful language reflects our paralyzing beliefs. Our thoughts control our words and our behavior, but they are not always reflected consistently into our language because the left brain speaks only from relative truth. Relative truth is the truth that is accepted by our negative, fearful mind and emotions and is reflected into our physical world as untruthful language.

The second major belief that has affected our language is, "I have only one life to live," and its source is religion. If we believe in only one life our mind is closed to change because we judge the value of life's opportunities as limited and beyond our reach. Our thoughts are judged by the belief and our perception of reality is limited by our denial language and our fear of change.

It is our belief that we have only one life to live that motivates us to create that life from negativity, fear, and an external reality. We cannot relate only one life internally to ourself because our soul knows that the belief is an illusion. Therefore, we externalize everything that we create because we find no relationship to our true soul and the religious language of our soul.

Our "one life" belief creates a language of desperation and despair and our thoughts reflect into our victim language as we expect ourself to fail the test of our limited time and space. Our sense of being inadequate and worthless in such a limited time is enhanced by our language of desperation and despair that expands the energy day by day. Our ego is winning our revolution as it formulates the language of illusion and it possesses our intellectual mind and our everyday language.

Our third major belief of "I know all of that" has its source in our intellect and ego and it has been enhanced by science. This belief is used specifically as the resistance and denial of our intellect and ego to seek internal knowledge of ourself. Our ego is fearful that internal knowledge will destroy its supreme role of controlling the externally focused intellect and its "factual" language.

Our internal language of "I know all of that" changes our ability to hear and allows our language to continue in the repetition of negative thoughts. If we believe that we already know what is being spoken, we will close our ears to hearing because we are in fear of our ego language being changed.

Our soul challenges us with opportunities to motivate us to grow and change. In experiencing the negative, fearful reaction to internal knowledge, we begin to realize that we have the freedom of choice in how we think, speak, and feel. Our ego arrogance will allow our language to be dictatorial and controlling as we close our hearing toward others' thoughts and language. The belief that we know it all is the most habitual of all beliefs and the denial and resistance that we live from the internal and external language of this belief is our fear that truth will be revealed and understood by our soul consciousness. Our ego limits our intellect because our ego conceals the language of truth from our intellect and creates illusion. Our ego language is designed to support our belief in supremacy.

When we deny and resist our ability to hear and to relate internal language to us, we are living the belief that we know it all. If we believe that we know it all we will be terrified for our thoughts to change because it is an indication of failure to our ego that fears the change of our internal language. When we choose not to hear the language our ego will shut down our hearing and use multiple forms of distraction such as ego trivia language to get its way.

Our ego stimulates our poverty consciousness by urging us to spend money in other places where we will not be exposed to knowledge. In experiencing the negative, fearful reactions to life, we begin to realize that we have the freedom of choice in how we think and feel. "I know it all" is a destructive and self-limiting belief that keeps our immature soul controlled and dependent on its fear language.

Our fourth major belief is "Man is made in the image of God" and its source is religion. This belief is the lesson of inequality, and especially the lesson of male and female inequality. The language of this belief has permeated our society and molded our cultures throughout the journey of our immature soul consciousness. Most societies have based their entire structure of family, government, politics, education, science, medicine, and religion on the language of this belief.

The language of "man" was extrapolated from the word "human" and the misinterpretation by the intellect and ego of our male, physical nature was normal for the times and the beliefs. God is both male and female. We are both male and female. When we believe that only man is made in the image of God we are learning the soul language of imbalance through living inequality. This belief rejects the female Divine Nature within us and allows our language to be discriminating, vulgar, profane, and sexist. Disrespectful language has controlled our businesses, relationships, family values, and other systems for over two thousand years. Discrimination and inequality toward the female has controlled the language and behavior of most religions from the beginning of religious thought. The refusal of many religions to allow women to play an equal role to men defines our lesson of inequality and establishes the religious language of suppression and worship.

Our fifth major belief as an immature soul consciousness is "Sex is love" and it too has its source in religion. In the early days of religion pleasure was considered a sin. Because sex was a pleasure to men it was necessary for them to believe that sex was love and therefore an honor to their wives. Sex was still considered a sin when it was not performed within a church-sanctified marriage. The urges for sex were considered to be part of the original sin that we inherited from Adam and Eve. This religious language of sex was of course superstition, but we were doing the best that we knew how to do at the time, and our ego has preserved the religions language as the foundation of our multiple religious and societies as moral law.

When we believe that sex is love all language and all words that are spoken in a sexual way are interpreted from the belief that the language is loving. This belief allows flirting, sexual attraction, sexual harassment, rape, and other sexual atrocities to be considered as the language of love in the mind of the perpetrator. The language of sexual ploys of any form always become an action that induces a reaction. Sexual language as overtures create feelings of rejection, scorn, abandonment, inadequacy, and worthlessness that must vent themselves in language of blame, judgement, control, and abuse. Judgement and accusations that have no basis of truth except in the language of the person who is creating the sexual abuse can cause pain, suffering, crime, and multiple other dramas in our physical experiences. All individuals who are controlled by their sexual language are living in the external, negative, and fearful immature soul level of consciousness and their sexual language is a constant reflection of their belief.

Our sexual belief that sex is love has been responsible for the tragic loss of many lives and the destruction of countless reputations. It is our belief that sex is love that allows courts to forgive "crimes of passion." Blame and judgement will be the language of the immature soul simply because love is not felt within the immature soul, which has created sexual language as the illusion of love. Our sexual language reflects the level of consciousness that the individual has reached and that is creating his/her reality. Our belief that sex is love creates the foundation of our sexual language in relationships and has been a major source of cause and effect in marriage, divorce, sexual scandals, rape, pedophilia, murder, and suicide. The language of sex is considered "manly" in our society and reflects our physical nature.

We can change our language and bring success into our life by re-defining many words and using positive language that allows us to communicate our thoughts with clarity. Positive language helps us to be more open with sharing ourself through our heart. We will gain the respect of family, friends, and co-workers who will learn by following our example if we choose to use positive language. Positive language allows us to respect ourself. Positive language provides a positive approach to all problem-solving. Our positive language becomes an example for others to follow. It allows us to be acknowledged as a positive problem solver when we use language as a leadership capability.

Positive language gives us the listening skills to evaluate life situations with an open mind. It gives us the freedom and the choice to concentrate and expand the positive qualities in intimate relationships, which has the power to neutralize negative language from another. Positive language magnetizes others with positive qualities into our life. It develops a closeness with family and friends that will give us an enhanced quality of support at all times. Positive language makes our life easier to live by removing the power from our repetitive, belaboring ego and intellectual language.

We can recognize our inspirations and get what we want in life if we are willing to seek the knowledge that our soul evolution requires. When we listen to the silence, we will become conscious of our internal language of inspiration. We can silence the ego trivia language by concentrating on our breathing. Spend quiet time with your internal self several times throughout the day. Breathe deeply, walk silently, think only positive thoughts, and invite your internal mature soul consciousness to communicate with you. Ask questions of your internal self and have faith in the language that you receive. Listen to the words, tone, fiber, and emotion of the spirit language. Eat and drink as close to nature as possible to support your cellular structure. Your cellular structure must be credible before you can sense acutely from your three levels of senses and become conscious of the language of your spirit.

Look at your beliefs. If you are attached to old karmic beliefs that internal voices are "evil spirits" or a sign of mental illness, you will be fearful of acknowledging what you hear as a supportive language. Follow your imagination which is your inspiration and pay attention to your ideas which are your knowing from soul memory. Both will lead your soul into a journey of growth. The language of our internal mature soul voice is at all times loving and supportive. If it is your ego language the information will come from a negative, external approach and you will feel fear and doubt as you listen. The language of the spirit is at all times inspiring and unconditionally loving.

Explore your memories of past experiences through writing about them in a journal. Look at your memories only to see what you were trying to learn as a soul. Do not judge, blame, or be critical of the experience. Everything that we experience is there to help us learn. Have no fear of change. The mature soul and spirit has a singular purpose of constant change and will repeatedly challenge us with the language of change. As an immature soul we will repeat our physical experiences until we get our attention and choose to change. Never judge or try to second guess your inspirations. Judgement and second guesses change the focus of the inspiration because the spirit language is filtered through the intellect and ego to be judged. When this occurs the language of inspiration should not be followed because it is no longer pure and may have expectations attached to it, setting you up for failure. The language of the ego is controlling, demanding, and fearful.

We recognize our inspirations by not being afraid to listen to our internal voices and their language. Our internal voices are always within our mind and constantly speaking to us with inspiration. It is our ego that feels competitive and resistant to accepting the language of our mature soul as motivation or the language of our spirit consciousness as inspiration. As we are living our transition, we have three distinct languages that are communicating with us. If we are in denial of our own soul and spirit, we will not accept these language communications. Frequently we will judge ourselves as being "mentally ill" when we become aware of our trinity of mind or our lateral soul mind speaking to us.

There are multiple ways that we can change our self-image and learn to love ourself. The first step in this change is unlearning all of the beliefs that are limiting our intellectual thinking and controlling our language. The five major beliefs that are reviewed briefly in this chapter color our language dramatically and control our self-image by controlling our thinking, emotions, and feelings.

POSITIVE LANGUAGE SUPPORTS CHANGE

Positive language will help you nurture yourself with silence. Eat as close to nature as possible to support health in your physical body. Spend time alone, nurturing your body with exercise, massage, manicures, pedicures, facials, swimming, walking, and whatever else makes you feel good about yourself. Take the time to read, journal, write to those you love, and to do other activities that give you a sense of freedom. Dress to look your best. Feel attractive to yourself. Set learning as a priority in your life. The more that you understand about yourself the better your self-image will be: Lower your tone of voice. Think before you speak. Choose only positive and meaningful words. If you normally chatter constantly as a way of distracting yourself, listen to your language. Become conscious of your attempt at distraction and the repetition that you find in your words. Listen to the dual meaning that you find within your own thoughts and words. A small number of negative words sprinkled among the positive words can change the intention of the thought and neutralize the language within your mind. Become conscious of your thoughts, words, and behavior and observe yourself to see if they are consistent. Be responsible for your own well-being and recognize denial as a way of avoiding truth and responsibility. Speaking your truth lovingly in all circumstances will change the respect that you feel for your integrity and commitment, which changes your self-image and the love that you feel for yourself.

It is only through knowledge that we can think differently about ourself, who we are, and why we are living as humans on earth. As our thoughts and language change we become more certain of our own wisdom, beauty, and magnificence. This knowledge brings about a calm, peaceful essense within us that changes our self-image and allows us to love ourself.

We can successfully approach change whenever we have the motivation and inspiration to create ourselves as a new being with a new outlook on living a peaceful, loving life of great passion. Life is a miracle and we should be passionate about living every precious moment of it. Life is to be lived in happiness and joy. When we have the inspiration and motivation to change our perception of life, we will do so with a great finesse by becoming conscious of every activity, behavior, and language that makes us who we are. We must be willing to release the language that is slowing down our growth. Make time for fun things that bring joy to your heart and you can proceed in the following fashion to create a new language to use for your journey home.

Set yourself as a priority of learning. Open your mind to new ideas, imagination, and perceptions about life. Examine your beliefs and see how they might be closing your mind to the ability to think, listen, and change. Listen with an open mind. Read from all disciplines of life, relating what you read to your own physical experiences. Share from the physical experiences that you have lived and the correlation that you find in what you have learned. Find people of like mind to help you validate your own growth through sharing. Never fear change. Accept that the unknown will become the known only through knowledge and experience. Use only positive thoughts to pattern a new self-image within and a new language for your daily communication. Never judge another person because when you do you are mirroring your own self-judgement. Consciously choose to speak positively and to listen positively with yourself and with others. Spend time with your family and get to know them as people.

Learn to think and speak quickly, accurately, and with inspiration and life will become very easy for you. Our negative language creates life as a challenge instead of enjoyment. Work isn't work when it becomes easy. Listen to how you speak and the language that you use. Are you always feeling sorry for yourself and considering your life hard, difficult, and full of work? Life is about enjoying living, not working. If we see our life as work we have two options. We can change our perception of what we do or we can change what we do.

Work is not work when you are enjoying it. Find employment and relationships that add joy to your life. Never allow old beliefs to get in the way of new ideas. Live in a partnership, function as a team, and enjoy each day. Never wait until tomorrow to complete what can be done today. Keep your mind clear. Don't block your thoughts with trivia. Follow your instincts and inspirations. If "piece work" is essential, make a game of it and be part of the team. Discuss ideas openly whenever they come to you or write them down so they don't get lost in the "memory bank" while on hold. Do what needs to be done and don't judge it. Judgement makes "mountains of work" out of inspirations. Positive thoughts and positive attitudes change the vibrational energy of any physical task.

We can always inspire ourself and other people to get the most out of a day's activities. We can inspire loyalty and joy into any situation by being an example of what we want other people to be. We can do this with ourself, in our relationships, in a family, with friends, and in business relationships. We cannot say one thing and do another and expect loyalty. We can teach "team play" in any situation by being a team player.

Participate in repetitive tasks that have a tendency to be slow if only one person is involved. Acknowledge equality. Never ask anyone else to do something that you would not do yourself. Share in activities that give equal pleasure in life such as cooking, cleaning, doing dishes, laundry, ironing, office coffee, grocery shopping, and running errands. Your intimate friend will love you and you will love yourself.

Release the old beliefs in roles and identities. Give everyone the opportunity to express ideas, take them seriously, and try them out. Never be afraid to try new ideas even if it means changing old beliefs or behaviors. Always compliment others rather than judging. Compliments will inspire everyone to do their best. Language is all that stands between judgement and a compliment. Choose your language wisely. Concentrate on the health of the person, never on the cost of a possession. This is very important when there is accidental damage where another person is involved. Let others know that you care about them as individuals. Speak positively, listen with an open mind, and set the example for what you want in all relationships with friends, family, co-workers, or intimate relationships. Live the Golden Rule: Do unto others as you would have them do unto you.

Our judgement comes from our language of expectations and it has the power to limit us and other people. We can learn to use inspirational language that will release our limitations and allow us the freedom to fly as an eagle flies without worry of failure. When we think and speak from a negative language, we can never reach our potential or appreciate ourselves or other people. Our fear of judgement controls every thought, emotion, and every word of language that we speak.

If we release all preconceived ideas about the outcome of events, time, or relationships and simply enjoy ourselves, we will be surprised to find how efficiently life works out the wrinkles. Our expectations are the ego's way of setting us up for failure with our internal and external language. Think positive thoughts to neutralize the ego language expectations of anger and rage. Our ego expects either reward or punishment as its perception of outcome. If we love ourself and live our self-respect by not abusing ourself with destructive thoughts, language, or behavior, we will feel a sense of lightness and well-being.

We must be conscious of our language and behavior to reveal old karmic beliefs that limit our happiness with unreal expectations. Relish the excitement of spontaneity and reach out to others socially. If we speak our truth without fear of punishment, truth will become our freedom. We always have the power to live in the moment and be in charge of our own thoughts and language.

When we appreciate our freedom of choice, we will resist control even when it is well intended. Some people mean well but they do not understand freedom when they use the language of control. Criticism, judgement, blame, control, and nagging are all languages of control, which reflects the insecurity and poor self-image of the person.

When we radiate the love that is within us through our language and without expectations of reward, our joy will expand tenfold. With our freedom we can release all attachment to our dependencies that exist as a way of life for us. We can act out our love instead of our fear and then we can watch other people changing their behavior to copy ours. Our immature soul learned conformity very well and we can make use of the habitual behavior and language of others to encourage change in them.

When we live with the free intention of being in joy and compassion it will become the language of our lives and surprise us. Our soul must unlearn old habits or we can simply accept the change by living it. Our freedom of choice, will, and intention are our strongest learning points in our thoughts and our language. When we open our mind to knowledge, and release all attachments to physical processes as our language, we will clearly see that it is our mind, emotions, and feelings that create our internal and external world of language, life, and relationships.

Our soul always learns best in loving relationships with family, friends, and intimate partners, but before we can learn from our relationships we must have a language of who we are and what we want our relationships to be in our lives.

Our soul is unique and we learn from our internal language first, and then we use our art of creation to make it real in the physical world. As an immature soul we have made everything, every thought, emotion, and feeling, real as language and behavior without being conscious of our art of creation. Once we understand our art of creation we can think our plan through mentally and emotionally before we decide to create it in language or as a physical relationship. Our consciousness of language as our first art of creation gives us the opportunity to test the waters before we begin in the relationship. We test the waters by communication as friends. Using the language of our heart, we share the truth of ourself.

When we live the kind of relationship that we want in our language with our family, friends, co-workers, and intimate partners, we can consciously choose to be with those who live the same way. Communication, compassion, and cooperation are the three Cs of a happy relationship.

We magnetize people to us from our own language essense. We must be conscious of magnetizing what we want in our life and not what we don't want. If a relationship doesn't feel good, back away from it immediately and rethink what you want in your life. The excitement and enthusiasm of our language is a strong magnetic force for our mature soul.

We must always live the life that gives us happiness, if we want happiness in our lives. The language and behaviors that respect us will be respectful and loving to others. Communication is the foundation of all loving relationships. If we refuse to communicate, we should not expect others to communicate with us. We must live what we want every moment of our lives. Verbal communication is a two-way language of speaking and hearing. Communication is a sharing of thoughts, emotions, and feelings through language and our physical body and behavior. In relationships our attitude and behavior are a form of silent language communication that can frequently speak a language louder than words. Don't be dependent on the other person to communicate with you first. If an attitude and behavior is making us uncomfortable, it is time for language communication. If we love ourself we will have no fear of being loving with our language in open communication.

We should always feel comfortable in reaching out socially and through language to those people that we enjoy in our life. Friendship and sharing are valuable forms of communication that express our love and caring in a simple and direct language. If we reach out to others with language and they wish to be our friends, they will communicate in return.

Everyone is good as a spirit consciousness. We are all equal as souls and we all live the same experience in our journey to the mature soul consciousness. We live the physical experience that our soul consciousness is seeking to help us understand our soul lessons. We can find beauty in all people, in all life, and in all of earth. All things interpenetrate each other and play into the lessons that are important in our life. In showing our love for life, we emphasize the good that we recognize in our family, friends, and other relationships.

When we joyfully express our feelings for others in loving language and behavior, we gift them with our loving consciousness. Love is the healing elixir for our soul. Love is also contagious. When we share our love, others feel the love and share it with someone else. Loving language caresses the soul and calms the most agitated of minds. Giving and receiving in this casual language has a deeper soul effect than can be detected on the surface. Speaking to another from the love within our heart can change the way the individual thinks about other people and can make an impression on them that will last a lifetime. Love is a gift of soul evolution. When we think positive thoughts, speak loving words, and live loving, compassionate behavior in all relationships, we are living our spirituality. Spirituality is living the consciousness of an advanced mature soul. Once we understand spirituality as the opposite of religion, we can understand that religion is a belief of our immature soul and spirituality is the language of our thoughts, emotions, and feelings, and the behavior of our mature soul. Returning to our core of being spiritual is the purpose of our soul journey. When we reach our mature soul, we have many levels of consciousness to learn and to live as spiritual beings. Our soul is equal as a male and female consciousness. It is equal as an immature soul living its physical nature and as a mature soul living its Divine Nature. We are learning balance, which means that we will live in our mature soul for the same period of time that we have lived in our immature soul. The difference between our dual souls is the attitude that we live and the language that we speak and hear. In our immature soul we live the perception that life is negative, fearful, and external. In our mature soul we will know that life is positive, loving, and internal, and we will communicate with the language of a cyclic trinity of minds and emotions.

When we accept that we are here to save ourself and not another person, we begin to acknowledge the power that is within us. We are here to support each other in our journey of being who we are. It is impossible to grow for another person. We save ourself by continuing our soul growth and change as evolution. Everything that we experience happens for the growth of our soul. Relationships with family, friends, and our intimate friends are the fiber that nourishes our soul and allows us to grow. Without the interaction with other people, we would choose death more frequently because we would feel stuck and we would have no one to mirror our reflection to so we could heal ourselves.

Acknowledging the support of our family, friends, and intimate relationships can help us see the value of our interaction. Sometimes we can only help some individuals by removing ourself from their presence. We never help another soul by rewarding inappropriate behavior. We can't change another person, but we can help them see the value of change by not supporting them in inappropriate behavior. Many times people will interpret our non-support as anger. Non-support should never be attempted in anger. Non-support needs to be lived with compassion and with total communication.

When we live our presence as an example that will help others learn to love themselves, we are teaching silently and lovingly. Living our freedom of choice, intention, and will gives us the freedom to be independent, equal, truthful, personally responsible, compassionate, cooperative, communicative, and loving, and we become a living example of a mature soul that is evolving. All of our relationships will add to our life when we are living as spiritual beings.

When we can be responsible for ourself, speak our truth language consistently, and behave through the knowledge that all people are equal, we will be living the language of spirituality in all of its many dialects.

SOUL AND SPIRIT EMBEDDED
IN PHYSICAL MATTER

As a living soul and spirit, the limbic system, endocrine glands, the complete nerve network, brain stem and spinal cord, the dual lobes of our left and right brain, and our posterior brain or cerebellum become our thinking, emotions, and sensory response which expands our consciousness. These specific parts of our brain and body control the dual soul as our thinking and emotions, our level of consciousness expansion, and our spirit senses in all three dimensions as our nervous systems that control the cellular function of our physical body. This is our tree of knowledge that is the "essense" of us as the trinity of our consciousness. In ancient Greek mythology this part of our body was referred to as the *"arbor vitae."* Our "tree of knowledge" that becomes the beginning of each new conception is a chemical laboratory beyond compare.

During the path of our immature soul, science has spent vast amounts of money, time, and thinking in an attempt to understand our brain. The missing link in understanding our brain is understanding the dual soul and spirit in relationship to our thinking, emotions, feelings, and our physical body. When science denies the dual soul and spirit, the brain and its functions will continue to remain a mystery. If the religious concept of our soul and spirit is used, the confusion simply increases because of the external, dependent focus on God, creation, and worship that does not include a definition of the soul, spirit, or consciousness.

Religion has created the foundation of our entire reality as we have lived our immature soul journey as an evolving consciousness. Because of our human need for "inequality" we have programmed our karmic ego belief systems with beliefs that continue to limit our perception of life without our intellect being conscious of the limitation. We have reached the point in our consciousness evolution where we must unlearn our dependent, fearful, and unequal behavior before we can continue to grow and evolve as a consciousness in a physical body.

It has been our "karmic beliefs" that have continued to hold our intellect in bondage and that prevent our intellect from recognizing itself as part of our dual soul. As we created our beliefs from our ancient superstitions, symbols, myths, and rituals, we were doing the best that we could. We created within our ego the addictive, habitual behavior of repeatedly reflecting our beliefs into each new physical life of our soul as we learned the art of creation. We have created our addictive beliefs as our physical reality and validated each of them as fact within our intellect. We are conscious of our "fact" only from the level of consciousness that our immature soul is living.

Our spirit consciousness never stopped its guidance of us as humans. There have always been some souls that are inspired to teach others with creative thoughts and universal memory of our soul journey. We have called this guidance "prophecy" and seen it as external to the individual relaying the messages. The consciousness level of the intellect, our internal fear, and our sense of inequality have allowed our spirit guidance to be interpreted externally as physical entities by our immature soul mind. Our external interpretation was frequently created into physical reality as a way to appease the "external Gods" that we believed were punishing us. This perception was normal for our childish immature soul that was doing the best it could with the limited knowledge and consciousness that it had reached. As we grow in knowledge and our consciousness evolves, we no longer interpret prophecy, science, or truth as we perceive it in our physical nature. We have always lived relative truth in our ancient immature soul consciousness. We will only understand truth at the level of our current consciousness which allows knowledge to be seen as "external fact" that does not relate to us. We evolve as a human species into our mature soul by the sensory response to our thinking, emotions, and feelings, which creates our consciousness. Our three dimensions of senses allow us to feel, our feelings stimulate our emotions, and our senses and emotions stimulate our mind to accept the inspiration of thought from our spirit consciousness.

If we look at the source of some of our most limiting beliefs we can see that our interpretations were the result of our fear and ignorance as we began life as "living souls" with no memory of our soul purpose or our previous lives. It is the purpose of our immature soul to learn the art of creation. As a childish soul learning about our physical nature, we have been learning the art of creation by creating every thought, emotion, and feeling as our life. The evolution of our dual soul creates the expansion of our consciousness through sensory stimulation.

Using the power of our dual soul and spirit consciousness, we created the pattern of our energy form and our physical structure as a living soul with a male and female consciousness. We chose to learn from the experience of living upon earth and experiencing all things upon earth. We chose to experience all of the elements of earth without becoming the element itself at individual levels of developing the pattern of our physical body. In this way we chose elements from all that was being created on earth and in nature as part of the fractal pattern of our physical body, which was designed as the living temple for our dual soul and spirit consciousness.

Using the temple of our physical body, the dual soul and spirit consciousness could live in matter and use the physical experiences of life on earth to understand its relationship to nature, earth, the universe, and each other in a direct and experiential way of expanding the spirit consciousness. In our journey as a dual soul and spirit, we created ourselves as a human species by using the perfection that we found in the chemical elements of nature, earth, and the universe. As a dual soul we must experience everything repetitiously until our dual soul lessons are learned in the opposite. Our lessons include all physical experiences of life as we act out its multiple images as our immature soul learns the art of creation. Our soul lessons of sexuality, religion, and science are providing the best societal lessons for us now as we see our beliefs about the religious hierarchy re-establishing their beliefs in the inequality of females. At the same time some religious males admit to prostitution, pornography, and pedophilia, and other religious males abuse women and children and commit terrorist bombings which kill hundreds of people. Other males and females in their physical nature bomb abortion clinics. All of these examples show how we live our lessons of control, judgement, blame, and rage by creating our physical experiences from our thoughts, emotions, and feelings at our precise level of consciousness.

Our living soul is divided equally into fourteen levels of soul evolution with an infinite number of levels that number seven times seven to infinity in each level. The first seven levels of our soul journey we are living within our physical nature and the second seven levels we are living within our divine nature as a soul focus of our dual mind and emotions. Multiple levels of learning are essential to support our multiple soul lessons of our spirit becoming human. All lessons must be learned in multiple images to expand our multiple levels of consciousness. We repeat multiple levels of each image of the soul lessons until our soul consciousness is understood. Each lesson that has not been learned in all twenty-eight images of the lesson will be stored as a karmic belief in our subconscious ego and will return with us as a lesson in our next physical life.

Each level of consciousness that we live adds to our awareness by reflecting our conscious soul awareness of mind, emotions, and feelings into our persona. We evolve as a soul into our infinite levels of consciousness through the physical experiences of our life. As we evolve our aware consciousness, we evolve into an understanding of our soul evolution. At this time in our soul evolution, we are attempting to understand ourselves.

Knowledge is divided as soul levels to include both awareness of knowledge and understanding of knowledge. These two levels of our dual soul evolution comprise forty billion years of physical time at each level. Spirit time moves with the speed of light, 186,000 miles per second or 11,160,000 miles per minute. We are presently completing the first level of aware knowledge and are transitioning into the second level of knowledge which will allow us to understand ourself.

We had a new beginning forty billion years ago as a dual soul, but it was not the original creation. This new beginning is the most significant time for us as a dual soul because it is the level of consciousness of knowledge from which we would transition into our mature soul. The immature soul is ending and we are ready to live all that we have learned and grow into our mature soul. We have reached the time of revelation for our dual soul mind and emotions. Without change we can also experience devolution if growth of the soul mind and emotions is denied and resisted.

Change is the free choice of our soul. Our addiction to worship as dependency, inequality, and conformity is the nemesis of our soul. During our growth, we have been fearful for our survival and we have created beliefs that we thought would save us. We have created each of our beliefs as our physical reality and we have believed that our beliefs are "truth." As the addictions to our beliefs have been lived generation after generation, we have created our fear beliefs as the foundation of our family, society, government, science, religion, medicine, and businesses. The magnitude of our "fear of survival" and "fear of change" keeps us from understanding the revelations of science in relationship to ourself.

We continue to follow our fears as our ritualistic habitual behaviors and externalize our knowledge. It is the externalizing or relating of our knowledge outside of ourself that keeps us from looking inside of our mind and emotions to understand who we are. Our external perception of ourself and our life keeps us from accepting our indwelling spirit consciousness and our dual soul as a male and female consciousness as the inte-

281

grated lifeforce energy that is embedded in the physical matter of our cellular body and head in chemical form. It is the chemical interaction that takes place in every cell of our body that combines with the chemicals that we breathe to produce energy. When we use or breathe chemicals that are full of excesses or deficiencies of chemicals we suppress our cellular energy response.

Creation as described in Genesis is the parable of how earth was created at the same time as man was created, over aeons of time, as we know time. Earth began from the ether, taking form very slowly, and in the creation of earth was the creation of the human species. Creation established the Doctrine of Two as the Spirit Consciousness created the Lord as male and female consciousness. The Doctrine of Two began the pattern of the opposites which became the soul organization of the Eternal Principles of Opposites: light and darkness, day and night, visible and invisible, land and water, morning and evening, heaven and hell, good and evil, birth and death, freedom and bondage, closed or open, right and wrong, fear and love, ignorance and knowledge, up and down, rich and poor, replenish or destroy, truth and untruth, happy and unhappy, descending and ascending, female and male, inhibition and excitation, and this eternal principle defined the opposites of our dual soul journey as the mind and emotional focus of our immature and mature soul consciousness.

There were seven specific levels of creation of Earth and of man as we created ourselves together from the chemicals of the universe. We began our creation as a spirit consciousness or an energy of thought. The ancient prophecy defines our beginning as an energy of thought as "the word." It was "the word" that designed our "tree of knowledge" or the *"arbor vitae"* and the *"elan vital"* as our lifeforce. The symbol of spirit on earth is our air. The symbol of our soul is water. The symbol of our physical body is fire as our "passion of life." Our dual soul as male and female consciousness each has seven levels of evolution. Our physical lives are lived in seven-year cycles. Each seven levels of our soul life cycle and the eternal life cycle of earth as we evolved has required 280 billion years.

The creation of earth, nature, and man required 240 billion

years, and in the last 40 billion years the earth rested and settled into its place within the universal system at the same time that our soul became comfortable with its male and female consciousness. After creation was complete we considered our work a "sabbath," which means it was put in place to stay. Both earth and man took a time of rest. We created a comfort zone within the physical creation of earth for the soul and spirit to know itself as a living soul in opposite energy form. It was our comfort zone of earth that we later called the Garden of Eden as the symbol of earth. All that we created is as it was, but we have changed our original creation to fit our needs as we have grown in the consciousness of ourself.

Since we are a part of earth that influenced the creation of earth and therefore the creation of ourself, change has occurred in the unity of the human and earth that does not support earth or us. Our level of evolution has changed one level at a time in cycles of forty billion years. Each soul level of forty billion years has brought about multiple levels of our evolution of consciousness. We now face our most important challenge as a dual soul consciousness in the level of knowledge because we must complete our level of awareness and move forward into an understanding of ourself. Our transition from an awareness of ourself to an understanding of ourself is the most significant level of evolutionary change that our soul has ever lived. We are changing from a consciousness of self-realization to a consciousness of self-actualization as our knowledge expands into understanding.

Spirit consciousness moves with the speed of light; therefore, what seems a long period in our intellectual mind is reduced dramatically when we relate time to the speed of light as a spirit consciousness. Man has been on earth from the beginning of earth time as a creation of our Spirit Consciousness. As humans we have not evolved from any species of animal or aliens from other planets. We created ourself from the chemicals of the universe with the brilliance of our fractal pattern as chemical life becoming our DNA. The DNA is the chemical pattern of our living soul and spirit as a trinity of consciousness embedded into physical matter.

As humans we evolve only as a consciousness of our dual

soul mind and emotions, which expands our spirit consciousness. Our dual soul was created by our spirit as "he created he them, male and female" and our male and female dual soul consciousness became the child of our spirit. Our body has been refined by our soul consciousness but the fractal pattern of our chemical design has not changed except for the mutations that we create as excesses or deficiencies for our soul lessons.

The Principle of Eternal Life is the organization and discipline of our dual soul and spirit in consciousness energy form. Our consciousness is energy and energy does not die but it must change form as eternal movement. As we live the Law of Continuation by repetition of soul lessons and the reincarnation of physical lives as a living soul, we are simply changing the energy form of our consciousness. We also change the energy form of our physical gender as we live the different male and female images of our soul. As our male and female consciousness begins its integration we are losing the physical differences of our soul mind and emotions that allowed us to think of ourself as unequal. Our physical body is choice and reflects the lessons of our soul into the daily creation of our physical reality. When the body dies and the soul and spirit change from physical matter to a gaseous or ethereal state, we must return to matter in three physical days because of the vast difference in the vibrational speed of our spirit energy form as it changes from matter to ethereal.

The parable of creation defines the difference between human and animal. The human species was given a sixth and seventh sense that allows thought and speech as communication to become "the word," which reflects into our physical behavior as language. This is the creation of the trinity of the human consciousness made in the image of the universal Spirit Consciousness or "God," and a dual soul mind and emotions that can communicate with "the word" as a male and female consciousness. Our language is intended to reflect the righteousness of truth as the spiritual ethical values within the mature soul consciousness and the wholeness or equilibrium within the spirit consciousness as the eternal image of ourselves as one unconditional love. The beauty and wisdom of our mental and emotional trinity bestowed upon us the power or dominion over other life within nature. The male and female were made equal within our dual soul and we were created as a chemical balance within the physical cells of our body. We were called HUMAN in honor of our Higher Universal Mana or Spirit Consciousness.

The parable of Eve as the Divine Spirit of female consciousness giving birth to Adam as our physical nature, physical body, and male consciousness is the symbol of our living soul descending into matter. In the creation of our dual soul mind and emotions as male and female, we reflected into our physical body as a gender-specific form of our male or female consciousness. Eve, as spirit, was androgynous and was reflecting the pattern of creation of the physical body for the human species as separate physical beings under the Doctrine of Two. Women today are searching for spiritual knowledge more quickly than most men because some women feel the magnetism of their Divine Spirit more intensely than some men. Hunting for and gathering intellectual knowledge is the focus of our physical nature. Understanding knowledge is the focus of our divine nature. Each of us has a dual nature of being physical and divine regardless of our physical gender. Our gathering of knowledge has not always been pretty or kind as we have lived our creation of physical experience from the primitive levels of consciousness that we had reached.

Adolph Hitler used his "political prisoners" to discover all that he could about the human body because he was trying to create a superior Aryan race of human life. He explored the human body in great detail and attempted to genetically engineer a master race through breeding. His work was looked upon as an atrocity toward humanity, but for decades his work has been used as medical knowledge that has saved many lives. This example shows us the constant of opposites in all physical experiences. The soul perception defines the good and the physical perception defines the "bad."

In our present time science is genetically engineering multiple forms of life and interfering with our fractal pattern and the fractal patterns of life that support us. Science genetically engineers babies in the womb and interferes dramatically with the soul lesson. Science genetically engineers our foods and mutates the chemical design of our body and mind. The drugs that we take can genetically engineer our chemical pattern and make changes in our fractal pattern that will follow us into our future lives. We are also mutating our genetic pattern through the pollution of foods, water, air, and our homes with toxic chemicals. While we perceive the good in some of our scientific adventures, the opposite is also true as a delayed "bad" reaction.

The Principle of Free Choice, Intention, and Will is the spiritual motivation of the Divine Nature of our soul and we have used it without an awareness of what we are doing. During our transition we consciously access our freedom of choice, intention, and will for the first time as we are motivated to seek the knowledge to understand ourself. In our physical nature we have been too fearful and controlled to recognize our freedom of choice as we have learned to follow and not how to lead. Our physical nature misinterprets fear and control for organization and discipline, which are inherent within our dual soul design.

As humans we were given personal responsibility to preserve earth and all that lives upon it, from plants, animals, fish, fowl and all other life. A pattern had been created in the creation of Adam by Eve as the symbol of our male and female consciousness that allowed the human species to live the Law of Continuation and preserve the life of the human species and all species. Eve as the symbol of our spirit consciousness gave birth to Adam as the symbol of the human species. We were specifically given the personal responsibility to replenish the Earth. Our spirit knew that the soul we had created could not learn to become aware of ourself without the physical experience of life. In choosing to be responsible for Earth and our own procreation of the human race, we accepted our responsibility for free choice even during the period of evolution when we did not have the knowledge to understand our choices. As an immature soul, our free choice was made by our mature soul as our internal soul guide.

Our spirit consciousness also knew that the evolution of our dual soul consciousness would take endless time. With the Law of Continuation giving us eternal life, our spirit gifted our soul with infinite time in which to learn through repetition. The parable of our dominion over earth has escalated to our destruction of earth by our ignorance. Our human responsibility to preserve the nature of earth for our own protection allows us to continue the human race through the Law of Continuation. Our evolution includes reincarnation through the dual procreation of the human race and the soul choice to continue with the consistent repetition of our lessons, until the Eternal Principle of Opposites and our Freedom of Choice are consciously learned. Our lessons are now our addictive beliefs that hold our immature soul mind and emotions in bondage.

Genesis symbolizes the Principle of Eternal Life, including the Law of Continuation of our eternal soul. All of life comes from the seed of Spirit Consciousness, and on earth all of life comes again and again from the seed of its kind. The human soul and body comes again and again from the seed of its dual kind to live forever through the tree of life as our chemical balance. This defines our genetic heritage as the heritage of our own evolving soul, as we reap what we sow. It is because of the fractal pattern that is found in each species of life that genetic engineering can bring us into devolution by destroying the integrity and truth of the hierarchy of our life design and the design of earth. Only the ego of our physical nature would presume to be more intelligent than our eternal soul and spirit.

As a living soul we created our body from the minerals of the soil, the oxygen, hydrogen, nitrogen, and carbon found upon earth and in nature. We were given the chemicals to replenish and preserve the living soul that we had created. We were given the breath of life as spirit consciousness and became a living soul of male and female consciousness. This understanding is of dramatic importance to us now as we begin the transition within our dual soul mind and emotions because we must create our body within a harmony and balance with nature. Our need for air, water, and the foods of nature to sustain life and our evolution of consciousness by balancing our body, mind, emotions, and senses is crucial to our transitional evolution as a dual soul. The breath of spirit life is our indwelling spirit consciousness which continually breathes life into our dual soul mind and emotions and our trinity of senses. Our dual soul as our male and female consciousness has "dominion" over our physical body as the elements of earth. Dominion is defined as our "freedom of choice, intention, and will," which was gifted to our soul from spirit as our personal responsibility for evolution. The trinity of our being as our dual soul and spirit consciousness is embedded into every cell of our physical body, creating us as body, dual soul, and spirit living as humans on earth. Without the energy consciousness of our soul and spirit we would not be human. As a trinity of consciousness we began as chemicals and we must stay in our chemical balance to live and survive in a human energy form.

Each moment that we live we must live the Principle of Personal Responsibility. As the spiritual principle of being the miracle of life and as a "living soul" of dual male and female consciousness, personal responsibility is our spiritual heritage. When we live our personal responsibility, we must live equally as a male and female and release our beliefs in the inequality of roles and identities. Our physical lives are divided equally between our male and female consciousness focus as a living soul.

It is our choice to focus our consciousness on our intellect and ego as our male physical nature for both the male and female gender. We live within our physical nature in a state of "sleep" or unawareness. When this state began we entered into the "land of Nod" and our spirit saw the wisdom of physically separating the two lobes of the brain. The physical magnetism, symbolized by the rib of emotion from our heart, was used to magnetize our physical nature to our Divine Nature. Physically this magnetized the male to the female as the image of our Divine female self as a way of continuing procreation as the Universal Law of Continuation, while simultaneously animating the soul memory of the love within the female soul.

As our trinity of consciousness separated the female Divine Nature from the male physical nature of our dual soul, both man and woman were committed to live life from their physical nature. The emotional magnetism of the symbolic rib gave woman the power to conceive, although we were focused mentally and emotionally on our male physical nature. This brought equality into our soul journey because both our male and female self would be using our male physical nature throughout the journey of our immature soul. This placed our male physical nature and our female Divine Nature in a state of mutual hostility or inequality as a male mind and female emotions, which kept both sexes focused upon their male physical nature and suppressed our love emotions. Both the male and female have remained unaware of their female Divine Nature until now.

This pattern shows us how we have been living from our physical nature as both man and woman during the immature journey of our dual soul. The sameness of the male and female is emphasized to show the equality that is important in the evolution of our soul consciousness. The woman was not allowed to stay in her Divine Nature but was given the gift of emotions and put into her physical nature to live equally with man. This symbolizes the female focus on emotions and the male focus on the intellect.

As we shared our physical nature, we have been living physical inequality as we created dual soul equality. It was necessary for the dual soul to bring recognition and acknowledgement of the physical equality of man and woman into our awareness by the art of creation of our physical life experience. Equality allows us to see that no one soul is better than the other since we have been living the same journey. We have lived our dual soul equality to avoid the worship of gurus, masters, graven images, gods, or either sexual gender as supreme. Despite our dual soul equality, we have lived the inequality of worship in the dark soul mind of our physical nature. This has allowed us to experience our inhibitions and our excitations as the opposites of our dual nature. Our control and superstition allowed man to see the female as unclean, inhuman, and incapable of intellectual growth for billions of years. The physical, mental, and emotional suppression of the female on earth symbolized the internal suppression of our Divine Female emotion of love.

Our dual soul has designed our physical experience to

emphasize our Principle of Eternal Equality, but our physical perception has been controlled by our ego. We have been slow to change our beliefs and look internally at our equality. As our spirit removed all memory and light from the intellect by the separation of the physical nature from the divine nature, we made man and woman of one mind and emotional focus, to be attracted to each other until the journey of the soul was learned. Both were naked in their truth and vulnerable to the physical nature within themselves. In the darkness of memory they were free of conscience and unashamed of the journey their soul had chosen. In the beginning the male and female knew within their heart that they were equal and magnetized toward each other. Loving communication and monogamous intimacy between the male and female in the physical experience symbolizes equality as the coming together of our dual soul as a male and female consciousness.

The twin serpents are the symbol of our dual soul as equality of knowledge in living. It represents the tree of knowledge of both our male physical nature and our female divine nature. At the time of our creation, we were tempted to live our path from the wisdom of our Divine Nature. The sense of vulnerability or nakedness we felt about ourself as we evolved in physical form caused fear to overrule our choice and we slipped into the abyss of unawareness. As we became engulfed in our ego denial, we created the true physical separation of our dual natures. We filled the void with dependency, worship, and the magnetism of sex as our emotional illusion of love to keep us drawn towards our Divine Nature.

As we gained in knowledge we began to see inequality as our own self-centered ego beliefs and we understood our free choice between good and evil as a way of living our life. Understanding the knowledge of our relationship to the universe, earth, nature, creation, and each other is our opportunity to transition from our physical nature to our Divine Nature within the focus of our dual soul mind and emotions. As we live in the transitional midline of the level of knowledge, we can realize that we have the freedom of choice to live our love. We can choose to relate our knowledge to our internal trinity of consciousness and live the good within us in the mature journey of our soul. This is the first time that we have truly been consciously aware of our freedom of choice between fear and love as our emotional natures. Good and evil or knowledge versus ignorance is the symbol of love and fear for our soul consciousness.

The further we have grown from the understanding of our relationship to nature the further we have grown from understanding our relationship to love as the truth of our soul and spirit power. We have acted out our lesson of inequality in the behavior of our physical relationships in each life. Our emotional soul has been reflected as our fear into our physical behavior and has been responsible for our emotional descent into depression. Once we transition into our female divine nature we become conscious of the truth and love of knowledge and we will know that we always have free choice of thinking, speaking, and behaving from our love and compassion. Transitioning from our male physical nature to our female Divine Nature opens our consciousness by allowing the male and female within us to balance us on our daily journey, giving us the choice of living truth as our goodness and love.

Our male physical nature has lived the immature journey of our soul with an awareness of external fear and a suppression of internal love because the intellectual linear mind does not relate love to its limited consciousness. Our soul sees the dark side of our sexual physical nature as its valley of death, because of our intellectual belief that we are finite and live only one physical life. Our subconscious divine nature has total faith in our internal spirit consciousness to provide the skill and knowledge as our art of creation that is essential to overcome the punishment and limitations of our physical nature. We live in our linear thinking, speaking, and feelings that are predominant in the fearful side of our immature soul mind. Internally our mature soul knows that we will grow out of our self-imposed valley of death with our dependency upon the intellect and ego. As our "factual" knowledge expands and we begin to understand knowledge as the absolute truth of our spirit consciousness, we will live our power of creation in our divine nature of love and wisdom.

The parable of the serpent being cast out of the Garden of Eden shows how we are to begin each successive reincarnation without memory of the knowledge and skills that we learned from the past lives in our descending soul path. The serpent, as our intellect, will feed itself on the dust, or gossip and judgement as "fact," for all of the days of its life. Therefore, as we come back into a new beginning our male physical mind will be as if it is asleep, totally unaware that it is repeating lesson after lesson in its fear of accepting knowledge as our truth. Once we begin the ascending journey of our mature soul, we will understand the knowledge of ourself, creation, God, and earth through the relationship of our female loving emotions and our eyes will be opened to the trinity of our consciousness. The internal passion, happiness, and joy of life motivates us in our divine nature. The negative, fearful, external beliefs of our physical nature that we have been living leave us feeling vulnerable and naked to the punishment of living only one life.

Our physical nature of fear focuses on the intellect and ego to control us and it predicts the soul's attachment to money, possessions, and all other physical obsessions as the curiosity and intellectual fascinations that we create in our physical reality. The deceit, dishonesty, control, manipulation, seduction, ignorance, dependency, and all other negative behaviors that we succumb to are being acted out as our art of creation to help us see our external focus of life, which represents our physical nature and our attachment to material possessions. Our physical nature will stoop to any kind of behavior and our intellect, which feels supreme, will justify in our ego mind the perfection of our self-centered choice for inequality. While this is mentally and emotionally our predicted negative behavior, we also ignore the importance of balancing our body with the elements of nature to maintain our health. We invite death by our thinking and behavior as a way of beginning a new life.

As the serpents represent the spinal cord and nervous system, they also symbolize our expansion of consciousness through the knowledge of our senses embedded within each nerve. The hostility that is established toward our divine nature is symbolized by the male holding the female as unequal to himself. The female feels the need for control, judgement, and punishment and the male feels the need to control, judge, and punish as we develop a mutual hostility toward our Divine Nature. The focus of our intellect and ego on the external reflection of our physical nature has colored our self-image in every aspect of our reality. Our addiction to our external physical sexual image is a key to change for our physical nature and to the importance of change for our Divine Nature.

Paradise was the symbol of delight in the living of life and the beauty of nature that was provided for the male and female as we were made into a living soul in physical form. Earth was provided for the living soul and spirit, and it provides within nature all that we need as humans to sustain us and keep our seeds fertile to provide for the generations of souls returning. When our pattern of life maintains its truth and integrity through the elements of nature, we will continue in life until we reach the level of spiritual expansion into our trinity of consciousness.

The tree of life is symbolized by the almond tree, which is a source of multiple minerals for our body. The tree of knowledge is dual. The immature soul is symbolized by the apple tree and the mature soul by the orange tree, which provides the plant chemicals that are essential to the balance of our soul mind and emotions within the alchemical vase. The balance of chemicals in our tree of knowledge is essential to our soul transition.

The parables of the tree of life and the tree of knowledge show us that we have been given all that we need upon earth to evolve from our male physical nature to our female divine nature. Our paradise is earth, which is symbolized biblically as the Garden of Eden. Earth was given to us as the way for us to replenish our cellular pattern through our biological needs of air, water, and the foods of nature. The perfection of the Garden of Eden is the perfection of earth and its support of the human body, dual soul mind and emotions, and spirit consciousness. As we destroy earth we destroy the Garden of Eden and ourselves as a living soul and spirit.

The Garden of Eden represents the joy that we can find when

we live close to nature and restore our bodies from the fruits of nature. The Garden of Eden symbolized earth as a tropical paradise growing within its breadth, depth, and width all foods that had been made by the Creator to sustain our human form. The breeze blew softly, gently caressing the body and face. The water ran smoothly, gurgling in harmony as it flowed from the four rivers meeting in the center of Paradise. The four rivers represent our eternal life cycle that we live as soul in four equal periods of time. The water of the rivers represents the harmony and balance that is inherent within our soul and that must be balanced in our body to sustain life. The rivers and waters of earth are symbolized in our body as our vascular system, which is designed as a fractal pattern of earth. The parable of the Garden of Eden emphasizes our personal responsibility to dress and keep earth viable for our own health and happiness. We have been living the chaos theory as an immature soul and when we change, Earth will change.

The Garden of Eden is the symbol of how earth will be when we create it as our "heaven on earth." The Garden of Eden was the parable that shows us how to live life as a delight and a joy, when we use the happiness of our integrated consciousness and consistently restore our body from that which we can provide for ourselves within the harmony of nature. The Garden of Eden parable symbolizes the importance of the foods of nature in maintaining the balance of our body, dual soul mind and emotions, and our spirit consciousness as the trinity of our consciousness from which we can use our power of creation. It symbolizes the importance of keeping the earth itself viable so that it will support us. The message of this parable is that everything that we need for life is on earth and can be found in the air, water and foods of nature. The tree of knowledge of good and evil defines how we will live from our physical nature as the "evil," or ignorance, as well as our divine nature as the good, or knowledge, and it shows us that our soul has the freedom of choice of knowledge or ignorance to use in our creation of life. The primary ignorance that is symbolized in our physical nature is the ignorance that we continue to nurture as we deny the power of our divine nature.

The four rivers that were found within the Garden of Eden symbolize the parable of our four stages or cycles of eternal life. The first river symbolizes our Cycle of Development in the crystals, minerals, gases, water, plant chemicals, animals, fowls, and fish; and the second river symbolizes the beginning of our living soul after our physical creation and our immature soul as we live the fear of our male mind and physical nature in the Cycle of Awareness; the third river symbolizes our Cycle of Understanding as we begin the mature journey of our soul into the goodness and happiness of our loving consciousness; and the fourth river symbolizes our awakening to the spirit within the heart of us. In the fourth cycle of life we integrate our dual soul, spirit, and physical self into the goodness, righteousness, and wholeness of our trinity of consciousness as we expand into our "Christ Consciousness" of unconditional love and "save" or heal ourselves.

Adam and Eve symbolize the creation of the human species as male and female in total equality both internally and externally. Genesis defines the creation of the male and female as the "Lord" of our physical nature and divine nature as our dual soul and formed a trinity of consciousness with the Spirit as the "Lord God" of life on earth. The trinity of our mind, emotions, and senses were being made in the trinity of consciousness of the physical form to symbolize our internal trinity. Genesis defines the creation of our body from earth and the reflection of our soul through our body. The third reference to creation shows how the choice was made for the soul to evolve first from the male physical nature into the female divine nature. The rib refers to the emotional rib of the heart as our magnetic connection between the left and right lobes of the brain, which was used to separate the two soul minds and emotional natures while maintaining the ability of attraction. In this choice the female divine soul became one with its male physical soul. This parable symbolizes the HUMAN creation as both visible and invisible energy and shows us the form, structure, organization, discipline, and our freedom of choice, intention, and will as a "living soul."

The parable of nakedness symbolizes the understanding of the spirit that we are vulnerable as we live in the ignorance of the dark side of our immature soul mind. The tree of knowledge symbolizes our dual soul mind and emotions and shows our ability to think in negative, external, and fearful judgement as our male physical mind that is our naked or vulnerable consciousness, and our ability to think in a positive, internal, and loving way when we become conscious of our female divine nature. We can only understand the relationship that we have to each other, earth, nature, and our spirit when we have transitioned into our divine nature. Our tree of knowledge of "good and evil" is found in the way that we think, speak, and behave in our evolving consciousness. Our "eyes being opened" symbolizes the level of conscious awareness that we have reached that allows us to continue searching for understanding.

The parable of Cain and Abel is the symbol of our dual soul and its chosen evolution as a descending, dark soul that must grow into the light. Cain symbolizes the dark side of our soul mind and his relationship with Abel and the murder of Abel is the symbol of the denial and abuse of our female divine nature by living in inequality from our male physical nature. This parable is a prediction of how we will succumb to our beliefs and create a collective consciousness within our negative, fearful mind to keep us in the bondage of our own ignorance as our "evil" behavior and believe that we are "saved" from the truth of the good of our divine soul and spirit mind.

Not only have we hidden from the good part of us, but we have suppressed our emotions as the symbol of our female soul and our feelings as the symbol of our spirit for trying to remind us of the good that is inherent within us. In our self-punishment of separating our male physical nature from our female divine nature, we have physically separated ourself by isolation, loneliness, and fear. This need for separation has kept us from living with a consciousness of who we are and the relationship that we have with nature, God, other people, and ourself. Because of our blame and judgement we deny sharing ourself with others. The fear of their blame and judgement of us as retribution and revenge for our "evil" ways leads us into our physical separation and loneliness. As we focus on our fear and judgement, we cast ourself in the role of victim and we feel the poverty of being unloved.

The story of the birth of Seth is the symbol of the knowledge that we learn and store, or record in soul memory, in each lifetime as an integrated level of our soul mind of female wisdom. Seth symbolizes the perfection of our mature soul that is good, and lives from the dutiful, faithful, spiritual values that we learned as we passed through the spiritual hierarchy. Seth lives his life in understanding, which symbolizes our subconscious and unconscious minds that remember and understand every mental and emotional response to our senses within the superconscious mind. Seth is himself the image of our advanced spirit consciousness as the core of the spirit community of humanity. He lives the communication, righteousness, and wholeness of our Trinity of Consciousness.

Although we have been given prophecy that has been recorded, we must take into account that all information that is handed down as mythology undergoes dramatic changes. The myths of our "Gods" are a perfect example. None is "truth," as believed, but truth can be found within the symbols of each parable when we understand our mature soul consciousness.

By examining these symbols we can find the lessons our soul has been learning as the child of our trinity of consciousness. We can see the reflection of our immature soul as we have struggled to explain ourself in our ignorance. We see our fear, control, anger, rage, seduction, and manipulation all being acted out as our dramas of life as we learn the art of creation. If we are brave enough to look carefully inside our own mind we can easily see how our fears are still with us today. We have the freedom of choice to change our thinking, emotions, and feelings.

The difference for each of us today is our ability to use our freedom of choice to change our beliefs with knowledge. Our evolving consciousness is no longer comfortable being stuck in our repetitive fearful beliefs of inequality. Internally we want to love ourself and live in the beauty and peace of a balanced society and earth. We want to respect and honor the wisdom and love of our soul and spirit that is embedded in each and every cell in our body.

THE ADDICTIONS OF
OUR ADVANCED SOUL

K armic beliefs are addictions of our advanced soul that are stuck in the revolutionary soul level which support our resistance and denial of change. Karmic beliefs challenge us to find the strength and courage to release our addictions without fearing change. Creating physical addictions is the way for our immature soul to get our immediate attention through self-abuse. Until we begin to abuse ourself we remain ignorant of the miracle of our own life that we are destroying. As we increase our internal awareness of ourself, we begin to see that our purpose in life is to learn to love ourself and the core of ourself as a spirit consciousness. Our immature intellect and ego creates physical addictions primarily because our ego fears change.

Addictions are the subconscious personality of beliefs and behaviors that we act out in the dark side of our immature soul mind and emotions. Every addiction has its roots in the fear emotions of our immature soul that are concealed from our conscious mind. Our addictive roots to fear have reflected the addictive mental and emotional consciousness of our beliefs and behaviors into every aspect of our immature soul evolution. In every grain of sand of physical experience, we are learning lessons of great magnitude. We have chosen to learn first what we don't want in our lives so that we can fully appreciate what we do want. In our immature soul we have consistently created our negative, external fears as our physical reality. As we get our attention with abusive physical addictions, we begin to see the value of what we want in our lives and our aware consciousness begins to change. Our abusive physical addictions are the physical reflection of the abusive beliefs that our soul wants us to consciously acknowledge and release. This relates to the quote "forgive them for they know not what they do" which tells us to forgive ourselves for our beliefs, as an internal forgiveness. We have externalized this parable to a forgiveness of other people.

Addictive beliefs and behaviors have given the soul a perfect way of suppressing our fear and supporting our illusion of not being an addictive person. Physical addictions create a momentary illusion of escape from the pain within our mind and emotions that we keep striving to repeat by repeating our addictive behavior. Without our attachment to fear we would speak our truth and have no fear of judgement from other people. Fear has existed for us in three distinct levels which has provided us with the opportunity to live the accumulation of our fears in every aspect of our lives. These three levels of fear have been the focus of our attitude, personality, character traits, and language as a reflection of our thoughts and emotions that we reflect into our behavior from our immature intellect and ego. The persona that we live is the energy from which we create our life as our consciousness reality. Self-abuse is part of our soul addiction at the present level of our immature soul consciousness.

Fear emotions exist in three primary levels of descent for our immature soul. When we are living in fear our first level is acted out as judgement-blame, nagging, control, manipulation, seduction, dependency, physical addictions to substances, and gossip. Our fear externally focuses on the lives of others, which distracts us from looking at ourself. In our fear we feel the need to worship someone or something external to us who will accept responsibility for controlling us, redeem us, or allow us to control and forgive them. Self-judgement, material wealth, possessions, education, and our perceived self-image compared to others has become a major focus of our external addiction. Our beliefs controlling our physical sexual self-image lead to multiple addictions from our self-judgement. Our language, tone, beliefs, and behaviors reflect our sense of failure in living up to the perceived image of others, which encourages the immature soul mind to create illusions of happiness. Judgement controls the system of law, medicine, politics, science, religion, and business at this time in our immature soul journey. We play into this judgement by lawsuits, material greed, competition, dependency on drugs, doctors, and religion, which erodes our own personal responsibility by focusing us on external worship. Judgement can be seen clearly in religion when the belief exists that only religion controls the pipeline to "God and salvation," plus many other religious beliefs that expand our fear and enhance our addictive dependency on external survival. Our entire immature soul journey has been lived by acting out our first level of fear.

Our second level is anger that is acted out as conformity attaching us to our fear beliefs and behaviors, which keeps us following someone else's path as our own. Conformity makes us want to copy the beliefs of another or the perceived image of another, denying our own inspiration. Conformity will only have an external physical manifestation of another person because the intention, love, and inspiration of another can never be known or copied. As our distractive addictions increase internally, we focus our attention externally on geography, relationships, or job changes in our attempt to find happiness. In anger we conform to lifestyle thinking, emotions, behaviors, and beliefs of peers we admire. We will smoke, drink, take drugs, try to be cool as an imitation of someone we admire, attach ourself to religious, scientific, and sexual beliefs, and we will accept these beliefs as the absolute truth of our reality. We pattern our personality from anything or anyone we are externally attracted to and can worship. We judge ourself by our self-image and conform to the latest information on any of our addictions with a fanatic, dependent obsessiveness that resists all change and denies all other information. Internally we will be suppressing extreme anger and depression because we are not being who we want to be. We are not living our truth and our anger will be suppressed but it will continue growing while concealed from our conscious awareness.

Our third level is rage, as our last primary level of fear triggers our internal rebellion. We act out our rage externally as we create a physical rebellion to accepted beliefs and behaviors, family values, cultural teachings, societal behaviors, and expectations. We will rebel externally with frequent changes of our physical location, jobs, and relationships. We will attach ourself to "graven images" as the image of someone else that meets our concept of perfection, and we may stalk or haunt every move the other person makes as we worship them. We see this behavior now in many sports activities as well as military images, political images, media images, sexual relationships, publicized roles and identities, career focuses, and other external focuses that capture our addicted immature soul mind and emotions. This is an addiction to being a follower and trying to live the life or behavior that we want to copy vicariously as our own. In our rage at our own boredom and apathy we blame and judge someone else for being the person that we would like to be. When we are in rage, we are making a desperate but foolish bid for love and attention. We will commit any criminal behavior to be noticed as we become involved in competition, war, violence, abuse, and critical judgement that we act out in the court systems with multiple lawsuits.

Rage also brings about violence and multiple types of physical abuse, which we then find the media conforming to repetitiously for purposes of greed, such as violent movies, books, and television. Killing becomes subtle until it is copied in rageful physical acts of violence. Repetition of violence expands violence and patterns the immature soul back into the primitive consciousness of past life memory such as torture, sexual sacrifice, and cannibalism, which repetitiously honors the addictive beliefs and behaviors of our primitive soul. This stage of rebellion creates the complete cycle for our immature soul rage which intensifies our primitive behavior and causes devolution. With this rageful level of fear, we shock our consciousness into the self-realization that change is essential for the survival of our immature soul as a human species. As we begin to change, we can evolve into our mature soul consciousness and live the love that we are seeking. All fears are accumulative for our immature soul, and when we reach the level of rage all of our fears will overwhelm us, creating destructive behavior and addictions throughout our family life, society, and the world.

A spiritual awakening is the only true cure for addictions as it allows us to evolve from the immature soul of fear to the mature soul of love. In a spiritual awakening we will transition into our enlightened mind of pure love which changes us, other people, society, and the world.

All fears are accumulative and will show up in our beliefs and behaviors towards every aspect of our life. Addictions create an illusion of reality that suppresses the truth of ourself, causing an expansion of judgement, anger, and rage, which are always self-directed but are acted out externally against someone else. Each level will support the soul in focusing externally on physical substances and behavior, allowing some lives to be totally controlled by our negative beliefs and addictions to alcohol, drugs, sex, food, and intellectual and physical competition. No one level of our fear is singular at this time, as we are living an accumulation of fears in the ebb and flow of our transitional soul.

Rebellion supports us in looking at ourself mentally, emotionally, and physically when it reaches a crescendo of pain and suffering. When we begin to see that rage has helped us learn as we have lived our fear in the dark side of our soul, we will stop blaming and judging other people in our fear and begin to change our thinking, beliefs, and behaviors into a positive focus. Without rebellion to our addictive beliefs and external physical behaviors, we would never accept change within our soul consciousness. When we accept the importance of change, we accept the beauty and wisdom of ourself.

We must ask ourselves these very important questions to awaken our mature soul consciousness. What is an advanced soul? What does an advanced soul mean in terms of soul evolution? Who is the average person?

An advanced soul is a soul that is at the crossroads of changing from the dark side of the immature soul mind and emotions into the light side of the mature soul mind and emotions. We

have been constantly evolving through the lessons of our immature soul mind and emotions since we began our journey as a
dual soul consciousness that was focused on our immature intellectual mind and fear emotions. We have kept the memory of our
immature soul journey and the lessons that we have learned
stored in the right brain of our mature soul memory but subconscious to our conscious intellectual mind. We have also kept our
universal memory unconsciously hidden in our spirit mind
because our intellect was not yet ready to accept the reality of
ourself and our dual soul journey of evolving consciousness. Our
immature intellectual soul consciousness does not acknowledge
our trinity of consciousness but sees the human being only as a
physical body and intellectual mind.

As we enter the stasis level of knowledge as a soul consciousness the average person has more wisdom within the
mature soul memory than we can imagine with our limited intellect. The human species and our world society is made from an
accumulation of multiple levels of consciousness found within
the immature soul of each person on earth. The masses offer us
an opportunity to see the many levels of consciousness that the
average person has lived as an evolving soul. When we are willing to look at the beliefs, behaviors, and addictions of people
throughout the world, we can see a composite mirror image of
the immature soul evolution of us as an individual. It is our subconscious mature soul knowledge and our unconscious universal
knowledge that we are seeking to access, which will heal the
immature soul in its journey into the light side of consciousness.
All addictions to physical beliefs, behaviors, and substances are
acting as an external resistance and denial of change for our
immature soul mind and emotions. We must understand ourself
as a trinity of consciousness before we can fully access and integrate our dual soul and spirit consciousness. It is our immature
soul that is addicted to staying the same and stopping our evolution into the trinity of our consciousness.

Our immature soul attaches itself to physical addictions to
get our attention and emphasize our need to change the focus of
our thinking, emotions, and feelings. Until the immature soul can

understand and accept the knowledge of who we are, we cannot find the strength and courage to stop the addictive behaviors or beliefs. We cannot evolve into the light side of our soul mind and emotions and at the same time continue with our addiction to beliefs, fear, and past primitive behavior as our external life. We are living beliefs and behaviors that are inappropriate and unacceptable for the mature soul. Therefore, the immature soul must understand the lessons of the mature soul before it can graduate and enter a class that is a higher form of knowledge and understanding. Once we evolve we see the beauty, magnificence, and wisdom of ourself as a dual soul and spirit and we are ready to accept who we are and the perfection of all the physical experiences that we have lived. Once we acknowledge our addictive fears, beliefs, and abusive behaviors, we can change as individuals.

When we are living as an advanced soul in the stasis level of knowledge we create addictions for ourself to keep us attached to the beliefs of the dark side of our immature soul as our fear of change. Addictions force us into a physical conformity that prevents change. It is our addictive beliefs that cause us to become physically addicted as a behavioral method of distracting our soul mind with fear, which keeps us from seeing the importance of loving ourself. As we focus on the physical addiction, we ignore the messages from our mature soul and spirit consciousness that are urging us to hear the wisdom of the voices within that are speaking to us. Addictions are used by our ego beliefs that fear the voices of our soul and spirit, which are advocating change and growth.

Our addiction creates the illusion of "fun" and "hell" as we alternate between our dual perceptions of our feelings and emotions. The distraction of addictions consumes us physically, mentally, and emotionally and keeps us from focusing on our consciousness growth. As the addictions suppress our mind, emotions, and feelings as our consciousness we totally shut out our mature soul and spirit. Our societal addiction to religious beliefs is a perfect example of an all-consuming addiction. Addictions cover up our consciousness of what is really happening in our lives and what our immature soul is attempting to learn. We see our fear beliefs and behavior as our salvation and we refuse to accept our personal responsibility to change as we conform in fear and judgement to the dependency and inequality of worship. Our intellect and ego are addicted to our dependent perception of life, and our fear of changing our dependency is overwhelming to us and causing our personal and societal devolution. We have the power to destroy all that we have created if we refuse to change our addictions and ourselves. We see examples of personal destruction happening with drugs and alcohol. Very few people understand that our addiction to religious beliefs is our immature soul addiction to inequality that must be healed before we can evolve into our mature soul of equality.

When we have addictions that we have been able to release it shows the growth of our immature soul consciousness. If we still have the addiction it indicates that we are stuck in the conformity of our soul revolution and we are denying our soul's wish to change and evolve its consciousness. When we deny our soul evolution we deny the love, wisdom, and equality of ourself.

Most addictions make us feel so confused and physically sick that we focus on our pain and suffering to ignore the lesson of the addiction. We subconsciously use our freedom of choice to indulge in the addictive behavior until we can realize the abuse that we are inflicting upon ourself. We can become aware that our addictive behavior does not support us and that it is self-centered and yet not have the strength and courage to be truthful and loving with ourself and stop the addiction. Pain and suffering symbolizes our immature intellectual soul desire to change and grow. The ego will urge us to continue our addiction because our ego wants to control us. Our ego sees change as its death and does not understand that it too will simply change its personality to humility rather than arrogance. As our immature soul wages a war between our intellect and ego with the ego addictions, we are trying to learn the most basic lesson of freedom and equality.

Addictions separate our thinking from our feelings and emotions. It is abusive to our soul consciousness to separate our thinking from our feelings and emotions. At this time in our immature soul evolution, we are attempting to understand the alchemical vase of our limbic system. We use addictions as our denial and resistance to naturally balancing our chemical consciousness. Our addictions not only separate our thinking from our feelings and emotions, but they separate us chemically within our chemical brain and our chemical cellular body. Addictions will physically separate us from our relationships. The physical relationship with our internal body and brain is denied when we abuse ourself, which is part of our resistance and denial of family, friends, and careers. When we become addicted to any chemical, including food, we are reminding ourself that we are a chemical consciousness.

Our left brain symbolizes our immature soul that focuses on our male physical nature and its sexual core, which is the unaware side of our mind and emotions. Our right brain symbolizes our mature soul that focuses on our female Divine Nature that is enlightened by our spiritual core, which is the understanding side of our mind and emotions. Our feelings symbolize our spirit consciousness and are used to evolve us through our dual soul consciousness as we live our multiple lives of external physical experience. Our alchemical vase is the master control system for the chemical factory of our body and symbolizes our trinity of consciousness.

All addictions are left brain attachments to old beliefs, behaviors, and habits that we use as obsessive protection to keep our intellect from becoming clearly aware of who we are. Our journey as an immature soul has taken us into primitive behavior and beliefs that are no longer appropriate for us at our current level of consciousness as an evolving soul. We are not being truthful with ourself if we treat addictions as a physical behavioral failure and stay in ignorance of our root beliefs that are the core of all of our physical addictions. Our soul is organized as opposites under the Doctrine of Two, which means that we live constantly from cause and effect as well as action and reaction. Therefore, all behavior is the end result of a belief.

Physical addictions of our immature soul mind are seemingly endless, such as street drugs, prescription drugs, over-the-counter drugs, alcohol, smoking, chewing, self-image, weight, sex, need to be loved, feeling worthless without love, need to conquer or compete, food, eating dead food, sugar, fats, starches, money, materialism, inequality, lying, possessions, work, science, religion, fear, beliefs, superstitions, depression, disease, control, dependency, anger, negativity, manipulation, externalization, seduction, rebellion, conformity, education, relationships: the list is endless. Our immature soul has always been addictive because it is ignorant of the miracle of life and our art of creation.

Beliefs are the oldest and strongest addiction for our immature soul, which then reflects our soul thinking, emotions, and feelings into our physical behavior. Addictive beliefs such as our fearful thinking, fear emotions, superstitions, rituals, negative attitude, personality, religious, scientific, disease, inequality, dependency, work, sexuality, education, materialism, money, possessions, and our physical image control us and our entire art of creation as our lives. Each of these addictive beliefs has been learned by our immature soul from our myths, rituals, superstitions, and addictive religious beliefs. These addictive beliefs became the foundation of our immature soul consciousness and are used as the governing moral laws of our society. Moral law allows each society to differ according to their addictive religious beliefs. All judgement is a learned addictive belief of our physical nature. When we judge others we are judging ourself as an external reflection of our beliefs. Judgement is a major issue in our society today because the immature soul feels that the end is near, and because of its religious beliefs it is seeking atonement for its sins to assure its place in heaven. The need for atonement allows hypocrisy to flourish as the immature soul seeks a redeemer for the sins of the masses. We are now living the identical beliefs, fear, judgement, and behavior that we lived at the time of Jesus.

In learning how to overcome our addictive patterns, we can learn how to transform ourself from a dependent personality to a free and loving personality. Our spirit consciousness is unconditionally loving. Our mature soul lives as a loving soul. Our immature soul lives in fear and judgement, and it has created its consciousness from our primitive ignorance that has become our addictive beliefs. Our addictive beliefs are predominant in three major focuses of our immature soul at this time in our evolution. These three addictive societal and personal focuses control our external reality and they are sexuality, religion, and science.

Our sexual addictions are an intense form of acting out our self-judgement, inadequacy, worthlessness, loneliness, rejection, abandonment, fear, control, anger, and rage. Our sexuality is our lesson of inequality, especially between the male and female. Our sexual addictions show us the importance of loving ourself first, which prevents the sexual abuse of others as we learn not to indulge in self-abuse, which is the lesson of equality.

Sexuality, which is the core consciousness of our physical nature that holds us in bondage by our reflected beliefs, is also attached to multiple societal beliefs involving our physical image, age, intellect, education, money, and family status. Our societal beliefs enhance our personal beliefs, such as sex without fulfillment, promiscuous sex as external searching for internal peace, identity that is found in our sexual image, a sense of worthlessness and loneliness if we are not receiving sexual satisfaction, sexual inequality, sexual roles and identities of specific genders, gender phobias, sex as love, self-abuse, and abuse of others as a way of self-gratification.

Addictive sexual beliefs that limit us are: I am nobody unless somebody loves me, looking for love in all the wrong places, love will save me, and sex is love. Because sexuality is the core of our physical nature, sex is always self-centered when we are living in our immature soul.

Some of our addictive religious beliefs, which have created the foundation of our immature soul consciousness and our society, are found in our religious hymns that hypnotize our mind and emotions by constant repetition. Our language is constantly used to strengthen our addictive religious beliefs in the same way that frequent church attendance is used as a reinforcement: "The old rugged cross. The emblem of suffering and shame. I love that old cross where the dearest and best for a world of lost sinners was slain. I will cling to the old rugged cross and exchange it some day for a crown." The verse of this hymn shows us how we reinforce our addictive beliefs without a consciousness of our actions. Our addictive religious beliefs of pain and suffering are symbolized by the cross which we hang ourself on each day with our perception of inequality, dependency, victimization, and poverty consciousness that controls our lives. The parable of the cross is the symbol that defines where we are in our evolving soul consciousness. As an eternal soul and spirit consciousness we are stuck in the revolutions of our beliefs. To see this symbol, image a circle with two lines dividing it into quarters. We have lived on this cross for fourteen thousand years as we are attempting to continue with our journey home as an evolving consciousness.

Other religious beliefs are: we have only one life, Jesus will save me, man is made in the image of God, blind faith is superior to knowledge. "Blind faith is superior to knowledge" keeps us in the darkness of our immature soul consciousness, allowing our addictive beliefs to create an illusion of righteousness in our fearful mind. Blind faith is the choice of our immature soul consciousness to accept ignorance as superior to knowledge. Blind faith reflects our fear of unlearning our addictive beliefs.

Other religious attitudes and beliefs that we are unwilling to look at are the ego karmic beliefs that hold us on our cross. Our addictive beliefs; our unwillingness to change our beliefs; our fear of retribution from God if we change the belief that Jesus will forgive our abusive behavior; our denial of evolution of the soul; our fear of damnation; our belief in right/wrong, good/bad; our fear of shame, guilt, sin and punishment; our fear of judgement; our expectations of roles and identities; our fear of failure, unworthiness, inadequacy, and separation; our belief in Jesus as a savior; our belief in inequality, dependency, and worship; and our ignorance of personal responsibility as acted out in blind faith: all assure us that we will stay on our cross and not evolve as a mature soul consciousness.

Our addictive scientific beliefs allow us to use science as our source of supremacy. We can never be supreme when we use linear or tunnel vision as a method of thinking. Each discipline of science sees itself as separate and it focuses on its information as fact without seeing the relationship of all knowledge to us. Our immature soul as our physical nature uses "tunnel vision." Our mature soul thinks in a "cycle," using our inspiration, knowledge, motivation, and creativity as the four parts of our "cyclic" thinking. It is the combination of free thinking, emotions, and feelings that we use in our "cyclic" thinking that lets us understand the big picture of who we are and the miracle of life.

Some scientific beliefs that are common in our society are: I know all of that, medicine will save me, if it can't be measured it doesn't exist, if it isn't based within scientific proof it isn't fact, science is superior to religion, science can stick to fact and not worry about emotions and feelings, each discipline is separate. Our scientific beliefs lead us into beliefs and behaviors that affect the perfection of ourself, each other, and the world. Our dependency on medicine and our belief that medicine can save us create fear. Our beliefs control our external image of disease, and our blame and judgement of external, genetic factors, and our fear of death turn us into victims. Our ignorance of the source of creation of matter, the patterning of our mind and emotions through the negative input that surrounds and limits our perception of reality, enhances our fear of living.

Addictive behaviors that we live as a reaction to our addictive beliefs have created societal attitudes as truth for our immature soul consciousness. Once we accept an addictive belief as a societal addiction it becomes a challenge to change. Two societal beliefs that reflect our external dependencies are: "Jesus will save me" and "Medicine will save me." Both of these addictive societal beliefs take away our personal responsibility to save ourself by changing our thinking, emotions, and feelings, which is the definition of our dual soul evolution as our expansion of consciousness. Both beliefs limit our thinking and produce a negative, external, and fearful emotional mind-set, which blocks our senses as our feelings, and we begin to automatically conform to other people's beliefs instead of thinking for ourself.

As we live through the duality of changing our thinking, we

can find ourself depressed, secondary to the diversity of our thoughts and emotions that are present in our dual soul. Depression is normal as our immature soul becomes conscious of its dual transitional emotions and the ego/spirit tug-of-war begins. It is the contrast between descending emotions and the ascending knowledge that we are living that allows us to experience depression. Depression becomes the normal transitional emotions as we ascend our mind from the left to the right brain with cross-fertilization and we allow our emotions to descend. Cross-fertilization can be called the internal genetic engineering of our consciousness. Whatever is happening internally, we make physical by the art of creation as a way of interpretation for our physical nature.

Knowing that we have free choice to focus our mind helps us to leave the fearful duality of thought and emotions and focus exclusively on the positive thoughts and loving behaviors that we want. To bring this change of focus about, we must accept personal responsibility for our attitude as our choice of thinking, emotions, and feelings. In choosing we release our addictive beliefs and our fearful emotions, and we evolve our consciousness to a higher level of total enlightenment. Enlightenment is the understanding of knowledge. When we are willing to accept the history of our addictive consciousness journey, we will accept the importance of our change.

Our addictive beliefs have become our habits and our behaviors, making us addicted to or slaves to our negative thinking and fearful emotions. Our primitive immature soul consciousness allows us to create the reflection of our mind and emotions as our physical life. Our karmic beliefs and our behaviors are created from our fears that we have learned in other lives. As we have lived our fears we have become addicted to our beliefs and behaviors and obsessively addicted to our fear itself, which makes us fearful of change because we fear punishment. All of our addictive fears, beliefs, and behaviors are karmic. Karmic defines the hidden accumulation of unlearned soul lessons. It is up to us to dredge up the fear through our physical experiences of this life and release it forever. When our fear is gone we will no longer need addictive beliefs or addictive physical behaviors as our protective devices and distractions. Without fear controlling us we will commit ourself to seeking the knowledge that will allow us to unlearn our beliefs. Our ego is a master of distraction and it will do everything possible to change our attention each time we want to commit to something new.

To change our addictions, we must change the image of ourself from unequal, controlled, dependent, powerless, and fearful individuals to equal, responsible, free, powerful, and loving individuals. When our thinking changes, we will know that we are evolving towards the core of our Divine Consciousness in our loving mature soul. Our spiritual awakening is the only true cure for all of our mental, emotional, and physical addictions, including our addictive personality. Change is our journey of soul evolution and as advanced souls we are prepared to change from left brain thinking to right brain thinking as we transition. Our dual soul consciousness is seated in the dual lobes of our left and right brain. Our immature soul consciousness is ready to integrate as a male intellect of our physical nature with the female loving wisdom of our divine nature. Our male and female consciousness wants to become one equal soul consciousness. Our addictive ego beliefs live as a primitive consciousness of electromagnetic energy which surrounds our left brain and limits our consciousness. The electromagnetic energy of our ego functions in the same manner that an electrical fence works to control the limits that our animals can roam. Each time that we try to step over the control limits of our ego beliefs, we are "shocked and fearful" and we return to our addictive beliefs and behaviors as our comfort zone. The energy of our addictive beliefs reflects into the physical body as depression, anxiety, stress, nervousness phobias, and inhibitions.

We can look at our beliefs and behaviors to tell if we are focused on the immature soul lessons in a lifetime or if we are focused on our advanced soul lessons. The physical addictions reflect the immature soul lessons of judgement, control, dependency, anger, and conformity. If we are attached to addictive beliefs from the level of sexuality, science, and religion, then we are continuing to work through the immature lessons of our soul and inequality, dependency, and judgement will control us as our fear.

When the immature soul consciousness is not evolved sufficiently to accept responsibility for its own actions as the means of saving itself, it will continue being dependent on sexual relationships, religion, and science. Anger as conformity behavior encourages us to copy the thoughts and fears of other people rather than thinking for ourself and allowing our inspiration to guide us. Conformity can be seen in our personal behavior, beliefs, relationships, sexuality, religion, and science, because we are afraid to be different. We are afraid to speak and live our truth because we fear others will judge us. Our fear is a reflection of our self-judgement. Many souls are now feeling different from birth, but the fear of "being different" prevents them from communicating their loving emotions and feelings. As they live in fear they devolve into more primitive addictive beliefs and behaviors.

If we live in total rage and rebellion, or release all of our beliefs regarding sexuality, science, and religion being our savior, we will trigger the soul lessons of our advanced mature soul. The advanced immature soul will take on physical addictions such as alcohol, drugs, and promiscuous sex to get our attention and encourage change. Using drugs or abusing ourself with alcohol or indiscriminate sex distracts the intellect from the mature soul and spirit and helps to keep us physically focused on the ego. In this tug-of-war between the ego and mature soul our ego will be brutal in its intention of winning. The sexual revolution that began several decades ago is part of our ego tug-of-war that does not want to change our sexual focus. Our sexual fears have a direct relationship to our addictive belief that "sex is love." In all addictions love, truth, and equality are the mature soul lessons that we are attempting to learn.

Our immature soul is learning many lessons by living through addictions. The soul can only grow and change by understanding the significance of the lesson that it is learning as it is lived out in our physical experience. The more dramatic the lesson the more determined the immature soul is to learn the lesson. Our lessons are always about our evolving soul consciousness and not about someone else. We always learn both passively and actively so we can learn from watching another person living their lessons, but we only learn passively when we can resist interfering. If we are determined to learn actively, we will create our personal dramas and crises, and we will repeat an image of the lesson in every aspect of our life through all cycles of our life until the lesson is learned.

If we externalize our focus and attempt to change someone else, we will not be internalizing the lesson to change ourself. No one can live another person's soul agenda. Each soul is unique and it works only on its personal lesson. If we try to blame the experience on someone else it is a lesson of interference that is being learned by both souls. In looking within our physical experience and fully understanding what we are learning from the experience of our soul consciousness, we have the power to change and evolve. There is nothing hidden in our soul consciousness that is not also a part of everyone's immature soul consciousness. When we feel guilt, sin, and shame, we are afraid to look at ourself. This is another ego attempt to keep us living our addictive, fearful beliefs. When we learn not to judge ourself, we will not judge others. As we become conscious of our thinking, emotions, and feelings, we must share them through communication with friends and relatives. Once we reveal our thoughts, emotions, and feelings verbally, we begin to realize that our need for secrecy or concealment was simply an addictive fear and judgement of our ego. As we speak our truth other people will relate to us and a healing occurs for everyone.

The power of our hidden addictions is immeasurable and insidious. We will continue to act out our addictions in our daily lives until we become conscious of how we are sabotaging ourselves with our abusive behavior. Our hidden addictions are primarily our concealed beliefs that control our behavior without our having a consciousness that the belief exists. Looking at the three major focuses of our immature soul as sexuality, science, and religion, we can find our hidden beliefs being acted out in our daily behavior as our personality. These karmic beliefs subconsciously control our lives as they subconsciously control our physical behavior. Looking within ourself and our physical experiences of life can help us discover our hidden addictions and will give us the power to release them. The biggest hurdle in changing our consciousness is to unlearn our addictive beliefs by learning new knowledge that lets us understand ourself. This is enlightenment.

Our immature soul, as our intellect and ego, is seeking reward, punishment, and pain and suffering with its self-abuse because our religious beliefs tell us that is our path to Jesus. Many of our physical life experiences are focused on the expectation of ego and intellectual reward or punishment. As an example, if we make a scientific discovery we will covet the Nobel Prize. If we make no discoveries our grant money is stopped. Our expectations of what we want in life cause our behavior to be controlling, dependent, manipulative, and seductive to meet our goal of physical and emotional needs. When we are immersed in this behavior we are working with our immature soul in a self-abusive way. Our addictions "of need" are controlling our entire physical reality and our perception of ourself, and we will be not only self-abusive but we will seek abuse from medicine, religion, and in our sexual relationships. The "need" for reward and punishment as well as self-abuse comes from old and well hidden religious beliefs.

One of the major addictive abuses that we have created as a daily habit is the way that we abuse our body with dead and polluted food. Adulteration of food allows us to paralyze our senses and hides our soul and spirit from our aware consciousness. Because we are a trinity of chemical consciousness as a physical body, dual soul, and spirit, we were designed with and were taught to use air, water, and the foods of nature to restore the chemicals within us, which balances the function and pattern of our chemical cellular structure and chemical consciousness of electromagnetic energy form. We have lost the conscious memory of our chemical origins and our biological need to replace these chemicals from the purity of nature. Our addictive belief that "all food is good food" and our greed for money have put us on an addictive path to self-destruction under the disguise of science. Greed and the savior complex of dependency play a tremendous role in this societal lesson for our immature soul consciousness.

We are holding our immature soul mind in bondage with our addictive beliefs and our addictive behaviors. Through the aeons of time our concealed karmic beliefs have formed a cosmic shell around our immature soul as a buried or concealed electromagnetic shield. This cosmic shell is what we call the ego because it will shock us in a violent and seemingly protective way whenever one of its beliefs is threatened. Our cosmic shell of beliefs holds our immature soul mind in bondage in the identical pattern that an embryo is held in the womb of a mother's body. Our spirit consciousness is giving our immature soul time to grow into an aware consciousness at its own level of awakening. Once the immature soul discards its karmic beliefs the cosmic shell of our ego dissolves into humility. As we experience the splendor and lightness of our open mind we cannot help but be in awe of our wisdom, truth, and magnificence. We feel the humility at the moment that we begin to understand the journey that we have lived with such ignorance and unawareness as our consciousness level. We must consciously open our immature soul mind and release it from its bondage of addiction by our willingness to seek truth and search for knowledge that feels true within our hearts. Our soul experiences a rebirth when we begin to live in our Divine Nature.

As we feel ourselves physically dependent upon addictions, we may begin to ask ourselves how to recover from our addictions. First it is important to realize that our physical addictions are reflecting our concealed addictive beliefs. We cannot cure our physical addictions until we are prepared to change our internal mind and emotional addictions.

Knowledge is the key to unlearning and curing all of our addictions. It is through knowledge that we begin to release our habitual and superstitious beliefs that hold us captive within our physical sexual focus of consciousness. Our beliefs have been created by our ignorance of the relationship of ourselves to earth, nature, and the universe. Because of our ignorance we came to our addictive beliefs as our relative-truth conclusions that we have accepted as fact and have refused to reconsider.

We have never understood that we created ourselves as a chemical consciousness with a beautiful design of energy form and physical structure that has an eternal organization and discipline as well as a consciousness of freedom of choice, intention, and will to guide us in our evolving consciousness. Despite the ignorance of our intellect and ego our subconscious mature soul and our unconscious spirit have always maintained the equality, truth, love, and integrity of our evolving consciousness. We have kept our intellect unconscious of our indwelling spirit because our addictive beliefs have led us to an acceptance that "God" is external to us and that "man" is made in God's image. This addictive belief defies the pattern of creation that we have lived within ourselves and that we have observed in nature, the animal kingdom, and other mammals. We are a spirit consciousness as the seed of a universal Spirit Consciousness and at our core we are both chemical.

As our immature soul has evolved through the levels of our soul growth it has done the best it possibly could to understand itself. It had to rely on its perception of reality and try to determine how the pieces of the gigantic puzzle of life fit together. All of our learning has occurred through the external acting out of our reflective thinking, emotions, and feelings in the reality that we call physical experience. Our immature soul has passed through aeons of levels of consciousness and it has now reached the soul level of knowledge. It is through understanding the relationship of our knowledge to ourself that we unlearn our addictions on a physical, mental, and emotional level.

As we have lived in our immature soul, we have looked externally from ourself and blamed and judged others, circumstances, and any number of other reasons for what has happened to us. As we learn to look within ourself, we find the relationship of what we have learned as the clever design of evolution for our immature soul. For example, medicine may blame disease on external germs, but when we look inside ourself, we will find a physical, mental, and emotional component that has depressed our immune system, which created an imbalance within us and made us susceptible to disease as an internal lesson that expands our consciousness. It is the disease that puts us in touch with how we are consciously abusing our physical body and how we feel mentally and emotionally about the value of life and our addictive fear of death. Disease is an internal lesson of our soul that forces us to experience our thinking, emotions, and feelings internally. Our knowledge about ourself will then motivate us into change that can give us a longer life or we will fall back into old habits and beliefs, increase our addictive beliefs, and learn nothing that will help us evolve. Because we are living our level of knowledge as a soul, and because we are transitioning into the second half of our level of knowledge, we must live our freedom of choice, intention, and will in our physical lives. We have evolved in our immature soul through our sexual magnetism, but as we recognize our equality we must consciously choose evolution by seeking the knowledge to understand ourself and live our freedom. It is only when we can live our freedom of consciousness that we become free of our intellect and ego addictions. Freedom relates to our thinking, emotions, and feelings and we interpret freedom as sexual because sexuality is the core of our physical nature.

We may become conscious of our internal challenge to acknowledge the wisdom of our mature soul. Our ego has limited the knowledge of our intellect by its addictive beliefs. To access the soul memory of our mature soul, we must remove the addictive beliefs that are closing our mind. We can also have a belief that we are accessing our mature soul mind when in reality we are accessing the primitive ego memories that are the subconscious and karmic lessons of our past lives that we are continuing to live. Disease always acts as a wake-up call to look internally at ourself and seek the knowledge to regain our health. An immature soul that is stuck in its addictive beliefs and gets disease will gladly put its life in the physician's hand without any questions being asked. An immature soul refuses to accept personal responsibility for its beliefs, lifestyle, language, and behaviors. Maturing souls with disease will seek knowledge and actively use their freedom of choice in treatment.

We acknowledge the wisdom of our mature soul by opening our mind to the reality that we have always created our life. Our ability to create what we don't want in life as disease, as well as what we do want in life as our health, shows us the wisdom of our soul as it seeks to capture our awareness. To open our mind we must be aware that the hidden addictive beliefs of our immature soul are the chains that keep our mind in bondage and closed to new knowledge and awareness. Opening our mind to accepting the relationship of ourself, each other, nature, earth and the universe allows us to live in our mature soul consciousness, which will continue to evolve our consciousness and our physical lives into a love of life.

We can ask ourselves, how do I live my freedom of truth? We may find the answer evading us as our ego tries to exert its control into our thinking and its fear into our emotions. If we give the ego its way, we will begin to feel depressed within a matter of minutes, hours, or days. This is simply our dual soul in its eternal struggle to evolve and grow. We have the freedom of choice to be happy or to be sad. We can speak our truth or we can lie. We can exercise free choice or we can conform as intimidation. No one can make our choices but us.

Living the freedom of our truth means that we must at all times speak our truth, live our truth, and use our truth in living as an example for other people. We have learned fear, judgement, anger, rage, inequality, deceit, greed, competition, war, and abuse as we have lived the physical experience of our immature soul consciousness. We have learned to suppress our true emotions, feelings, and thoughts, and we have chosen to speak from our expectations of what someone else wants to hear. We have learned conformity to our addictive beliefs that have been abusive, unequal, unloving, untrue, and deceitful, and we have innocently repeated them in our ignorance.

As we face the most important time in our evolution as a soul consciousness, we must be aware of our loving emotions, feelings, and our truth in thinking. We must honor ourself by the honest communication and expression of ourself and our feelings. As we seek knowledge in our search for truth, we will discover who we are. In speaking our truth we exercise the freedom of our physical experience, mind, emotions, and feelings. This is the awakening of our immature, addictive soul to the spirit consciousness of our mature soul, and it is our cure for all addictions—physical, mental, and emotional.

THE RELATIONSHIP OF PSYCHICS, SOUL GUIDES AND SPIRIT GUIDES TO OUR EVOLVING SOUL

In studying Metaphysical Philosophy from the alpha to the omega or the beginning to the end of our evolution as a spirit and dual soul consciousness, we will explore the mysteries of concealed knowledge, the mystics or ancient prophets, and the magi or seers of old. First and foremost we will study the fractal pattern of our spirit and dual soul consciousness and its integration into our lives as a physical being and discover the relationships that exist personally within us, the universe, earth, nature, and all other people. As we explore both the visible and invisible aspects of our physical body, dual soul, and spirit, we begin to understand that our physical experience has changed as our soul has grown and that our experiences are all perfectly normal for our soul journey of evolution. All of the levels of consciousness that we have lived have been perfect for our dual soul.

To understand the influence of our immature soul mind as our psychic mind of the intellect and ego, our mature soul mind as our soul "guide," and our spirit consciousness as our spirit "guide" helps us to know the precise mind that we are using in our daily lives. To understand that all communication with our dual soul and spirit is internal can help us change our external focus of reality. It also helps us to understand how we take information from other people and we analyze and evaluate it externally in relationship to what we think. Unless we understand the trinity of our mind consciousness, it is impossible to see the "evil" or "good" influence that we inflict upon our own lives from the focus of our thinking, emotions, and sensory stimulation.

When we perceive all communication of our soul and spirit as external entities, we then judge ourselves as inadequate and unequal to others. Our mature soul mind motivates and our spirit mind inspires us on a moment by moment basis, but we frequently refuse to listen. When we have only an external perception of our reality, we will miss the joy of soul and spirit communication within our own mind. Without an awareness of how our soul and spirit communication happens and how the level of communication can be recognized, we won't use the internal power that is there to be used, and we won't recognize that we aren't using our power. Our intellect and ego will create the illusion within our immature soul mind that we are spiritual and it will resist further growth by using the "I know all of that" belief.

In understanding the mystics or ancient prophets, we begin to understand where our beliefs and behaviors originated. We have created our beliefs, through our perception of mystery, from the symbols that we were conscious of existing and the superstitions that we took to heart when we attempted to understand our relationship with each other, nature, earth, and the universe. It is important that we never blame or judge ourself or other people, but instead always remember that we are our own ancestors. In our primitive lives we were doing the very best that we could do as we attempted to expand our aware consciousness into an understanding of our purpose in being spirits that are learning to become human. As we are ready to transition into our mature soul from our immature soul, we are moving into our Cycle of Understanding and leaving our Cycle of Awareness. It is our soul growth in consciousness that is causing our ego to have a temper tantrum and deny all change for the soul. In the immature soul, we have lived the parable of the Ark of the Covenant. In our primitive lives we took prophecy and made it into a self-fulfilling physical process or "thing" by learning the art of creating our beliefs as physical to make our beliefs real. Our attempt to expand our consciousness of the prophecy expanded our belief in our own interpretation. In essense we have been creating our reality from our fear, negativity, and our external interpretation of events throughout our immature soul consciousness. Our spirit consciousness has always been heard by a few people, but our interpretation of the information has always been external and fearful because we are ignorant of who we are as a trinity of minds, emotions, and feelings.

The Ark of the Covenant is the parable of what we have done with our immature soul intellectual mind as we have confined it in a box of ego beliefs. We have sealed our mind and then covered it repeatedly with our beliefs as the illusions or veils through which we perceive life. We are challenged to remember the gold spirit light that overlays our intellect and the crown of jewels as wisdom that waits for us as we open the Ark of the Covenant to the Ark of the Testament, which symbolizes the Cycle of Understanding of our mature soul.

When the parable of the Ark of the Covenant was given as prophecy to Moses the Egyptian, we, as primitive man, proceeded to build a physical Ark of the Covenant that we then worshipped as a sacred physical object. The beliefs that we attached to this prophecy through our ignorance were multiple superstitious beliefs that are still with us today. The religious priests were put in charge of the Ark of the Covenant and believed that if anyone other than a priest touched the Ark of the Covenant they would die from their sin.

This religious belief was the beginning of our karmic belief that "death is a sin." Because we believe that death is a sin rather than a new beginning for the soul, the churches and medicine have competed with the soul to maintain life even when the choice of the soul to begin again is obvious. Our belief that death is a sin also allows us to see disease and the infliction of pain and suffering as the punishment of God because of the sin of impending death.

We lived the Ark of the Covenant by believing that religion was responsible for the moral law and control of our immature soul. This belief created our attachment to the Antichrist teachings of Paul. Paul collected the "laws and ritual beliefs" from

325

many religious cults which became the Christian laws of life and death. Paul created the belief that worshipping Jesus as the Messiah was the way in which religion was protecting the mystery of our immature soul. The only mysteries that exist in our lives are those which we create from our ignorance.

The primitive part of our mind that has created these negative beliefs about religion, creation, birth, death, man, and woman is our intellect and ego. Our intellect and ego is the "child" mind as our immature soul that has been trying to find logic in a new situation. The more we hide our intellect in the Ark of the Covenant, symbolized by the cosmic shell that covers our ego beliefs, the more fear we feel and the more dependent we become.

When we are confused about life, we can become dependent on "psychic" information from another person. Psychic readings come from the intellect and ego cosmic shell of our immature soul mind. They will be fearful, negative, external, and full of physical dramas. They can fulfill the dependent addiction that we have to drama and help us feel protected in the physical world, but they can also create dependency and addictions that can keep our immature soul from growing.

Ancient mature soul and spirit prophecy has many merits, but the ignorance of our primitive minds led us into misinterpretations of the prophecy. When the ancient spirit prophecy is read with an open mind, we find the perfect story of our immature soul and the attempt that our spirit was making to help us understand that we were learning and gravitating toward our mature soul. We will know that our transition has occurred when we stop living our "hell upon earth" and we begin living our "heaven upon earth." We are not living our spiritual self until we stop judging, perceiving ourself as superior or inferior, living in fear, being negative, looking externally, lying for any purpose, being unequal, worshipping others, and living our old addictive beliefs.

The beauty of spiritual prophecy is that it helps us understand what we are now living. If we are attached to psychic prophecy, we are wallowing in our ego cosmic shell of primitive beliefs and our intellect as the parable of the Ark of the Covenant. If we are living our love, freedom, equality, and truth, we are living in our Ark of the Testament, or the mature soul of the right brain, where we share equally in communication of truth with everyone. In the mature soul we never think of ourselves as "knowing it all": instead we are in total awe of what we have not yet learned, and therefore, seeking knowledge is the purpose and intention of our life.

The soul journey that we have lived as a trinity of mind and emotional consciousness is our miracle of life. The aware consciousness that we have slowly developed through billions of years is now allowing us to begin to understand ourselves. The miracle of transition of our mind and emotions is the level of our soul consciousness that we are living at this time. It is during this time of transition when the dual soul is experiencing its dual visions of life that depression is a plague for society. Depression occurs because of the contrasting realities of the immature soul mind and the emotions as our consciousness moves back and forth from fear to love. Love challenges our ego and enhances our fear, causing depression, phobias, stress, separation, panic attacks, addictions, and total desperation. Each of these fear behaviors is our ego acting out in our physical attempt to avoid change. As we have ascended our mind we have descended our emotions, creating our emotional depression.

To begin understanding ourselves, we must first learn to see ourselves with a different perception than we have used until this time. Throughout the journey of our growth we have believed ourselves to be only finite physical beings, which has kept us ignorant of the energy of our dual soul and spirit as our source of life. In our obsession with our physical body, we have stayed in ignorance of the trinity of our mind and emotional consciousness which is the eternal energy of us. Religion has taught us to suppress our emotions because it has taught us fear, judgement, wrath, and inequality, which has slowed down our transition with repetitious and unequal beliefs and behaviors. We must live our emotions equally with our intellectual mind before we can accept and live our mature soul mind of wisdom and our love emotions. Our mind and emotions must seek balance in our immature soul before we can move into our mature soul. We must learn the dance of life as our mind and emotions embrace in total harmony and rhythm as the double helix of our soul.

We are made as male and female in the image of the Christ Consciousness as our living soul, and the image of the "God" Consciousness as our indwelling spirit consciousness. Our male and female consciousness is the Lord of our living soul. Our spirit consciousness is the internal good within us. As physical beings we are a trinity of the living dual soul and the indwelling spirit consciousness as an eternal trinity of consciousness that is embedded in every cell of our physical body, while living its journey of consciousness expansion as its evolution. If we look at prophecy with these points as an internal image within our mind instead of an external image of God and the Lord, we begin to see the beauty of ourselves and our ability to communicate with our trinity of minds and emotions. As we change the focus of our consciousness, we will also interpret prophecy from a different perception.

We live the persona of our living soul by focusing on the precise level of consciousness that our soul has reached. Our living soul is our dual mind and emotions. The consciousness of our dual soul is symbolized as the left and right lobes of our brain. The left lobe of our brain is the male consciousness of our physical nature that is our psychic mind. The right lobe of our brain is the female consciousness of our divine nature that is our soul memory that acts as our soul guide. We wear the exact level of soul consciousness that we are living as our "coat of many colors." Our soul consciousness changes levels multiple times in each lifetime as it is expanded by our sensory stimulation, emotions, and knowledge.

Our indwelling spirit consciousness is focused within the posterior brain of our cerebellum and it is the sole source of inspiration for our dual soul minds. Our spirit is our thoughtform or inspiration. The inspiration of our spirit is distorted by the cosmic shell of our ego beliefs which filters our inspired thought. Our immature soul persona becomes the fear, controlling, and judgemental behavior of our intellect and ego soul mind and emotions after our inspiration has been distorted by the ego. It is our ego beliefs and behavior that manage to dispirit or remove the spirituality from our physical lives as our ego beliefs distort and conceal the inspiration of our spirit.

Our physical body is made from the chemicals of earth and nature. "For dust thou are, and unto dust thou will return." As the soul and spirit leaves one physical body, because it is no longer productive and creative for the soul and spirit, it creates another physical body through conception by another male and female within three days. The trinity of our consciousness continues to live and to grow subconsciously and unconsciously even though our conscious mind and emotions has not learned to understand who it is or how the different levels of our minds and emotions function. Our immature intellectual soul remains captured in the Ark of the Covenant as the cosmic shell of our ego beliefs. Our intellect is "struggling in pain and suffering" to free itself of the veils of illusions that our beliefs have used to conceal truth from us.

As we evolve as a soul and spirit consciousness into an understanding of who we are, we will choose to create love, peace, and joy in our lives. When we were first created as a living soul in physical matter, our male and female consciousness chose to live equally within our physical nature. Now, as we are consciously evolving as males and females, we are both transitioning into our divine nature. Because we were placed into our immature soul as both males and females, we immediately began our lessons of equality by living inequality as the constant physical experience of our daily lives. In our immature soul we have lived our lessons by the mirror or opposite reflection of what our mature soul wants to learn. Because of our reflection into the physical world, we live what we don't want, to create a consciousness of what we do want. Our psychic ability develops as we become conscious of the primitive memories in our cosmic shell that our intellect reflects itself into as a mirror image of our beliefs.

Because Paul hated females he advocated the moral law of inequality and submission of the female to the male when he began his universal form of "Christ" worship. Christ means savior or messiah. Paul learned this law of female submission in his Hebrew beliefs, in his polytheistic focus in the pagan religion of Hinduism, and from his worship of the Persian pagan god Mithra. Buddhism, Confucianism, and multiple minor religious sects also taught the law of submission of the female to the male. Zoroasterism, Judaism, Hinduism, and Buddhism were the four primary religions at the time when Paul was structuring the laws of Christianity. The Greeks of the time also followed a mixture of Hinduism and Greek philosophy. Paul was born a Jew and was later attracted to Hinduism and other pagan forms of worship because his soul was experiencing past life memory of lessons he was attempting to learn. Paul's many psychic experiences created an obsession with the creation of Christianity. Therefore, Christianity became a blend of Judeo-Oriental and pagan laws, which have been adopted as Christian beliefs and worshipped for nearly two thousand years. As we have worshipped our revolutions of superstition, symbolism, and rituals, we have become addicted to our beliefs and we fight against change. Paul's psychic experiences are now being repeated by millions of people who are feeling obsessed with the creation of new religions.

As our immature soul has been living its intellectual and ego revolutions, we have been living our physical revolutions of warlike behavior as we experience primitive memory. Our wars were fought "in the name of God" as the lesson of inequality for our intellect and ego-focused soul mind. Our wars began in our personal relationships and spread to include societies and nations. Inequality is the lesson that we must learn as humans before we can bring the male and female soul consciousness together as one soul consciousness within our mind and emotions. We cannot become spiritual until our male and female consciousness is integrated and lives in the love, truth, and equality of our divine nature. As long as we are hypnotized by our psychic attachment to our primitive soul lessons of beliefs, we are not open to change because we think that we have fulfilled our expectations and reached our destination.

The interpretation of inequality in the Christian laws and

beliefs, the influence of Mithras, Hinduism as nature worship, Buddhism, and the influence of the Hebrew and Muslim laws have molded our societies and our world in our immature soul journey. We have passed our influence down through generation after generation as truth. Religious laws and beliefs have their foundation in the primitive interpretation of spiritual prophecy, which requires submission and inequality for the female. It is our belief in the inequality between the physical male and female that clearly reflects the level of growth for our immature soul consciousness. Religions are based upon worshipping the male image of God. Buddhism and Hinduism taught and continue to teach guru worship as pagan worship and submission. Christianity worships Jesus as its savior. Hebrews worship God or Yahweh. Muslims worship Allah. Worship creates inequality. Religion, as worship, creates inequality between the male and female. When we can acknowledge that the foundation of our societies is held together by primitive religious beliefs that came from the primitive interpretation of spiritual prophecy by multiple individuals, it becomes evident that all prophecy should be examined with a new perception and knowledge.

Prophecy has never been given as information to be worshipped. It has always been given to reveal truth, and it has been given in the level that man could understand at the time of the prophecy. The level of prophecy interpretation had to fit the times or it would have had no value to the people. All true prophecy changes in meaning as our consciousness level changes.

Worship is the symbol of inequality that our descending immature soul has lived. We have attached ourselves to the Ark of the Covenant with our chains of inequality, deceit, and fear, and we have worshipped relentlessly without the knowledge to rise above our own ignorance. We have worshipped in near identical revolutions for four thousand years because we have shut down our thinking, emotions, and feelings. Worshipping creates the essense of inequality in every aspect of our life. As long as we interpret prophecy as our need to worship an external God of some venue, such as male or female, Christian or Hebrew, guru or pagan idol, and sex over mind and emotions, the longer we will cling to our belief that we "need to be saved." Religion means worship and prophecy has never been given for the purpose of worship. Prophecy is given as revelation, but when it is interpreted by the intellect and ego it is distorted. Once our beliefs began to conform to the religious interpretation, we became caught in the web of illusion and could not escape.

Because our male soul mind and emotions has not been capable of memory from one life to another, we have entered into each new physical life with our intellect being a blank slate for us to fill with information. Religion has continued to be an integrated focus of our personal beliefs, family life, society, and the world, and it has always been there with its laws and rituals to repattern us in each lifetime. As we die we store all that we have learned in each lifetime within the right side of our soul mind and emotions, which we cannot access from the focus of our intellect because of our ego cosmic shell of karmic beliefs. When we try to reach our mature soul without the appropriate knowledge of our dual soul and spirit, our linear intellect becomes caught in our ego cosmic shell of past life memory and we feel we have reached our mature soul consciousness.

Religion has never been stored within our mature soul mind and emotions because worship is the primary lesson of inequality, which we now must learn and release before we can change. Many individuals have assumed they have learned the lesson of religion and the assumption has led them into the intellectual spiritualism that is flourishing today in religions and in New Age thought. Until we understand our dual soul, we are not aware of the capabilities of our trinity of consciousness and of the limitations of our intellect. Worshipping a modern day prophet, career, leader, religion, or relationship still qualifies as worship. When we worship intellectual spiritualism we are worshipping the limitations of our intellect and ego illusions.

The karmic lessons that we have not learned are brought back into each new life as our cosmic shell of beliefs and are waiting to be acted out in our lives and learned. Our beliefs are primarily the lessons of religion that our soul is continuing to work on as our physical experiences of fear, judgement, control, dependency, abuse, deceit, anger, rage, and inequality. We have been crossing into the psychic subconscious mind of our cosmic shell of karmic beliefs for millions of years and we are still struggling to understand what is happening to us. It is the worship of our primitive memories as our psychic soul that creates it as the illusion of our spirit. Worshipping a relationship, our physical body, a guru, medicine, science, or our intellectual memories is no different than worshipping a religion and the lesson is always inequality. Each focus of worship that we have keeps us from loving ourself and opening our mind and emotions to the knowledge of who we are as spiritual beings. When we focus on worshipping our psychic mind, we are putting ourself in the bondage of our cosmic shell.

Our cosmic shell of beliefs surrounds our intellect and literally imprisons our immature soul mind and emotions with the restrictions, limitations, and denial of our ancient and superstitious beliefs. Our beliefs become the ego perception of our reality from which we live each physical life as we chip away at our beliefs with an accumulation of knowledge. Until we can chip away enough of our ancient beliefs, we continue to be held as a "victim" of our immature soul mind. Our ego cosmic shell of karmic beliefs is the "demon" of our primitive mind. It is our devil, it is evil, it is our satan, and it is that part of our intellect that holds us captive in ignorance and fear. When we have fearful thoughts, we are living a primitive level of consciousness that is our subconscious ego mind. We are living the physical prototype of our art of creation.

When we act out our fearful behavior, we are acting out our concealed ego karmic beliefs. At this time our ego beliefs are being chipped away by knowledge and we are drifting into our primitive cosmic shell which makes us feel we are psychic. Because we are exploring our primitive beliefs, our behavior becomes more primitive as a reflection of our beliefs and we begin to act out the karmic superstitions, myths, symbols, and rituals of our past life memories. We return to ancient beliefs and behaviors and innocently think we have become spiritual. Our belief in inequality between the physical male and female is a

direct reflection of the primary lesson of inequality for our immature soul. Ancient societies lived inequality. Therefore, many of
the primitive beliefs and behaviors are being acted out in our
male and female relationships on all three levels as individuals,
society, and the world. Any and all beliefs in our sexual inequality proliferate into an infinite number of unequal behaviors in
every facet of our sexual relationships. Many times we live without an aware consciousness of our unequal behavior as primitive
behavior. Our belief in inequality has its basis in the primitive
interpretation of prophecy that has led us into the religious belief
that "man is made in the image of God," and woman was made
from the rib of man, which makes her unequal to man. This
belief defies the truth of creation as we have lived it. This specific belief has created all religions as the Antichrist consciousness in our world. It is the psychic primitive memories of the creation of moral law and female inequality that we are now living.
It is the psychic memory of inequality that has allowed religions
to repeat the old resolutions of female inequality as the moral law
of today's society.

It is the internal lesson of equality for our male and female
soul that we are learning as a dual soul of male and female consciousness. When we learn the lesson of equality for our dual
soul, we will live that equality with truth and love in every aspect
of our lives. We are seeking equality as a dual soul to evolve into
the equality of our spirit. Our psychic or religious focus is opposite to our mature soul and spirit focus for our thinking, emotions, and feelings. Equality will rid us of our beliefs in sexual
inequality, roles, and identities, such as our "I know it all" concepts, our "need to be saved," "death is a sin," our "sex is love"
attitude, our need to be "right" and our fear of being "wrong."
In addition to dissolving these primary fear beliefs, we will also
dissolve all of our external beliefs, which will then stop our fears
and negative behaviors. When our negative beliefs are gone, we
will begin living our loving behavior in every aspect of our lives
as we transition into our mature soul memory of our divine
nature.

When we begin living our loving behavior as a reflection of

our loving actions, language, and thought, we have the power to create a completely different society which will focus upon love, truth, and equality toward every human being on earth. As we transition into the divine nature of our loving soul mind and emotions, we begin to realize the loving potential that is within us as human beings. The prophecy of John the Divine in the book of Revelation shows us the journey of our immature soul and the levels that we have lived. Revelation also shows us the journey of our mature soul and the beauty and wisdom that we are becoming.

The "apocalypse" does not mean that the world is coming to an end but rather that truth will be revealed to us. We reveal information in science, living, and prophecy as our normal methods of self-revelation. Apocalypse means "a prophetic disclosure or revelation." Armageddon symbolizes the final war between our ego and spirit as we are caught in the midline within our dual soul where our left brain and right brain must come together before we can understand the beauty of our male and female consciousness as one. The war that is being fought is the war between the "evil" ego and the "good" spirit as our ego denies the change that is occurring within us. We have lived the battle of good and evil as we have believed that blind faith as evil is superior to knowledge as good. Our male physical nature is the symbol of evil as the worship of ignorance, and our female divine nature is the symbol of good as a seeker of knowledge and wisdom.

Even those who have blind faith have struggled to balance their knowledge with their religious beliefs. During the past nearly two thousand years we have lived our revelation as we have felt the ignorance within us melt away and we have dedicated ourselves to the search for knowledge. Christianity began nearly two thousand years ago with Paul as the symbol of the Antichrist who structured the belief in Christianity from the exact opposite focus of the teachings of Jesus and taught Christianity as blind faith conformity in ignorance.

Jesus was a prophet and a philosopher who came to show us through his own teachings and living what was waiting for us in the Ark of the Testament within our mature soul. Paul was not a prophet, but he was a psychic who experienced past life memories during his epileptic seizures. He was given the mission of being the Antichrist who led us through our blind faith into the intellectual realization that our fear, anger, wrath, control, judgement, manipulation, and seduction is the ignorance of our evil self. Paul stimulated our lessons of truth, love, and equality into our consciousness as he created the moral laws and dogma of Christianity from his own untruths, inequality, rage, anger, control, manipulation, and fear. We magnetized our beliefs and behaviors to his beliefs and behaviors, which provide us with an opportunity to live the opposite of the knowledge that our mature soul was seeking. The moral laws of Christianity became the dogma of religion as the dogmatic and dictatorial teaching of our male physical nature.

Each introduction to the writings of Paul spells out the untruth of his teachings when it states, "Paul an apostle of Jesus Christ by the will of God, according to the promise of life which is Christ Jesus." Paul was never an apostle of Jesus and never saw Jesus in the flesh, but he was a self-appointed apostle as the Antichrist and his anger towards women was his anger towards the female Divine Nature of our internal God. There was never a Jesus Christ or a Christ Jesus. There was Jesus of Nazareth. The Christ dwells within each of us as our Christ Consciousness. It is reaching the consciousness of our mature soul and spirit that saves us by our integration as a dual soul. God is the good within us and that is the freedom of choice, will, and intention of our mature soul and spirit consciousness.

To understand how we have created the focus of our immature soul mind and emotions within our fearful, negative, and external intellect and ego for so long, we must look at the prophets that have guided us through these last several thousand years. We can learn more from a different interpretation of the old prophets than we can from the beliefs of Paul. Prophets have always tried to help us understand ourselves, but we have interpreted the prophets according to the superstitious beliefs of our psychic mind.

In addition we have clung to these superstitions with a vengeance because our ego is terribly fearful of change and it does not want us to focus on any part of our soul that it cannot control. Our literal interpretations of biblical prophecy conceal the truth of the prophecy under the veils of our ego and intellectual mind. Our ego and intellect fears for its survival as the superior mind of our immature soul.

Every individual that has interpreted prophecy has used, by necessity, the precise level of soul consciousness that they have reached, which coincides with the beliefs of the day. Those who consider themselves prophets can only use the specific consciousness of the soul mind and emotions which they live in their daily lives. If the information is indeed true spiritual prophecy it can still be distorted by the consciousness of the individual's belief system. This is not a conscious but a subconscious distortion.

We can begin to understand the degree of distortion that occurs within prophecy when we look at the way the prophets lived and acted out their beliefs through their behavior. Another primary distortion occurs when the prophet knows that the information that is being given cannot be understood by man at his present level of awareness and the prophecy is concealed in the parables of the time. This is why Moses of Egypt, Moses de Leon, Jesus, and other well known prophets all had to speak in parables. For prophecy to be understood, it had to be spoken in the beliefs of the time and stories were used so that the audience could relate the information to themselves. It is only now that we are able to accept the love within us. During the days of Jesus they were "changing money in the temple" with the intention of business and greed in the same way that we do today. The perception of their lives was external, negative, and fearful and followed the identical revolutions that are experienced by some immature souls today.

Because of the personal distortion in prophecy, many psychic prophets reveal only their intellectual spiritualism or unlearned past life memories instead of the story of our creation in the purity of our spiritual consciousness. Psychic information is always distorted by the ego beliefs of the psychic and the beliefs of the recipient, and both levels can readily be defined in the personal behavior. If a soul prophet is not living what he/she teaches then they are teaching the duality of the soul as a psychic and not the unconditional love of their spirit consciousness as spirit prophecy.

From the beginning of our creation as a living soul, we have always been conscious of a supreme being. Our consciousness of a supreme being has been intentional as a part of our spiritual guidance from within our trinity of consciousness. Having the internal sense of a supreme being has kept us consistently focused externally in trying to discover who the supreme being is and what its relationship is to us. As we have lived our lives trying to understand the "supreme being" we have focused externally in our search while living in our physical nature because the external perception of reality is the normal focus of our intellect and ego soul. If we focus on information from the external guides of our immature soul, we are accessing the past life memory or subconscious psychic intellect. If we access past life memory we are not yet living in our integrated soul mind with the influence of our spirit consciousness. If we see God as an external being and speak to God externally, as in prayer, we are living in our intellect and ego immature soul mind and emotions. It is in believing that the "supreme being" is external to us that we reveal the conscious mind and emotions that we are living as our immature soul.

As we move into the divine nature of our right brain, we begin to look for that supreme being internally, which is the normal focus of our consciousness in our mature soul mind and loving emotions. Once we begin to search internally for our supreme being, we discover that each of us has a "supreme being" which is our indwelling spirit consciousness. This realization helps us to understand that our supreme being of spirit consciousness has been guiding us throughout our journey as a dual soul. Our dual soul, as a dual mind and emotions, is the child of the supreme being of our spirit consciousness. As we transition into our wise, loving, and mature soul mind and emotions, we are growing into the adult phase of our dual soul life as our divine nature. Once we begin to live in our mature soul, the "knowing" or stored lessons of our mature soul begins to guide our life.

In our physical lives we live three dimensions of consciousness with multiple levels of consciousness in each dimension. This makes our physical life a fractal pattern of our trinity of consciousness of our three dimensions of mind and emotions. From birth to 50 years is the physical nature of our physical life, from 50 to 100 years is the mature divine nature of our physical life, and from 100 to 150 years is the spiritual nature of our physical life. The more spiritual we become as a human species the longer our life span will become. We live our constantly changing reflection from the trinity of our mind and emotions when we plan on long lives as a means of evolution. As a mature soul consciousness we have the free choice to plan a short life or to experience death as a new beginning at any time that we feel we are no longer growing in creativity and consciousness in our physical life. A balanced and healthy mature soul mind and emotions can create a balanced life both mentally and emotionally with a long, healthy physical life.

All of the knowledge and lessons that we learn in a physical life is taken with us into our next lifetime as part of our mature soul mind and emotions. If we are strongly attached to our physical nature and deny seeking knowledge, we will usually not live very many years past our fiftieth birthday. The immature soul has a fourteen-year or two-cycle window that it will sometimes use as an opportunity for change in our second dimension of life. If we continue to deny change during the period from fifty to sixty-four, we may choose death as a new beginning or we can totally lose our mental and emotional consciousness as a way of living our death without a consciousness of life. We bring these changes into our life by creating a chemical imbalance in our mind, emotions, and cellular structure, which paralyzes all of our senses as feelings and stops the consciousness expansion. By living our death as a suppression of our thinking, emotions, and feelings we can learn the lesson of revolution and how we have been suppressing our mature soul consciousness.

When we can understand birth, life, and death as a cycle of expression for the dual soul within our eternal life cycle, we can more easily understand how our mature soul and spirit is constantly guiding our childish immature soul along its journey to accept the supreme being of our spirit consciousness. Once we are born we spend one life cycle or the first seven physical years in our spirit consciousness. With the negative influence of society on children today, we can close our mind down to our spirit consciousness at any point. The average child will totally close their mind by eleven years if the influence of their life is negative. Negative, for a soul, is being constantly exposed to a level of consciousness that is more primitive than the level of consciousness that the soul wants to live.

"Knowing" internally on a cellular level that we have a trinity of consciousness as a dual living soul mind and emotions of male and female consciousness and our spirit consciousness sets the stage to help us understand prophecy within ourself and from our ancient ancestors. Knowing intellectually that our male intellect and ego fear consciousness is our physical nature, our female consciousness is our mind of wisdom and love as our divine nature, and our spirit is the universal mind and unconditional love consciousness, we can begin to see the diversity that is possible in prophecy. Each dimension of our mind and emotions has multiple levels of consciousness that we are constantly using, but we are not aware of them intellectually and therefore we totally deny their existence. We can also clearly see that God is not made in the image of man, but "God" is a trinity of spiritual energy and we are a trinity of spiritual energy as males and females. As humans we are made in the same trinity of consciousness energy as God; therefore, all humans are made in the image of "God" as a trinity of consciousness.

In each dimension of our mind and emotional energy we have zillions of memory nodes to focus upon. Because of the number of focuses that our mind and emotions can choose, no two people could ever be absolutely identical. This shows us how each immature soul has its own personal agenda as the physical experience it wants to live and to evolve within. It also

340

shows us why we have a diversity of prophetic information that has been handed down through the ages of time, and why that information has similarities but it is never truly identical.

Prophecy is given for the time and the people living when it is given. The collective focus of the majority of immature souls during that specific time will be able to grow into the information if they choose to do so. During each "time" as past, present, or future, prophecy can be given from any memory node that exists within the trinity of consciousness of the individual. The difference will be first recognized in the emotional level of the information as it moves from fear, love, and unconditional love. As humans evolve and our knowledge expands, we get different pieces of the puzzle of creation which eventually gives us an accumulation of prophecy that creates a more complete view of exactly who we are, why we are living, and what the purpose of life is all about.

We frequently hear about psychics and the information they present to people. Psychic prophecy is information that is given from the left brain intellect and its ego cosmic shell of beliefs. Psychic information generally deals with physical information which can come from memory nodes within the ego cosmic shell and can take on the persona of an individual who lived in some ancient time period. This information might be validated by an identity, occupation, language, character traits, personality, attitude, and it will reveal the level of information that is being received by the persona that is being acted out.

An example could be: the information will be coming from a physical entity who is using vulgar language. "God" as our Spirit Consciousness does not use vulgar, negative language. The issues that the psychic addresses in the communication itself will usually deal with the physical aspects of life as expectations and destinations. As an example: You might be told that you will be buying a new car or meeting a new lover. You might even be told of something physical that is going to happen, an earthquake, accident, your marriage ending, or losing your job. You may be given initials, dates, times, physical characteristics, first names, or any other type of physical data that will attract you to a person, place, or thing. This type of information leads you into a self-fulfilling prophecy, and you will do anything within your power to create what you have been told as your truth.

Psychics normally access the cosmic shell of the ego that exists in our subconscious ego mind of our past life memory nodes. The past life memory nodes that are present within the left brain are lessons to be learned. Psychics also draw on the sentimental concept of relatives as entities because that is a vulnerable emotional control point in the psychic's relationship to you. If the psychic knows that you are religious they may "get in touch" with saints. All of us have had religious experiences in our past lives and this provides a vulnerable emotional connection for the psychic with our psychic memory. Psychic information is easy to fulfill as prophecy because the information is taken from your own attitude, personality, character traits, and thoughts as your energy persona. By nature we attract the same energy to us that we are working upon. It is either the same energy as ours in terms of our "coat of many colors" or exactly the opposite to what we think that we are living but is the hidden reality of our immature soul energy.

Memory nodes that are within our cosmic shell are there because we have not learned the lessons of those lives in our present physical life. In reality, getting information from the cosmic shell does not give us knowledge that will help us but it triggers us to repeat the experience, which does give us an additional opportunity to learn the lesson. Normally a psychic will speak of our physical roles and identities, which will be emphasized verbally and which we will act out through our physical behavior. A psychic reads the energy of the physical traumas and dramas of our intellect and ego. Since our ego and intellect are external, fearful, and negative, frequently a male role or an extremely fearful and angry female role, which the ego will attach itself to, will be found as a memory node.

Many psychic claims are made as a means of "fortune telling," which is primarily focused upon money and not on helping the person. Many psychics claim an element of external possession by an identified physical entity or communication with a dead physical entity. Psychics frequently have the ability to read your left brain mind and to tell you exactly what you want to hear. Psychic information is normally fearful, negative, external, judgemental, controlling, manipulative, seductive, and crisis-oriented. Since we are addicted to drama and crisis in our immature soul, psychic information fulfills our need to be dependent.

Psychics will also want you to be dependent upon them. This method of control is at times a dual dependency, first for the daily life guidance for the seeker, and the psychic's dependency is for a rich and steady flow of money. The more the psychic talks to you the more "on target" the information will be, as the information can be read more easily. Psychic dependency is rampant within the New Age community and it is the opposite of Spiritualism, as it is an external addictive dependency that relates to the "I need to be saved" belief.

Soul prophecy is information that comes as insight and knowing from the infinite memory nodes found in the right brain of the mature soul mind and emotions. This is a more ethereal vision of prophecy than the psychic can manage. True soul prophecy will always be positive and focuses on the lessons of the soul. Our mature soul will not deal with physical realities in a definitive manner, but will offer more attitude and personality changes to look at within yourself. Our soul is our mind and emotions and our physical world is created from our intellect and ego focus at this time.

Soul prophecy will frequently use the identities of angels as a way of making the information more acceptable. When this happens in soul prophecy, we will frequently relate the name of the angel to a known religious angel. This relationship is the interpretation of our intellectual mind. At the true core of us, we are angels as our spirit consciousness. When the focus is upon accessing the memory nodes within the right brain as the lessons that we have learned, we will frequently see the memory node in its ethereal context. The mature soul will use only a first name, as any further identification creates a role and identity which may have been used in that lifetime. Because our vision may see the image of ourself in that lifetime as "good," we make the angel connection as something other than ourselves because we see ourself as "sinful." In learning a lesson we store the knowledge in the essense of a "good" energy or angel consciousness. The interpretation frequently externalizes the image because that is the belief of the intellect which will distort the interpretation from an internal energy to an external entity.

True soul information normally comes from the dual source of our male and female lives, which increases our belief that our information is an external communication from angels or Saints in the "spirit" world because of our belief in only one life. Our belief in "only one life" and our belief in "needing to be saved" leaves us interpreting our communication as an external "spirit" entity or "angel" entity because we are unconscious of our multiple male and female lives. We might consider that we are experiencing an external possession of our physical body by a "past life soul" or "spirit" entity. Our left brain intellect frequently refers to our right brain soul prints as external angels. These soul prints are positive consciousness energies that we won't claim as our own when we are still unaware of the dual soul as our internal dual mind and emotions. During our transitional journey our intellect will hear the voice of both our immature and mature soul speaking and can experience confusion and fear from the ego reaction.

As individuals we frequently have flashes of soul memory that guide us personally, and this comes from our mature soul mind and emotions as we cross-fertilize our knowledge. We may see ourselves in another lifetime living with people that we know now, and within our vision or insight, we will also find the lesson within the experience. The closer we move towards transitioning our focus of consciousness from our immature to our mature soul the more frequently we will be conscious of our personal soul guides and how they are trying to help us.

We will sense our soul guides as we were in different lifetimes more frequently than we will sense the soul guides of other people, unless we shared the lifetime that we are sensing with a relative or close friend. We will frequently sense ourself with family members or spouses and even very close friends because these individuals are usually from the same soul family and we share many lifetimes with them. Spouses are frequently sensed as a soul guide, and so are children or other family members such as a mother or father. We are our own ancestors and it is good to remember this reality.

Our immature soul always has the freedom of choice to communicate with our internal soul guides, but it will usually choose those who are the most involved with our evolutionary lessons of the time. We should always be open to our internal soul communication because it is there to guide us. It occurs on a regular basis during our sleep period when our conscious mind is working with our mature soul and spirit consciousness. On awakening we usually have no memory of the interaction. If it is important that we remember the team work of our trinity of consciousness, we can convert the information into dream symbols to impress our intellect and ego.

The soul prints of our own immature soul will also be available as guides in both an awake state and a sleep state. These parallel soul prints are essentially our "guardian angels." Each physical life of our soul has an investment in our soul's evolution. Many times these soul prints will guide us by their physical image being seen, the voice being heard, the love being felt, and the message clearly received as it triggers multiple senses within us. Our senses are all part of our spirit consciousness. Our past lives are the cheering section for our immature soul as we struggle through our beliefs and behaviors every moment of our lives. Our soul guidance from these ethereal soul prints, which are a consciousness from an internal soul memory node, provide constant internal guidance. At times the soul consciousness will create a vision or voice sound as a way of letting us know that we are not alone in our search for change. In understanding how we have changed, we have more faith in our ability to change. We use the many mansions of our mind in multiple ways as we live our lives.

Parents are physical soul guides for children. An agreement has been made between the souls of the parents and the soul of the child. The child is coming back into life with a blank slate for its intellect and a perfusion of ego karmic beliefs that are surrounding the intellect as a buried electromagnetic fence. The parent always has free choice to repattern the soul of the child in its organization and discipline, which in our physical world means personal responsibility for ourself. The parents can repattern the soul in either a negative or positive manner. If the parent is attached to the physical processes of life, he/she will frequently repattern the child's soul in the physical nature. If the parent is attached to knowledge, the pattern will be more compatible with the mature soul or divine nature. The child, as a soul, also has the freedom of choice to take on the pattern of one or both parents or to live and believe the opposite. The soul's free choice, intention, and will can be acted out as rebellion when the parents and child are focused on different intentions.

Children choose their parents as their soul guides with a full spectrum focus, which means they accept all that happens. Many times the child chooses examples in the parents that show what patterns the soul wants and those it doesn't want. In seeing the dual patterns of the soul in the parents, the child's soul can have its freedom of choice made very clear as the child is growing into adulthood. Living in their dual personas creates the souls of the parents as actors on the stage of life for the child's soul. The freedom of choice for our soul is never taken away but the conscious intellect and ego is oblivious to its freedom of choice, will, and intention until the time of transition of our soul. It is at the time of transition that we become aware of our dual soul mind and emotions and begin to understand that we always have freedom of choice in every aspect of our life. By living our freedom of choice as a child, we will live "rebellious" behavior in the minds of our parents if we do not conform to their beliefs.

Frequently we will be given guidance from the dreams that we have when we are conscious of either ourself, or ourself with others who are friends, family, and spouses. The symbols within the dream will show us our mental and emotional level within that lifetime as well as our attitude, personality, character, and behavior. These will be reflected into the circumstances, such as the location, geography, weather, drama, and ambiance of the dream. In the morning we may only remember the emotions of the dream as fear or the warmth of love. This is a soul message to look at our emotions that are being suppressed.

Frequently these soul guides or memory nodes that come to us in dreams are showing us the level that we lived during a past lifetime and the level that we may be living now. Many times the mental and emotional texture of the dream will show us stasis or our growth while it also shows us the harmony and balance of our mind and emotions or how they are not balanced. The energy essense of the dream is usually more important than the people who are in the dream. Dreams are at all times symbolized for our intellect in the waking state, if the internal communication of the mature soul and spirit is not understood by the intellect during sleep.

Seeking personal prophecy from others is a path that can help you open your own inner knowing, but it is more important to listen to yourself. You may want some spiritual guidance from someone in the interpretation but make certain that the individual is truly spiritual and is not coming from the intellectual spiritualism of the psychic perspective. Understanding a dream or personal prophecy will generally move you forward another level in your soul evolution by expanding your conscious awareness.

Intellectual spiritualism occurs when people want to be spiritual and the ego and intellect tells them they are, despite their behavior reflecting the immature soul beliefs and fears. Spiritualism is the way that we live our unconditional love, truth, and equality in every aspect of our life to become a spiritual being. If we are fearful, angry, revengeful, suspicious, focused on our pain and suffering, worshipping, abusing our body with chemicals or chemically grown foods, and living addictive beliefs, our ego may tell us that we are spiritual but in reality we are not living a spiritual life. Our intellect and ego is controlled by the sexual core of our physical nature and it is guided by fear and a "I know it all" belief. If our focus is primarily on our physical sexual image and our "need" for a relationship, we are stuck in our immature soul of intellect and ego. Our mature soul is focused upon the love, truth, wisdom, and equality of our divine nature and it lives the love of itself. Intellectual spiritualism is involved in multiple forms of external worship such as physical processes, ancient memories, crystals, rituals, superstitious beliefs, physical possessions, status, and money. Religion is the opposite of spiritualism.

We must live our love in a balanced and harmonious way for us to truly be spiritual as a mature soul. The mature soul mind and emotions can experience a definite level of spirituality because the light from the spirit enlightens the mature soul. The ego and intellect live in the dark without the enlightenment of the spirit to guide them. The darkness is created by the ego cosmic shell of beliefs, which prevents our awareness of the trinity of our mind and emotions. Therefore, our intellectual awareness is limited to the ego's perception of our soul and spirit as external entities.

Each person has the soul and spirit as part of their trinity of consciousness. We have not been taught that we can listen to our soul and spirit speak to us, because our ego is protective of what it considers its "turf." This does not keep us from spontaneously receiving true soul revelations through a knowing, or through visions as seeing, dreams as sensing, or through hearing voices or tones. The three dimensions of our seven senses were given to us to guide us into an expansion of consciousness and it is through the touch, taste, smell, hearing, seeing, thinking, and speaking that our soul and spirit is constantly guiding us into our mature soul evolution of consciousness.

Understanding our spirit and soul senses and the role of our physical senses is important in the same way that understanding our biological needs of air, water, foods of nature, and sexuality is important. We must always ask "why" as our first question. Children ask "why" naturally and insistently. The foods that we eat provide the chemicals that are important to our mental and emotional balance, which opens our intellectual mind to our mature soul and spirit minds. We need these chemicals to fill the alchemical vase of our limbic system, which allows the electromagnetic energy to enhance our brain synapses as well as our physical cells.

Depression is the direct result of not having these chemicals within our brain to help us integrate our male and female soul mind and emotions. Depression then becomes the normal transitional emotions for us when our dual soul is attempting to integrate itself. The chemicals provide the electromagnetic energy to help us transition. The phytochemicals that we need at this point are those that are found in raw vegetables, fruits, and herbs. In our Cycle of Development these phytochemicals helped us to develop our consciousness of ourself as we passed through the plant kingdom.

Our dual soul, as our dual mind and emotions, is seeking to bring together the male and female consciousness within us to allow our trinity to be unified and function as a cyclic mind and love emotions. Our mature soul has always been guiding us through the magnetic power of the minerals to subconsciously allow us to use both of our minds as the lessons of equality, love, and truth. Many times during periods of crisis, which may or may not include the death of someone that we love, we will be conscious of the energy of another soul being with us, talking to us, showing us the beauty that is our mature soul realm of consciousness energy. Our sensory response will not be as acute in our life experiences if any of the chemicals are missing or in excess in our brain and our cellular structure. When we are chemically imbalanced we may not be conscious of our internal soul. Souls are intimately connected in various ways. The soul family members frequently return to the same physical family for many lifetimes, to repeat the lessons of balance as a soul family. This is essential if abuse is tying the soul family together. Abuse can happen because of a chemical imbalance which limits and distorts our immature soul thinking, emotions, and feelings.

A soul generation is 30 years. It normally takes a soul 7 generations or 210 years of life to work through a single image of one lesson. If abuse is a lesson for a physical family the immature soul may choose to return to the specific physical family to continue supporting the family in learning the lesson. The scales must be balanced for the soul, and frequently the soul can only be precisely balanced by that individual who it abused. Therefore we can become our own grandchild, for example. Our mature soul always has the freedom of choice in life, although our intellect will hold that information subconscious to itself, and it will hold the spirit guidance unconscious to itself, because of the ego cosmic shell of beliefs which thinks that "we only have one life" and "our intellect and ego are always supreme." The soul information is always known by the soul despite the intellect being protected from the information by the ego.

Our ego feels that it is "supreme" and "knows it all," which is the funniest of all beliefs because our intellect holds less knowledge than a drop in the ocean compared to the knowledge within our mature soul. The ego prefers blind faith to knowledge. This belief creates the follower mentality and the fear emotions that the ego uses to control our intellect. Knowledge is the level of evolution that we are living within our dual soul. We must understand the knowledge of our soul and spirit before we will willingly accept our internal soul and spirit wisdom. Knowledge is the only level of our dual soul evolution that is divided between the immature and the mature soul. Therefore, it is through knowledge that our immature soul becomes mature, which is reinforcing our dual soul intention of balancing the excesses and deficiencies of chemicals that control the brain energy.

The subconscious and unconscious guidance of our mature soul and spirit has been the internal consciousness behavior to help the immature soul evolve to this point of our transition. The voices that we hear internally can come from any memory node of our dual soul as well as the universal mind of our spirit. It is the emotional magnetism that has allowed us to evolve despite our beliefs and behaviors of dependency, control, fear, anger, abuse, inequality, deceit, and ignorance.

All that we learn is stored in our mature soul mind at death. The more we learn the more we evolve in our next lifetime on earth. The mature soul and spirit vibrates at a frequency that is extremely high and that is closer to the speed of light. At death our soul and spirit must enter into a new physical conception within three days. Therefore, within a three-day period the soul and spirit is conceived and resurrected into a new developing physical body with a new image of its soul agenda. The fractal pattern for the creation of our new human body is stored in the soul and spirit memory. Therefore, each conception begins with the soul and spirit consciousness as the lifeforce energy that resurrects the physical design of the body from the soul pattern of the DNA.

Our mature soul and spirit guidance that occurs without our conscious knowledge is constantly designing new physical experiences for the immature soul as a way of learning and expanding its aware consciousness. Our mature soul and spirit never forsakes its child of the intellect, but it will create multiple opportunities to try to communicate with us through the emotions and senses that we have been given. There is no limitation to the methods that our mature soul and spirit can use, but each of our physical experiences will be perceived from the external immature soul consciousness of our physical senses and not as physical guidance from our mature soul and spirit consciousness.

Because of the complexity of the dual soul design, prophecy by another in relationship to our mature soul is best understood from spirit prophecy. Our spirit is our internal prophet and spirit guide who will make us aware of our past lives when it is important to see the relationship between our past and present life. Until the mature soul relationship is important to our immature soul, the information will be used as an ego distraction.

Spirit prophecy has been received by many souls living upon earth from the beginning of time as a way of trying to keep the soul magnetized toward its evolution. The ego and intellect has fallen into the abyss of physical processes, myths, symbols, superstitions, and rituals repeatedly as it has lived its journey as the immature soul mind and emotions. Spiritual prophecy has been given multiple times to advanced and mature souls to create a different level of consciousness in the physical journey of our immature soul. Spirit prophecy sows the seeds of inspiration within our imagination and ideas to continue inspiring the immature soul to seek knowledge and grow.

For forty thousand years, especially since the physical nature of the male declared itself as "made in the image of God," we have wandered in the wilderness of superstition, ritual, and worship. This is the parable of Moses wandering in the wilderness for forty years as they searched for the promised land. In the promised land they found fruit that was too heavy to carry, which symbolizes the love, truth, and equality which man finds a burden to live as our immature soul. The impact of religion declaring that only the male was created in the image of God brought our lesson of inequality out of the abyss of our immature soul and put it directly in our lives to be lived. As we began to worship the male as the image of God, we sank to the very depths of our descending emotional soul. Giving up our attachment to inequality, lying, and fear is a burden for our ego, which has to shed its beliefs of superiority before we can continue with our consciousness evolution.

Spirit prophecy is given to be understood at the time that it is needed. It is always given a few levels above the average person's soul mind and emotions in an attempt to magnetize the mind forward into the more expansive concepts of reality. We have clung to the old primitive interpretations of prophecy that was given for the primitive mind nearly seven thousand years ago, and we have taken the information literally instead of understanding the parables that were used. A few souls are always chosen to trigger the soul memory of the masses to open their minds and expand their consciousness. But soul growth is a slow process and we must move forward one baby step at a time until we are changed with each step and learn it well enough to live it consistently in our behavior for eternity.

Our spirit is the originator of all inspired thought. Once the thought leaves the spirit consciousness it moves into the left brain, traveling in a clock-wise motion, and in the left brain our thought becomes captured within the left brain cosmic shell and it is then distorted by our ego belief system. Our ego belief system turns our inspired thought into ego/intellectual thought which is based on externalization, negativity, and fear. As the intellectual mind fills with knowledge, our knowledge begins to force open the shell surrounding the intellect and our perception of reality begins to change. Ignorance holds us captive and limits our consciousness when we refuse to change our beliefs and see our spirit prophecy as our true spiritual guidance.

Once our immature soul mind and emotions begins to integrate with our mature soul mind and emotions, we begin to lighten the journey that we are living and our physical experiences of life become easier. We can throw away our old, primitive beliefs that are creating a needless burden in our lives and see the beauty of our spiritual self. The spirit is the light within us. It is the essense of our electromagnetic energy. It is our unconditional love. Our spirit is found in every cell of our body. The spirit consciousness of unconditional love is focused primarily on the inspiration of knowledge and understanding to open the mind of the masses by opening one mind at a time. The minds of the people that understand first will be the prophets who will write and teach spiritual prophecy as they live their truth, love, and equality at the time of transition into our mature soul.

Each and every person has a spirit consciousness and a mature soul consciousness as well as an immature soul consciousness. We are each equal in the design of our trinity of consciousness energy. Some souls will be moving at a different pace than others during our transitional period. The speed with which we grow has to do with the age of the soul and the beliefs that capture us in our ego mind. Old souls that have advanced can come into life with a focus upon their mature soul and spirit consciousness. Their dual soul minds will be open, integrated, and enlightened. New souls are those souls that have been created at a later date and that are not as advanced and open in their consciousness as an old soul will be. New souls can also be those who maintain a closed mind and resist growth during multiple lifetimes. For the soul, being old is a symbol of wisdom. Being a new soul is a symbol of ignorance.

Many infants are being born today that are coming back as very old and advanced souls with their minds open to the light of their spirit. It will be a challenge for many of these old and advanced souls to keep their minds open for their entire lifetime. Because of the expansive number of old souls that are now returning it is important for parents to understand the trinity of the mind consciousness and the pattern of the soul to support the open mind of the souls of their children who are living their soul integration. The most challenging part of our life is to walk to the beat of a different drummer in childhood without understanding why others think differently than we do and knowing no one who can help us understand why we feel different.

Old souls should be worked with in the uterus of the mother, consciously and lovingly through telepathic communication, reading, music, eating, and lifestyle choices. This will allow the left brain to be filled with the knowledge of the right brain. There are techniques for working with old soul minds that can be rewarding to both parents and child. Teaching your children an awareness of their trinity of mind and emotional consciousness from the time of conception will avoid beliefs and behavioral problems in later years.

Rearing a child to consciously understand themselves as a dual soul and spirit consciousness is a gift to the child and to ourself. Just because we have never been taught about our internal consciousness of dual soul and spirit does not mean that it is productive to continue to ignore this knowledge. When a child comes into life with an open soul mind, the child will experience many unusual situations that relate directly to the soul and spirit, which cannot be answered by the beliefs of today.

Every child has these experiences, as do adults, but without a consciousness of why the experience is occurring we begin to doubt our own sanity at any age. When we believe that we are "different," we increase our self-judgement and depression. When we have consciousness experiences as adults that are foreign to our belief system, we will also become depressed. Depression is the precise emotion that allows us to understand that we are in the transitional stage of our dual soul. It is our essense of "not knowing" that pulls us back into our old primitive beliefs and behaviors and convinces us that we are mentally ill.

Our beliefs and behaviors have traveled a long and dusty road within our physical experience. In the past fourteen thousand years we have begun to realize that it is time for us to change. But fourteen thousand years ago we were still trying to discover the relationship between ourself, the universe, earth, and nature. During that time we looked at everything in life that we were conscious of and we worshipped it as our "God" of life.

As primitive beings we began what is loosely described as Nature Worship. We didn't worship any specific aspect of nature, but we worshipped all aspects of nature, earth, and the universe and our "Gods" became our symbol of seeking knowledge. The functions of the body, the sun, the moon, the stars, the earth, the seasons, the snow, the wind, the water, the trees, plants, fire, animals, and all else that came into our visual field we made into a "God." At that time we believed that all "things" had a dramatic "spiritual" effect upon man. In many ways we were smarter then than we are now because this concept held many truths.

Our polytheistic concept of worship was extremely important in the development of our consciousness and it led us into the first science of Metaphysics as we studied the energy of our own body in relationship to the universe and nature. This was not what we would call a "double blind" study of scientific merit, but it was an expansion of our consciousness that was in many ways far more expansive than we are now experiencing in our "double blind" studies. Today we have a thick cosmic shell of belief systems that limits our consciousness in a way that it has never been limited before. Because of our cosmic shell, we have been revolving at tighter levels of fear, control, and judgement in the past two thousand years than we have ever lived before. Our revolutions of beliefs have restricted and limited our consciousness as our external perception. Our internal perception of our soul and spirit self became vehemently denied as we focused on "hard" science. Because our intellect returns into life without memory, the soul and spirit as our internal parental guides have been forgotten and replaced with an external god.

From the beginning of time we have had the supreme energy of spirit on earth within our trinity of mind consciousness. As the children of "God" we have always heard the voice of our indwelling spirit consciousness and our mature soul consciousness guiding us. When we were more primitive, we heard the voice more clearly than we do now, and we always knew from the knowledge within our internal voice that there was a supreme being and that we were a part of that supreme being. The more we have descended into the depths of our immature emotional soul the less consciousness we have maintained of our internal soul and spirit consciousness and its relationship to our daily life because of our fear. As we have learned to shut out our soul and spirit voices that have been guiding us, we have become more dependent on the worship of our external "God" to save us because we feel helpless and hopeless to save ourselves from our depression.

For nearly the past two thousand years, we have entered into the Antichrist consciousness with our restrictive fear beliefs and behaviors, which have shut out the acceptance of our internal soul and spirit communication. Our depression has reached the emotional pit of our immature soul, and for two thousand years we have been addicted to our religious beliefs as our perception of how we can "save" our soul. Because of our beliefs we frequently assume that anyone who speaks of spirit or soul is of an "occult" mind. Occult means "hidden," as in the Ark of the Covenant of our immature soul mind that is addicted to its fear and worship. There are no mysteries connected to our mature soul and spirit consciousness, except for the mystery of how we have worshipped ignorance for so long as the "evil" immature soul within ourselves. Once we open our mind to the knowledge of our internal dual soul and spirit consciousness, we can no longer worship ignorance as a "mystery" and we will no longer live our control, judgement, inequality, deceit, and fear as our religious beliefs. We will use cyclic telepathic communication within our trinity of consciousness as our normal way of living our thinking, emotions, and feelings. We will not think that our soul and spirit is guiding us because we will accept our dual soul and spirit as us.

When we were created in human form we spent eighty billion years simply learning to live by eating, drinking, and breathing and learning to love by having sex and children. The consciousness of the Spirit Creator was always near at hand to coach us, but never to do our living for us. The spirit energy was made

our indwelling spirit guide and for billions of years the prophecy came from the spirit of the female. It was not until man began
to think of himself as made in the image of God that males began
to be used on earth as prophets. When women were labeled as
disdainful and unequal, men were no longer willing to be guided by the female soul and spirit. The wisdom and understanding
of female prophets taught many of the Greek philosophers as
late as 300 B.C. The male would not historically acknowledge
the female prophecy and always accepted the credit for prophecy as the right of the male. Therefore, there is very little docu-
mentation of the great and adventurous female prophets of
ancient times.

Approximately ten thousand years before the sinking of a
large part of the continent of Pangea, known as Atlantis, man
began to become self-centered and self-focused and to see God
as made in his image. At this time God was inspired to send more
physical males prophecy from the spirit consciousness to capture
the attention of our physical nature. We had begun to be in total
disdain of the divine female nature and to treat females unequally, which led men and women alike to deny female prophecy.

Despite the denial, not all prophets were sent as males
because the physical nature could not have survived without the
interaction of the female divine nature. To live the example of
integration of the male and female consciousness, females were
sent to be prophets together as consorts, or equal teachers, and
within marriages with a male. The intellect and ego of the physical nature continues to have a limited imagination, and a closed
mind, which restricts its ability to hear the voice of the spirit consciousness within. When the male physical nature was given the
ability to hear the internal communication it was then distorted
by the cosmic shell of the belief system, which enhanced the
already present restrictive beliefs. The male interpretation of spirit guidance as prophecy has become the foundation of our present day religious cultures.

The Christ Consciousness of the mature female soul was frequently used as a means of prophetic inspiration, but it too could
be and was distorted by the beliefs of the cosmic shell in the male

consciousness of our physical nature as interpretation took place. The cosmic shell of beliefs was gradually formed and thickened with each day of living as an immature soul in our physical nature. As the belief that man was made in the image of God was solidified, it happened because the ego of man was seeing God in his image. It was through this mirror image of the primitive energy of man that the external image of God was imagined and created to be controlling, judgemental, angry, wrathful, abusive, and fearful. Man himself had adopted this precise immature soul persona as his image of God because of his belief in inequality that he lived externally as the suppression of the female. With each passing day the soul of man that is captured in its physical nature becomes angrier and more controlling as his belief in inequality suppresses his own loving female emotions.

These beliefs were gradually imposed into the nature worship over many thousands of years, and with time man began the worship of himself as law. During this time the Christ Consciousness known as Hermes had spent many lives and fifty thousand years living on earth as a teacher of humanity. As the ego strengthened, the many spirit prophets of both male and female gender were being inspired to listen to the voice of the spirit within themselves. It was during this time that a universal message was being sent out from the Spirit Consciousness: "Let he who hath an ear, hear."

The first accepted prophet on earth to hear was the prophet Zoroaster from the Spitama family of Iran. Zoroaster was born in 5893 B.C., although historians have tried to place his birth in 1200 B.C. Zoroaster heard the message of freedom of choice, intention, and will. He understood the duality of the soul as evil and good. He was taught the equality of the male and female and the importance of living a good life of conscious righteousness. He understood that we had free choice to live our hell or our heaven. He was taught the resurrection of the body and our personal responsibility for salvation. Zoroaster heard, but his interpretation was colored by his own superstitions and the hell of fire became an idol for his worship.

Zoroaster's followers worshipped the God of fire, which

became a dramatic influence on the Hindu religions that were being organized as part of the Nature worship of the Sun God. Later the Buddha (Siddhartha Guatama) was also influenced by Zoroaster's teachings. Slightly changed versions of some of these teachings, such as the hell of fire, also became the foundation of Christianity under Paul's influence as he borrowed teachings from Judaism, the Persian pagan god Mithra, and Hinduism. Many of these teachings came from the voices of past life memory and not from the physical experience of Paul's life. Paul's teachings were interpreted by him and those who used them and therefore were frequently opposite to the meaning of the voice he heard when he was given his initial mission. Power and Paul's hatred of women became very influential in the foundation of Christianity and were adhered to always by the Church as they adopted Paul's belief in the female as unequal to the male.

When Zoroaster began to teach he was shunned by family and friends alike as his teachings were opposite to the beliefs of the time. He wandered destitute and alone for many years, talking to those who would listen. Just when he felt that he should forsake his teachings, he was called into the presence of the King and asked to perform a miracle on the King's favorite horse who was dying. All other forms of healing had been tried on the horse without success. Zoroaster healed the King's horse and was from that time on living in the King's favor.

It was only after this time that Zoroaster's teachings were accepted as prophecy from the voice of "God" and he could stop his wandering. The information that he was given regarding the savior of God within us was interpreted to mean that a savior would be coming. All prophetic communication is given for the times and will be given in parables or will be interpreted by the level of intellectual consciousness available. Zoroaster's message of the internal Christ Consciousness influenced those who were willing to change. His inspired thoughts were recorded in the hymns of the Gathas and the Avesta Holy Book.

The next prophet that was given spirit prophecy to guide man was Moses of Egypt in 1650 B.C. The universal spirit mind of Moses related to him the aeons of creation and the prophecy of the organization of our dual soul. The imagination of the left brain could not conceive the infinity of the prophecy and those who later interpreted the work reduced the beauty of the story to the limitations of the ego of our physical nature. The prophecy of Moses became the story of creation as the first five books of the Old Testament and also began the "Laws" of Judaism. At the time it was considered by some that Moses may have plagiarized the teachings of Hermes, whose information was much the same and had been handed down as myth for fifty thousand years. Since the interpretation was different to fit the times, the similarities were soon forgotten. Hermes was the same soul as Jesus of Nazareth and his prophecy was always directed towards the love and power that we concealed within ourself. Zoroaster taught a philosophy that was to teach those involved in Nature Worship about the supreme being living internally within all of humanity. Judaism was to focus upon the religious law of Moses and expose humankind to the fear that it had been living. In the law of Moses the inequality between the male and female became a living force and man saw himself as equal only to the external God and supreme to the female soul and spirit as well as the physical female. The symbols and superstitions of the earlier Nature worship, Persian paganism, and Hinduism became intertwined with the law of Moses and the beliefs of Judaism took on a rigidity and warlike force that set one man against another.

Many men after Moses were known as prophets. This became a role that was adapted from the Hindu Shamanism, and those who were called prophets had many times inherited the role from a father or were appointed as the revered head of the largest tribe. These false prophets tarnished the image of the true spiritual prophets and caused persecution to flourish.

The next spirit prophet that has been very influential in the journey of our soul is the man called Jesus who was born in 7 B.C. Jesus came to earth as the Christ Consciousness to show man how to live a spiritual life of equality, truth, and love. The time had come in the journey of the immature soul where man must accept personal responsibility for his own evolution to integrate with the mature soul. Jesus lived the consciousness of his

360

mature soul as his Christ Consciousness, but only a handful of people were truly open to his teachings.

Jesus lived a spiritual life on earth, giving the people of the day an opportunity to see how we must all teach and live the spirit within us to evolve into our mature soul. His love was not welcomed and he made many enemies. After thirty-seven years on earth Jesus returned to the unseen energy of spirit. He had become whole within himself and found it a challenge to remain in physical form.

Jesus stayed on earth unseen and unknown for another twenty years until he returned to the trinity of his pure spirit consciousness. In A.D. 43 Saul of Tarsus, now known as Paul, was traveling and had what was thought to be a sunstroke. During Paul's period of epileptic seizures he had a psychic vision where he related that he saw Jesus. After that experience he set about creating a church but seldom related the church to Jesus and did not use the teachings of Jesus. Rather, Paul created his own laws and began to teach his own beliefs to the followers of Jesus, which were the same people that he had been persecuting.

Paul's laws were: Justification of faith rather than works, salvation through the mercy of God in Jesus Christ as savior, persecution on the cross with pain and suffering as the glory of God and the source of man's redemption, and the reconciliation of all men in the superiority of their Godly image. Paul brought to his church a full theology of sacraments such as dispensations, forgiveness, baptism, communion, redemption, marriage vows, and all were to be governed by the law of God through the grace of the church.

Paul began his teachings without a great deal of support. He was teaching the exact opposite of what Jesus taught and he was living opposite to the way Jesus lived. He was not a prophet, but he was a man on a mission that had been chosen to be an interesting example of inequality and fear. Structuring his church upon the opposite to the teachings of Jesus as the Christ Consciousness cast Paul into his universal role as the Antichrist.

Although Paul had been born and educated as a Jew, he didn't get along with his own culture much better than he did with the Gentiles that he had been persecuting. His church was a religion for the Gentiles that was being influenced by Paul's interest in Hinduism, the Hindu god Mitra and the Persian pagan god Mithra, and Judaism. Paul had fallen out of favor with his own people and had been attracted to the pagan and polytheistic religion of Hinduism. Mithras was a popular god in Rome at the time of Paul and was in high favor with his own Persian cult that was passed down from Zoroaster.

Classical Hinduism had grown from Vedic religion which had grown from the old polytheistic religion of Nature worship. Classical Hinduism was popular from about 500 B.C. to around A.D. 500. With the Persian god Mithra and Hindu god Mitra being of interest to Paul, he also borrowed beliefs from many other sources which were to become of primary importance in the new religion that he wanted to become the universal church. Paul structured his holy days from the Hindu feast days, using the exact dates but relating them to Jesus instead of the Persian god Mithra and the Hindu god Mitra. It was Paul's role to show the Gentiles and all of the world what they didn't want as he taught them pain, suffering, punishment, fear, inequality, control, and the untrue stories that he based his version of Christianity upon. He took his role as the chosen "apostle" seriously and lived it despite being called the Antichrist, devil, and satan by both Gentiles and Jews.

Even the name "Christianity" was borrowed from the ancient Greek Philosophers who were practicing Christianity in 350 B.C. and continued to maintain many followers. The ancient Christianity was based upon the Metaphysical philosophy that our spirit was at all times indwelling within our physical body and was held captive there until our time of death when it would leave and return again to continue its journey as a soul in a new physical body. What was seen as truth by the great philosophers of Greece is true today. We continue to have a living soul and indwelling spirit consciousness as the trinity of our consciousness which returns as the lifeforce of soul and spirit into our next physical body.

Jesus was a philosopher who lived as a teacher and prophet

with a clear realization of the social customs, beliefs, and behaviors of the day. His focus was to create a new way of thinking within the masses and to help people understand their power of creation. He did not "preach" hell fire and damnation or the end of the world. His approach was to allow people to recognize their freedom of thought and to find the strength within themselves to control their daily thoughts and behavior. It was his intention to teach the "kingdom of God" as our indwelling spirit consciousness and dual soul consciousness. Jesus was attempting to prepare people for the transition from the beliefs and behaviors of fear, control, war, and inequality that were accepted as the normal lifestyle, to a new way of thinking, emotions, and feelings that could be lived as support for equality, truth, and love.

Those individuals who followed Jesus were open to new thought and were not troublemakers, dissidents, homeless, or uneducated, but they were the opposite as scholars, businessmen, and large numbers of females. Jesus was astounded by the diversity of human lifestyles that culminated into the same fear and unequal beliefs and behaviors, which had no respect for the dignity, honor, and value of human life or society. During Jesus' life primitive beliefs, sacrifices, hatred, meanness, lying, inequality, and fear created the fabric of the societal and family life. The only sense of balance that existed was the ancient teachings of the philosophers who were dedicated to searching for an understanding of the soul and spirit within man. Only those who were seekers of knowledge would agree to hear the words of Jesus.

It was primarily scholars, women, and children who were followers of Jesus. The men who were followers were fewer in number because it was more challenging for men to face the release of control, anger, inequality, deceit, and warmongering than it was for women. Women were being forced to live in humility by the societal, religious, and family mores that were inflicted upon them, which allowed them to understand the teachings of Jesus on a completely different level. With the change in the women and children within a household, the men would sometimes follow suit and find themselves listening attentively to the words of Jesus. The teachings of Jesus spread by word of mouth, and the groups became more frequent and larger in number as people sought an internal balance that would help them cope on a daily basis with the chaos of the religious wars and an unstable society.

The followers of Jesus did not worship Jesus. They accepted him as their teacher and found his teachings refreshing. Nothing was too complicated to receive an answer. Each answer was given to define the relationship of the question to the questioner. Jesus would use every nuance available to him to help his listener understand the relationship. Some answers were parables, some were cynical, some were humorous, some were philosophical, and most of all they were loving and honest. Jesus was not above poking fun and using the antics and behavior of others to help clarify his point, but his jesting was done with so much love that his followers found no offense. Jesus helped his followers see through his example that the way we live is the love and learning experience for our mature soul.

Jesus saw himself as a practical teacher who could explain life from the basic experience of how life was lived and at the same time show the soul and spirit philosophy that was being learned and why it was important. His manner of teaching was to share observations equally and he frequently used himself as the object of his own cynical approach, reflecting the illusions of his students back to them. He lived the equality that he taught and his example freed the female in particular from the submission that she was expected to live at home. The impact of Jesus' teachings on society came from the female to the male as a change in the strength and courage of the female in refusing the role of submission. Equality, love, and truth were not only the foundation of Jesus' teaching but they were his way of life as he lived the Christ Consciousness of his mature soul and spirit.

The social unrest that was predominant in Galilee was due primarily to the religious wars that were being fought between the Greeks, Romans, and Hebrews in an attempt to determine the power that would rule. The inhabitants were tired of the struggle for power, the bloodshed, and the dramas that went with the lack of respect for the lives of others. The emotional climate of the day made a certain group of people ripe for the teachings of Jesus, as his cynical philosophy changed the emotional response of the female to the male. Although Jesus' followers learned from him, they never worshipped him. He interacted with them equally, always assuring the group that he was equal to the least of them. The intention of Jesus was to help people understand that "the kingdom of God" is within all people as their indwelling spirit consciousness.

Jesus came at the time when humanity had to learn the trinity of its own consciousness as the internal "God" of man. It became very obvious early within Jesus' teaching career that man was not ready to learn, which would have meant changing the old beliefs of worship, female submission, human sacrifice, and inequality. War was the way of power, the phallic symbol of our physical nature, and it too was based on human sacrifice. When Jesus left earth his group of students understood that the lesson of the Antichrist was a lesson to be lived by the masses. They knew the fabricated stories of his "death" missed the power of creation within his mind, which was the lesson that he was teaching them. It is because we have intensely lived our Christian worship of inequality, dependency, fear, pain, suffering, and control that we have learned what we don't want as the opposite of the teachings of Jesus.

Christianity has focused on the human sacrifice by "God" in his judgement and wrath in the same way that man has focused upon the human sacrifice of war and inequality. Our spirit has never been judgemental or wrathful toward the human species. We are children of "God." But because we perceive "God" in the external image of man, we have bestowed the identical characteristics of man upon our image of "God" and thought of ourselves as the sacrificial lambs of our external God. Jesus taught that the Kingdom of God is within us, and that is a perfect description of our spirit consciousness and mature soul mind and emotions. Having believed the teachings of many prophets that have taught us inequality as religion, and having sacrificed ourself to the pain and suffering of inequality, we are now able to recognize the difference. In discovering the love within us, we can move forward into the integration of our dual soul mind and emotions, and live our equality, truth, and love as Jesus lived his while he was human.

Living our equality, truth, and love as our daily consistent behavior is being spiritual, and it is using our intellect and mind of wisdom with the unconditional love of our spirit consciousness as our inspiration from our spirit source. All religions share a belief of worshipping the male image. Worship is the living behavior of inequality, which represents the "evil" or ignorance within us. To enlighten our living soul, we must integrate the dual soul into one soul mind and emotions of our male and female consciousness and live our equality, wisdom, and love. In living our soul knowledge, equality, truth, and love, we will be living our Christ Consciousness and using the Trinity of our Spirit Consciousness from which we can access our Universal Mind. Our indwelling spirit and male and female soul consciousness have been our internal guides from the beginning of creation. Our mature soul and spirit will continue to guide the immature child of our soul until it embraces the wisdom and love of itself as an equal male and female on earth.

CHOICES OF
OUR EVOLVING SOUL

Every aspect of our physical life from birth to and including death is a choice for our mature soul. Our choice is not a conscious intellectual choice of our immature soul consciousness but it is the choice of our subconscious, mature soul. If we can't accept what our dual soul is and what its overall goal is in being a living soul, we will not understand that all of our life is choice. It is our soul choices that have kept us learning and growing as an evolving soul consciousness, despite our attachments to old superstitions and rituals in our intellect and ego.

Our intellect and ego are both a part of our immature soul that lives in its fear emotions. Our intellect is the "blank slate" mind that we return with in each lifetime. Our intellect is our conscious mind that we use to gather knowledge. Our intellect is our forager and gatherer of information for our immature soul. Our ego is subconscious to our intellect and it is formed by old karmic beliefs, which are unlearned lessons that our immature soul is continuing to work on in each lifetime. It is our ego that forms a cosmic shell of beliefs around our intellect by its electromagnetic energy that limits the linear thinking of our intellect. Our intellect is the "floppy disc" of our soul and our ego is our internal program, such as DOS or Windows. Our mature soul consciousness is our mind of wisdom and loving emotions. Our mature soul consciousness acts as the "library" for our intellect as it stores everything that we learn at death. Our mature soul functions like the files stored on the hard drive of your computer. Our spirit consciousness can be compared to a mainframe computer or a server unit. Our spirit has universal memory that supports our dual soul. We now have free choice as to which we want to use. Until we understand our dual soul and its evolution we remain ignorant of our freedom of choice during our transition as we live from both our left and right brain.

We have always been internally conscious that we have a soul and spirit and yet our addictive religious beliefs have given our soul and spirit the illusion of mystery because of the control that our ego has over our intellect. The knowledge that we absorb is limited by our addictive ego beliefs. Within our intellect and ego we have reflected our consciousness externally and have lived in fear of the shadows created by our ignorance and superstition. Shadows within our mind are created by information that exists because of our beliefs but does not fit the design of truth. The illogical beliefs that we accept as fact do not fit in our mind and therefore they cast shadows of doubt when the design begins to reach completion. Our external reflection of the beliefs about our soul and spirit, which is at the core of our being as a human species, has kept us from understanding the truth about ourselves. If we do not perceive the truth of our indwelling spirit, we cannot conceive that we have a living soul, what that soul is, how it functions, and the purpose of that soul in our daily physical lives.

Because of our religious beliefs in an external God, our living soul and indwelling spirit have been shrouded in mystery. Mystery is the very substance of our own ignorance. There is no mystery when we have the knowledge to understand any subject. There was a time in our evolution as a soul when we did not understand gravitation, motion, balance, thermodynamics, engineering, genetics, space travel, chemistry, computers, and many other concepts that are common knowledge for us today. The more knowledge we have the better we understand the mystery, and the mystery is then resurrected into simplicity and we accept the new knowledge as part of our reality. Our old karmic beliefs are the superstitions that create mystery when we close our mind to expanding our knowledge. But when we open our mind the most shrouded mystery becomes clarity with the light of expanded knowledge. Once we expand our knowledge into understanding our soul and spirit as an integrated energy of every cell within our body, the pieces of the puzzle begin to fall in place and we can see our relationship as a living soul to earth, nature, and the universe. As a physical body, dual soul mind and emotions, and an indwelling spirit consciousness we are part of nature, and as we observe ourself and life we can easily understand our soul evolution.

It has been acceptable to open our intellect to external knowledge and to deny opening our intellect to internal knowledge. Yet within each of us is an indwelling spirit that contains all memory within its universal mind and our dual soul mind and emotions that is being used to expand our consciousness. The trinity of mind and emotional consciousness energy that lives within us creates a supraconsciousness that is our true internal image of God. Our intellect and ego mind has danced to our addictive beliefs and fears as it has descended into our immature soul. As we have been evolving through our descending emotional soul we have been saving all that we have learned within our mature soul mind of wisdom and love. Our mature soul contains all of the memory of our physical experiences that we have learned through the aeons of time. Our ego contains all of the addictive beliefs and superstitions that we have hung on to as immature soul lessons, which we have not yet completely learned.

The purpose of our living soul is to allow us to experience other souls, nature, earth, the universe, cultures, and everything that exists in relationship to ourself. We must have and live our physical experiences to expand our knowledge and understand ourself as a trinity of consciousness. Therefore our immature soul has a purpose of sensing self through the relationships that we experience with others, earth, nature, and the universe so that we can expand our consciousness as an understanding of ourself. Until we learn our lessons and can see the wisdom of turning loose of our old addictive beliefs, we hold our intellectual mind captive with our fear emotions. Living in fear is repeating the emotions of the immature soul mind and emotions throughout the journey of our immature soul. In effect, we have been like mushrooms growing in a dark cave as we have covered up the light of our love.

We are at all times an expanding consciousness as human beings. Our expanding consciousness occurs through the choice of our physical experiences that are designed and created by our living soul and indwelling spirit consciousness. We began as spirit consciousness and we created our living soul as a dual consciousness of male and female that would learn through the physical experiences that we call life. We also created matter in which our living soul and indwelling spirit consciousness could live. Our dual soul and spirit are ethereal or a chemical consciousness energy, and this energy needed a physical tool from which it could experience physical life. Only our physical body is finite. Our dual soul and spirit consciousness are eternal as chemical energy.

Our dual soul as "Lord" and our indwelling spirit consciousness as "God" designed our physical body to use as the living soul, which would allow the soul to further the expansion of consciousness of the spirit. Our dual soul as our dual male and female consciousness is the "Lord" of our body, having been given dominion over our physical matter as our living soul. As we think and experience our emotions as a soul and our feelings as the senses of our spirit, we reflect that precise level of consciousness into our physical reality as our moment-by-moment creation of life.

Our living soul was designed by its male and female consciousness in unity with the spirit creative consciousness as a dual consciousness of mind and emotions that would reflect the opposite aspects of itself into our physical life. Therefore, our male consciousness became the consciousness of our physical nature and chose to use sexuality as its core focus. Our female consciousness became the consciousness of our divine nature and it chose to use love as its creation focus.

The consciousness of our living soul as a dual male and female energy and the consciousness of our indwelling spirit created a trinity of consciousness energy that would always be present in matter as a way of expanding itself as consciousness energy. When the trinity of our consciousness chooses to leave the physical matter, which it created from the elements of earth, those chemicals of physical matter will return as chemicals of earth and the soul and spirit consciousness as an eternal chemical energy will choose another physical life as a conception within three days of physical time.

The trinity of the dual male and female soul and spirit consciousness always ascends from the physical matter with total animation and generates a new creation of physical form from the memory of the fractal pattern it has developed as the design of its physical life. In three days of earth time the soul and spirit consciousness chooses to resurrect or regenerate the memory of the physical form of the living soul and it begins as a new seed or conception to recreate itself into a new physical body. In life we go through seasons or cycles of expanding our consciousness in the same way that we do as a soul and that all of nature goes through as the seasons of earth.

Each new beginning of life as a birth is a free choice of the soul. Each and every moment of life is free choice and our death is free choice. The reality of our not being conscious of this cycle of expression of the soul and the choices that we make is simply due to our choice still being subconscious to our intellect as a choice of the divine nature of our mature soul. We have not yet learned to be conscious of the trinity of consciousness within our supraconsciousness, although as we transition into the right brain of our mature soul we will become truly enlightened by the direct influence of our spirit consciousness.

Our living dual soul became our left and right brain of the human form of energy and in each lobe of our brain we are dual as a mind and emotions. We live with a dual focus of our physical and divine nature, an external and internal perception, a negative and positive attitude, both fear and love emotions, and a male and female consciousness. In our immature dual and

371

opposite soul minds and emotions, we function consciously and with fear as our physical nature is predominant and we subconsciously suppress our female divine nature of loving emotions. The dual living soul, then, has a physical focus within the left intellectual mind with fear emotions being prevalent, and a divine focus within the right brain with love emotions living within a wise mind. It is the perception of our mind and emotional consciousness that we reflect into our physical lives as a living soul. The way that we live is the choice that we make as a soul to reflect the mind and emotional perception into our physical reality as our art of creation. It is the reflection of our level of soul consciousness that creates our physical reality. It is easy to change our perception of reality once we are no longer attached to our addictive beliefs and create a different lifestyle.

Our living soul is dual in every aspect as male and female, negative and positive, external and internal, physical and ethereal, closed and open, fearful and loving, darkness and light, descending and ascending, physical nature and divine nature, and dual mind and emotions. It is dual within itself and dual within its opposite selves, and it always has the freedom of choice in its beliefs, behaviors, and its emotions. Until our immature soul mind and emotional consciousness expands to the level of our balanced mature soul, the physical nature of our immature soul remains unaware that it has the freedom of choice. Our mature living soul as our dual mind and emotions has the freedom of choice at all times. But it is the consciousness of knowledge about ourself, as a dual soul and spirit, that we lack mentally which prevents our conscious use of free choice. As we begin to seek knowledge we become aware of our freedom of choice.

Freedom of choice for the living soul means we can believe what we want to believe, behave as we want to behave, have the attitude, personality, and character that we choose to have, and resist and deny change until we see the wisdom of change. When we expand our soul consciousness as our mind and emotions and grasp that we are a living soul, and that we create our living reality, we will have a consciousness of our freedom of choice to focus on our loving soul instead of our fearful soul. An advanced level of understanding ourself will change the intimacy of our sexual relationships as well as the relationships with our family and friends.

As long as we are focused externally and blaming others for our life, we are acting out our denial and resistance to changing to the internal focus of thinking and emotions for our mature living soul. We are in effect fighting internally against accepting our loving self as our core self because of our beliefs in the sexual core of our physical nature. We have lived aeons of time in the physical nature of our immature soul and we adapt to the habitual beliefs and behaviors of our thinking, emotions, and perceptions of truth. Our belief that "sex is love" acts as the strongest physical denial to our immature soul choice of change.

Now we are faced with leaving the focus of our descending emotional soul and moving into balance with our ascending mental soul and our ego is in a temper tantrum of resistance and denial. We are refusing to accept the knowledge to understand ourselves as an evolving dual soul and spirit consciousness because of our addictive ego beliefs that are suppressing our soul emotions of love and the physical female as the symbol of our mature soul. As we refuse to change our beliefs, we are asking for help from earth, nature, and the universe to allow us insight into our own resistance. And at the same time our intellect and ego is busily attaching itself to the external processes and primitive memories of our ancient beliefs to distract our descending emotional soul from forward movement and growth.

Our indwelling spirit consciousness is at all times guiding us with its internal voice, which we accept as our inspiration. But until we have a consciousness of our living soul and our indwelling spirit being a part of our physical body, we refuse to hear. Throughout the book of Revelation there is a repeated quote, "Let he who hath an ear, hear." This quote is telling us that those who have developed a consciousness of the indwelling spirit can hear its voice and they should consciously choose to listen to its message.

Our living soul as a physical nature doesn't want to hear, but the living soul of our divine nature will motivate us to listen to the indwelling spirit. Our ego is into resistance and denial of change so that it will use multiple distractions to avoid hearing the voice of our indwelling spirit. Our ego sees change as its death because it identifies itself with supremacy not humility, which it will become when we choose to change within our soul. When we are willing to listen it shows that we have given up the beastly and controlling ways of our physical nature and have become innocent and pure in our divine nature of love. Change becomes our first lesson of freedom of choice as a mature soul. Our society has been acting out multiple examples of the struggle between our immature and mature soul for us on a daily basis as we deny and resist change.

Since we have chosen to revolve mentally in the same superstitions and beliefs, we have lived our identical behaviors as a descending emotional soul. Changing our view of ourself is a major change, and yet it is the intention of our soul and spirit to motivate and inspire us to consciously make this change as our free choice. We can dig in our heels and distract ourselves for many lifetimes, but we will eventually change from our revolutionary state either consciously by accepting change and evolving or subconsciously by denying change and devolving. Change is a major choice that our soul is facing today that is of great magnitude. Many souls on earth today have begun their devolution by living deceitfulness, judgement, war, killing, and worship. As our mind fills with knowledge and we suppress our emotions with our religious beliefs in inequality, we create a dramatic imbalance. Sex does not create an emotional balance with our mind.

By accepting change we are living the lesson of our freedom of choice and the lessons of equality, truth, and love as a mature soul. For our soul these are all lessons of transition which allows us to evolve from the descending emotional soul into the balance with the ascending intellectual soul. As human beings we are unconsciously living the transition of our immature soul journey into its mature soul journey. We can accept this transition by seeking the knowledge to understand ourselves or we can deny the transition by closing our mind to knowledge and staying addicted to our old karmic beliefs and behaviors. During our periods of denial the ego will create distractions of external physical sexual focus and will mimic the voice of spirit to create the illusion of growth and change. The living soul will reflect the level of growth that we are truly living into our behavior and will frequently focus upon illusions of spiritual consciousness as an intellectual choice.

We are energy and we can only live in the inertia of revolution for so long a period as a living soul. We have reached the end of that period of emotional descent; therefore, we change by choice and begin our emotional ascent or we change by default and devolve mentally as an immature soul. The difference in devolution at this point in our immature soul growth is significant because it goes beyond the devolution of a single lifetime and becomes the accumulation of the soul's choice to stay attached to addictive beliefs, ignorance, and fear. If we choose to resist change, we are subconsciously choosing to devolve. In the past we have devolved by going one step backwards and two steps forward, but in this level of our immature soul we must evolve or we will devolve backwards into our Cycle of Development and begin our evolution over again. It is our choice to either change and continue with evolution or not to change and slide backwards into devolution. No one else can create our change for us. Change is the personal responsibility for each individual soul. The story of Lot's wife symbolizes this choice of our soul. When Lot's wife was leaving the burning cities of Sodom and Gomorrah she was told not to look back and dwell on the sins of the cities. But she chose to look back and she was turned into a pillar of salt. The first level of our Cycle of Development was lived in the crystals of salt.

As we look closely at our society, we can see the beginnings of change and evolution, and the beginnings of true devolution. Seeing the duality of our soul during this period of transition is normal for us because it shows us that we have choice. If we choose not to be conscious of the fact that we are currently living our dual reality as a society, we will not choose to accept our freedom of choice. As our beliefs and behaviors create our living the opposite realities of our dual soul, we become conscious of what we don't want and can consciously choose what we do want.

Many individuals in our society are choosing as evolving souls to seek knowledge and the love within their hearts. Others persist in living the superstitions, symbols, and rituals that our physical nature created as its addictive beliefs and behaviors, and in so doing they choose not to change and they are devolving. As we transition, we move from our descending emotional soul of fear and negativity to our ascending soul of love and positive living. Our future depends on the force of the soul consciousness that becomes predominant within society. If the majority of the collective consciousness remains fearful of change, the Law of Motion will force us into devolution. If the majority of the collective consciousness changes into loving and positive energy, then the Law of Motion will let us begin our ascending path into our mature soul.

Isaac Newton (1642-1727, English Physicist) defined this physical law of motion which comes under the Spiritual Principle of Equilibrium, and it is a Universal Law that does not change. It applies to all energy within the universe and it can be understood on a physical level as Newton understood it, or on a soul level, which explains our soul evolution as we are now living it.

Newton's law of motion was defined as a physical law, but in reality it is a reflection within the physical of a law of motion that is the fractal pattern of the Universal Law of Motion. When we realize that our soul has been at rest and revolving in place for the past fourteen thousand years as our "sabbath," we can then understand that the greatest force that is applied upon the collective consciousness of our soul will determine the movement of our soul. If the strongest force comes from the negative, fearful mind we will devolve or decelerate, but if the strongest force comes from the positive, loving mind we will evolve or accelerate. It is only at this point in our soul growth that we have enough knowledge to understand that we have free choice in how we think and behave, which will determine what happens to us as our choice is made. It is our thoughts and our behavior that act out our choice of contribution to the collective consciousness as an energy force that will move our soul in one direction or the other.

The design of our soul goes one step further to support this law of motion as the Principle of Equilibrium. In 1915 Albert Einstein published his General Theory of Relativity which dealt with acceleration and gravity. This fundamental principle of the nature of space, time, and gravitation is the perfect explanation for the evolution of our dual soul. In the space of our inert consciousness and within aeons of time our soul has continued to gravitate toward the loving side of its dual self.

Our gravitation has allowed our soul evolution as acceleration despite the basic inertia of our aware consciousness. With our mind and emotional focus being solely directed in the linear direction of our intellect and ego, we have been able to ignore our emotions, feelings, and forward movement without understanding how our growth as evolution was taking place. The focus of our intellect within the singular concept of our physical nature has allowed us to look for evolution within our physical body and not within our mind and emotions as our dual soul consciousness. The gravity of our evolving soul was part of our sexual design, which created our magnetic arc of gravitation.

It is important to have an aware consciousness that allows us to recognize the daily choices that we make as a soul. If we respond automatically by an immediate reaction of our ego, we make choices that frequently do not serve us long-term. As our ego lives its temper tantrums, our ego tug-of-war becomes evident in all of society. Crises and chaos seem to be happening in every aspect of our physical lives.

All growth within us internally and externally is a repetition of the fractal pattern of the Creator. Fractal geometry has shown us the unlimited ability of our soul design to change itself by showing us the unlimited changes that can occur within a mathematical equation. The chemical pattern of our physical life is a fractal pattern of our soul life and our soul is a fractal pattern of our spirit. As a soul and spirit we are a fractal pattern of nature, nature is a fractal pattern of earth, and earth is a fractal pattern of the universe. The universe is a fractal pattern of our Spirit Consciousness as a Chemical Consciousness.

This understanding of ourself shows us the wholeness of ourself and the integration that we have with nature in particular. Because we are made from nature, we must have the pure chemicals that are found in the water, air, and foods of nature to maintain our chemical cellular viability. What we eat is our choice and we make that choice multiple times each day. Our self-centered, addictive beliefs and habits get in our way of choice and we innocently eat foods that are destroying our physical cellular body and interfering with the function of the electromagnetic energy of our mind and emotional consciousness to stay balanced.

The ability to understand ourselves is already within our soul wisdom if we allow our soul mind to be open to sharing the knowledge. Our universal mind of spirit consciousness understands exactly how, why, and for what purpose we have chosen to become an indwelling spirit and living soul experiencing through physical matter. Our choice of foods, water, and air as the essential biological chemical supports that are in nature to protect us can only be made wisely through knowledge of ourself and nature.

Each moment that we breathe we live the reality of our art of creation along with the reality of what we create. We cannot separate the two. When we think in terms of separation, we close our mind to new thought and new emotions and the only choice left for our soul is repetition and devolution. Our physical life is created by us as the choice of our soul to expand our level of consciousness. Our intellect has used separation as its creation of mystery, and in doing so it has kept the pieces of the puzzle from uniting into an understanding of the beauty of us. What we think and the emotions that we live are the first in a very long list of choices that we make as an evolving dual soul.

Souls interact with each other, allowing the choice of one soul to capture the attention of many souls. Because our soul has the intention (inspiration) and will (motivation) to change, it will make choices now that it has not made in the past. The choices of our soul are frequently made as a way of capturing the attention of the world. Whatever choice the soul makes is the perfect choice for the soul. The physical experience may not appear to be a perfect choice to those who are watching, but it is the perfect choice for the soul that is living the experience.

Each experience reaches out to trigger the memory of the soul within each person that is touched by the soul's choice of behavior. During each day as we come in contact with family, friends, co-workers, people that we don't know but that we may have contact with in driving, shopping, dining, celebrating, etc., we act as an example for them of a specific level of soul consciousness. If we are loving we can make anyone's day better. If we are judgemental, controlling, arrogant, cold, rude, angry, and abusive in our language or behavior, we can bring the other person's day into a state of depression, saddness, or fear. Our attitude and behavior are both choices of our soul.

Making the choice to cope with all of our life in a loving and productive way allows us to be happy, creative, and to have wonderful relationships. Our human relationships are falling apart today because of the difference in the levels of consciousness within our dual soul perception. When one person is focused into the negative and fearful soul and another person is focused into the positive and loving soul, they will have nothing or very little that is commonly shared, which will include the definition of words in the language that is being used. When two people have an opposite soul focus mentally and emotionally, we can still have a sexual attraction. But that attraction will usually fade within about three months and each person may wake up one morning and say, "Why am I in this relationship?" Our relationships are the choice of our dual soul and there are many lessons that the mature soul designs into each relationship.

If we have no understanding of our mature soul and how it makes its choices, we certainly won't understand the physical relationship. If we do understand the soul, we will see that within the relationship there is a lesson. Maybe it is a lesson that we need to be reminded of as a soul but also one that we can learn fairly rapidly and not have a dramatic "physical need" to belabor the chaos for a long period of time.

379

When we understand the dual soul, we will understand the interconnection that is always there with other souls and how important it is for the soul to connect with another soul to complete a lesson or to challenge itself to see if it has learned the lesson so that it can go on to the next lesson. As souls we are cleaning up our lessons, which means we have more lessons that we are living at this time than we have ever attempted to live before in any one lifetime. Most of us do not connect our beliefs, thinking, attitude, personality, character traits, emotions, and behavior with our soul. Yet each of these physical attributes reflects the precise level of our soul consciousness. There is no mystery surrounding the soul level of growth once this reflection is understood. We live who we are as the choice of our living soul.

The way that we live our daily life comes from these seven elements of ourself. The level of these elements is used by our immature soul to create every moment of our reality by guiding the choices that we make as a soul. There is never a mystery about our soul because we wear it as an energy cloak, in the identical way that we wear clothes. We change the accessories of our energy cloak daily as we control, manipulate, and seduce ourself and others with the addictive beliefs of our sexual core and its physical needs. At this time the soul is aware of its duality and is making a conscious choice to focus either into its physical nature or its divine nature. Every addictive belief that our intellectual soul holds near and dear to its ego has its basis in our sexual core. Our beliefs have changed to fit the times, but each belief began as a sexual belief which evolved into religious beliefs and has consistently been supported by family, cultures, science, and religion. Because of the changes that our beliefs have undergone, we no longer recognize the wolves that have been redressed in the innocence and purity of the lamb's white wool. The image change of our beliefs has been essential to the security of our ego cosmic shell, and it has put the scientific and religious seal of approval on superstitions, symbols, and rituals that are bizarre in the mind and emotions of many people today. When we are focused in our physical nature our immature soul will choose to follow the beliefs and superstitions that are familiar and comfortable.

Every day we experience twenty-four hours of living and every day we make countless choices without recognizing that we create our reality of life. When we are not aware of the choices of our immature soul, we will blame and judge others as being responsible for what happens to us as we distract ourselves from personal responsibility. When we blame and judge others, we create the lesson of inequality within ourselves and see ourselves as a victim of the other person's choice. Dependency is a choice of our evolving immature soul and it is used as an ego distraction from personal responsibility. Religion, medicine, and our sexual relationships are all based on dependency, control, and worship, and these addictive beliefs of "need" have a long and repetitive history within our immature soul.

We are always able to choose as an evolving soul if we can think and speak. If not, we are operating only from the sensing realm of our five senses and we are suppressing the thinking and speaking. There are souls who freely choose the path of non-communication out of fear and refuse to think, speak, and to freely express their emotions despite the ability of the physical body to do so. Our soul's choice is frequently unknown on an intellectual level, although communication is an inherent gift of our mature soul and spirit consciousness and is natural within all human beings. If we damage our "tree of knowledge" as our soul and spirit consciousness, we can paralyze our body and some or all of our senses. If this happens to us there is always a lesson for the soul, and the lesson can also be a societal mission of revealment to the world. No one else is ever responsible for the choice that our soul makes.

When we refuse to use our free choice during several lives as a soul, we will choose a life where independence is forced upon us as a young child and we will not have the opportunity to stay dependent. When we are intellectual with a closed mind for many lifetimes, the soul will choose to return into a life of limited intellectual ability and focus the life on emotional expression. Each life of our soul is chosen to give us the needed experience to learn the lessons that the soul wants to learn for its evolution.

We may not be intellectually conscious of the lessons that our soul has chosen, but we will subconsciously live each lesson repeatedly until we consciously learn the lesson, or we will get stuck and we won't learn the lesson. When our mature soul realizes that we are terminally stuck and mired in the lesson of our immature soul, our mature soul will choose to begin a new life. The soul always has a choice to begin a new life through the physical experience of changing its focus, or it can begin a new life through a change of the physical body as death. Death is always a choice for the soul, and it gives the soul time to regroup and confront the soul lessons again from a different image of physical experience.

Our soul does not choose to come into each lifetime to die of old age. The internal mature soul has the freedom of choice to make the design of our physical life exactly what is essential for the immature soul consciousness. If we need to come back as a soul to learn only one detail of a lesson, we can do that. We can choose a very short life and return as a soul into many short lives before we again choose a long life. Our freedom of choice as an evolving soul allows us to touch the lives of many of our soul family and gives us the ability to be present as a mature soul that is living in our spirit consciousness, which can lead to some intense telepathic communication between the mature souls and spirit consciousness of both the mother and child. The mother may be totally unaware of the intention of the visiting soul, and normally the father is not conscious of the visit happening. The soul is never limited in its choice and it does not respond to the expectations of interference. The soul is clever in its choice of design and it will not accept interference that is not of choice, and this includes abortion.

When we recognize that we have freedom of choice as a soul, we begin to get serious about consciously creating exactly what we want as our physical experience. Understanding our freedom of choice in living removes us forever from the belief that we are a victim of life, anyone else, or any circumstance. We accept personal responsibility and we accept our responsibility joyfully, willingly, and creatively. When we can accept our soul's choice, we begin to laugh at ourselves. This brings us to a new choice of living in a loving and positive way. Our physical experiences will continue to contain the lessons that we must learn as a soul, but we will cope with each lesson with a new perception of our soul choice.

Our lessons began for us when we first became a living soul and indwelling spirit consciousness in a physical body. As a trinity of consciousness energy that had chosen to expand itself through the physical experience, we knew we would have a lot to learn as we moved further and further away from our conscious memory of spirit. Because the pattern of our physical body was designed as a fractal pattern of our soul and spirit, we maintained subconscious and unconscious memory but our conscious memory, as the intellectual focus of our mind, became a blank slate with each new life. The more evolved we become as a soul the more memory we have access to as our mind opens itself to its wisdom. As we approach the energy influence of our mature soul, we are conscious of our freedom of choice in every aspect of our being. In understanding that all of our reality is choice, we begin our ascension. When we began our physical focus on the inequality of thought, gender, and race, we became aware of our freedom of choice as an evolving immature soul. We always choose our parents for the role they will play on our stage of life. If we look at the relationship with our parents and the beliefs and behaviors that we are being patterned to repeat, we will know why we chose our parents. We choose our parents in three distinct dimensions of lessons. We can choose parents who show us the duality of our soul by the parents being focused on opposite consciousnesses. We can choose parents that are both focused within the negative, external, and fearful concepts of life, or we can choose parents that are both focused on the positive, internal, and loving concepts of life.

The design of the fractal pattern of our soul consciousness meant that we would need to have the blank slate of our intellect repatterned each time that we came back into physical life. This allowed the soul to use its freedom of choice in choosing the perfect parents to support our soul lessons. It was essential that our soul be repatterned into those soul lessons that it had designed into the physical experience, and therefore it was appropriate for the soul to choose parents that would support that memory. The lessons do not come one at a time but rather in multiple images that exist within levels. The primary levels will contain the most intense lessons for the soul. But other lessons exist in levels of seven times seven to infinity, which means that all accumulated lessons may be addressed during any one lifetime that is lived as an evolving and transitioning soul. The lesson may be so brief that the intellectual consciousness will have no awareness of the lesson since it can be as simple as a chance meeting of the eyes. An instantaneous lesson can be remarkably profound and can be for the soul like the loose threads that are left on a garment by a seamstress.

In choosing our parents we will communicate with them telepathically to reach an agreement and be certain that our life design is fitting their life design patterns. We can choose parents to teach us exactly what we want, or what we don't want, or we can choose parents to teach us both as each parent becomes an example of the dual soul. The same parent can teach us the dual concepts of lessons, and both parents can play that specific role. We can also choose parents that will abandon us, abort us, kill us, teach us fear and abuse, or that will love us, support us, nurture us, and teach us all of the wonderful sharing that is available in our lives. The parents that we choose will offer our soul exactly what it wants. Our parents of choice will agree to play the role that we asked them to play on our stage of life, and without that agreement we wouldn't choose them as parents.

When parents agree to accept the role of parenting a child they subconsciously and unconsciously understand that role, but each parent can choose to teach the child in a negative or positive way. This supports the choice of the parent's soul and allows everyone involved to learn from the physical experience. Parents and children can learn together or choose not to learn together. No one soul wants to stay stuck in negativity and fear, although some souls cannot find the strength and courage to change. The form, structure, organization, discipline, free choice, will, and intention of the soul are to be repatterned within the first fourteen years of life. It is the choice of the evolving soul and its family as to how the repatterning takes place in the physical experience.

Parents can always teach more by example than through words. If the words and language say one thing and the behavior relays a different message, the duality will also serve as a lesson for both souls. Roles reverse within parents and children and may reverse several times during a lifetime. Parents and children are always in the roles of teachers and students and students and teachers. Those who recognize this interaction early in life will consciously use the soul life more effectively.

Each soul has the fractal pattern of its unique pattern of lessons. No two souls have an identical fractal pattern because the physical experience can never be identical for two souls. Our perception and the lessons change the unique fractal pattern of the soul as it creates a unique thinking, emotional, and feeling response to the physical experience. The lessons can be fairly similar for many souls, but the perception and response to the physical experience will be lived differently. For example, all members of a family could be sharing many of the lessons within the family but the difference in the perception and physical experience of each lesson within each person's soul will create the lesson in a unique way for each individual soul according to its personal soul choice of evolution.

The response to the family can be closed or open, and the choice is always dependent upon the willingness of each soul to expand its consciousness. The lessons that the soul wants to learn will be lived and reflected through the beliefs, thinking, emotions, attitude, personality, character traits, language, and behavior of each individual soul. Living and wearing the cloak of our immature soul persona helps us flaunt our lessons through our behavior, which consistently reminds us of what we are supposed to be learning. The intellect will not be conscious of its lessons because the ego cosmic shell will be controlling, manipulating, and seducing the intellect into its sense of superiority or inferiority. This keeps the duality of the soul alive and well within the intellect and ego despite the ego's subconscious state.

The lessons that we repattern with our parents are those lessons that are going to follow us into each and every relationship that we have in our life. Our immature soul consciousness is intent upon living the lesson; therefore, each lesson will be brought forward and played out in its many images in each type of relationship. Sometimes we may choose to live our lessons in a dual fashion, having some relationships that are a challenge and others that appear fairly balanced in our life. This gives our dual soul an opportunity to see the value of balance as we experience both harmony and chaos.

As an example, we can have friends that we are more in tune with than we are with our intimate relationship. Our friends may be in harmony with our negative, fearful soul and our intimate relationship may be more loving and positive and as such would be opposite to the energy of our own soul, which would make us uncomfortable. As we experience the dualism of our soul being acted out in our relationship, we could choose to change the intimate relationship and find someone else who is more in harmony with our negative and fearful soul focus. And the opposite could also be true, where we can find ourselves comfortable with only those who are close to us and feel pain and suffering when we are around negative and fearful energy. The soul will always have free choice of being in or in leaving a relationship. When our intellect is unaware of our freedom of choice as a soul, we will be indecisive, confused, and fragmented as we move back and forth in our thoughts and emotions.

When we can understand the reason for our choice of relationships, we will see the lessons that we are living with clarity. If we are captured in blame and judgement of our relationships and the other people who are involved, we will have no perception of the lesson our soul is attempting to teach us. We will repeat the physical experience over and over again in our life and in the multiple physical lives of our soul until we understand the lesson that is to be learned. Each lesson is learned through twenty-eight primary images that are lived as the fractal soul pattern of seven times seven to infinity within each image. Because of our fractal pattern the number of times that we are destined to repeat a lesson is endless. As we begin to understand how the pattern of our soul is organized and the Universal Laws that act as our soul organization and discipline, we can move more quickly through our consciousness evolution as a soul.

Life is the Ph.D. of our soul, because our lessons are piled high and deep in each and every relationship. Every moment has meaning for our soul. We never work on simply one lesson in life and we never approach a lesson through just a singular approach or person. The lessons of our soul are chosen collectively in every aspect of our life. We will change the images slightly in some aspects and in others we will work with the lesson in the identical image that we use with everyone else. Our intellect and ego can live multiple lives over aeons of physical time and never develop a consciousness that it is choosing to learn about itself by blaming and judging everyone else in its life. We choose others as a mirror to see the image of ourself. Frequently we feel that it is the other person that is being judgemental when it is in fact us. Since we choose to see the image of who we are in others it is important to realize how our soul reflects our persona and begin to look at ourself to explore what lessons we have been living.

Taking the "sins" that we see in others and seeing how they are being lived in our own lives is the beginning of exploring the chosen lessons of the soul. Never judge another person. Look at yourself instead of them and explore your own thinking, emotions, and feelings to see why you are being judgemental and controlling. Our soul is telling us a lot more than we are willing to hear when we constantly blame, judge, and criticize someone else. Focus on the other person's good points and it will reinforce your good points. This allows you to balance your energy and begin to love who you are as you also increase your love for the other person.

Look within the relationships that you have to see if you are attempting to control another person. Do you manipulate or seduce others to get your way? Is getting your way a self-centered focus for you? Do you feel that you are perfect and everyone else needs a lot of work? Do you feel better knowing within your own mind that someone "needs" you? Do you feel that you are better than or less than any other person? Do you always speak your truth? Do you find yourself telling lies when the truth would serve you better? Are you conscious of your duplicity as the words come out of your mouth? Do you understand why it is your choice to lie when the truth would serve you better? Asking yourself these questions will help you begin to understand yourself and your relationship with other people. Use these questions to explore your internal feelings as you journal.

The immature soul of the intellect and ego will be living unequal, lying, deceitful behavior, and abusing self and others at this time in the soul journey. The mature soul of wisdom and love will be living equality, truth, and love in a peaceful, joyful life. Look at yourself to see the lessons that you have chosen for this lifetime. In looking you can understand why you have chosen your parents, siblings, lover, friends, and career contemporaries. Do not be afraid to look into your own mind and emotions as an evolving soul. Each physical experience has tremendous value to our dual soul.

As we identify the lessons that we are learning, we gradually change the focus of our consciousness through the cross-fertilization that occurs within our thinking, emotions, and feelings. Cross-fertilization of our dual evolving soul creates activity in both our male and female consciousness of the left and right brain. The more we cross-fertilize our male and female souls the less we can identify differences between the persona and the physical body of the male and female. As we come together as male and female evolving souls, we will be true to our physical gender preference because we will understand why we think, have emotions, and feel as we do. Expanding our consciousness of understanding ourself is the primary way that we become loving, spiritual human beings. If we are afraid to release our old confining beliefs, we will not change our thinking, emotions, or feelings. But we will repeat each experience until we capture our attention and decide to look internally at who we are.

Each relationship that we have in life has a meaning for our soul and the lessons that we are learning. Nothing in our life is without a lesson at this time in our soul evolution. The difference between now and the past is that our consciousness of ourself and our relationships is changing and expanding as we change and expand. Be conscious of how the change shows our growth as a soul.

To see the lessons that we are learning we must look at our reactions to other people. As we look at the behavior that we live in our everyday life in total love, truth, and equality, the repetition of our soul lessons begin to reveal themselves.

Am I angry, rageful, resentful, revengeful, abusive, judgemental, controlling, critical, nagging, manipulative, seductive, dependent, and irresponsible? Am I self-abusive? Do I have dependencies on relationships that allow me to be controlled? Am I abusive in my language or behavior with others? Do I have addictive beliefs that control me? Do I have addictive behaviors that control me? How am I acting out my addictions day by day? Am I willing to change my attitude toward life? Am I bringing my opportunities to fruition in life? Am I living the love of myself?

Go into your relationships through your memory and look at your feelings. Journal as you think. Start with your first cycle of life from birth until seven. Record everything that you can remember thinking, feeling, emotions, beliefs you learned, and your behavior. Leave nothing out. List the people that you can remember from that time. When you finish with the first cycle go to the second cycle of your life and repeat the exercise. Never judge anything that you discover. Simply write it down and continue. Continue with the seven-year cycles of your life until you reach the present. This exercise is the best that you can use to identify the precise lessons of your soul. You will find a pattern being created in the first cycle that will continue into the present cycle. Be especially conscious of the pattern of lessons as only positive experiences for the evolving soul. Our mature soul does not indulge in self-judgment. Once you finish your life's review, date a new journal entry and begin again.

As we begin to understand ourselves we will begin to understand the choice of our birth, such as singular, plural, or multiple. At this time in the evolution of our soul the way that we come into life reveals part of the lesson that our soul is working with in this lifetime.

We can look at our birth to identify our birth opportunities. If we chose singular, twin, or multiple births when we came into life there is a soul lesson that is symbolized by the number we chose. If we chose a singular birth as an only child in a family then look at the lesson of separation. Many of these children chose separation as a way of life and might be involved in a career that has a separate focus or that allows isolation in the method of work. If we were one of several children we can look at the relationship that we have with our siblings. If we came into life as a twin look at the type of twin. Did we choose to be identical, fraternal, or opposite sexes? Twin births help the soul with the image of its duality and clearly shows that the soul will be living both sides of its duality as a male and female consciousness in this lifetime. The types of twins allow the soul to see the lesson of duality from a subtle perception of loving self, a dual perception of self, and an opposite perception of self.

Triplet birth energy is showing us the trinity of our consciousness being reflected into the physical. This will show exactly where the energy is focused for the children as well as the parents. Each triplet birth will reflect different images of consciousness for each soul and show how each soul works within the trinity. At least one soul within a trinity will be reflecting the spirit and the others will reflect the dual soul. This reflection can be found in the lessons of the soul and the levels that are being worked with. Triplets can also be simultaneous lives or reflections of different levels of soul growth. There is never any predetermined concept for any birth, as each soul has free choice.

Multiple births can create different focuses for one soul or multiple souls with individual focuses. Multiple souls can be fragments of one soul that has many lessons to cover in this lifetime. These souls can represent different levels of the soul or the same level of the soul and can be seen by the interconnection that becomes evident in the personality, character traits, behavior, beliefs, attitude, thinking, and emotions. The primary lesson that is being learned for multiple births, twins, and triplets is the lesson of unity and integration. It takes "team work" to participate in a multiple birth. Multiple births have already acted out unity in their behavior of birth. There is also the capability of the soul to choose simultaneous lives as multiple births, or to return with the lessons of parallel lives as new souls to complete many soul lessons in one physical period. Each soul can also choose to simply return with other souls from the primary soul family.

It is also important to recognize the role of the family and the interactive lessons: If we think our mother or father are controlling then it becomes very important to look at our own behavior to see the pattern that we might be either repeating or consciously avoiding. If we recognize the controlling behavior or other judgemental behavior in another family member, then chances are we are learning the same lesson in the same or in a different image. We must not be afraid to look honestly at and then truthfully acknowledge what we find in our own behavior. Perhaps our parents will show us the opposite, with one parent focused on loving us unconditionally and the other focused on control, manipulation, and seduction. One or both parents could also be teaching the lesson of independence by what could be felt as rejection or abandonment. Multiple lessons will be seen in the choice of each soul, and the children in a family can be total opposites.

When we can look at our family with absolute love for the support that we are receiving, our soul lessons can be truly healing for the entire family. The lesson of unconditional love will frequently appear as crises or adversity as we are living it. Our evolving soul lessons are examples of love, truth, and equality that can be manipulated in a negative or positive way by parents or other family members.

Do I manipulate truth? Do I lie even to myself because I am afraid to look at the true image of myself? Do I feel that I must save other members of my family by convincing them that I am right and they are wrong? Do I use lies to manipulate, seduce, and control others? Do I make family members dependent upon me by trying to control their thoughts or activities? Do I become angry if a family member doesn't do exactly what I want them to do? Do I feel shut out of family activities? Do I isolate myself from my family or other people? Do I comfortably discuss what is on my mind with family members? Do I expect the family to become angry if I want to discuss a family problem? Am I embarrassed to share my personal thoughts, emotions, feelings or behaviors with family and friends? Do I take the time to nurture and love myself?

Lying creates inequality and fear in all relationships and is especially toxic to our soul emotions, our beliefs about family members, and our ability to communicate openly and freely. Control, manipulation, seduction, and fear all originate from the lesson of inequality, and when we are learning that lesson we will lie to help ourself appear and feel more equal. We will also want people to be dependent upon us because it makes us feel important, in control, and worthwhile, which creates the illusion within our ego of being worshipped. When we are living the lesson of truth we will make our lesson physical by lying to ourself as well as other people. To our ego this is a form of superiority which creates inequality between ourself and others. Any communication or behavior between us and others that creates any form of lying as inequality also creates untruth and fear.

Families are always unconditionally loving of each other on a soul level. This may not be the total reflection that is seen physically because the reflection of the immature soul can deny the mature soul connection and its love. When we are able to recognize our "coat of many colors" that is reflected through the energy of our persona, we will sense the untruth in relationships even when the immature soul is ignorant of the image it is reflecting. The immature soul is frequently flying on blind faith not knowledge, and blind faith ignores the fact that our soul and spirit is internal and therefore consistently visible in our behavior.

The unconditional love of the family members can pick up where it left off years before and be as beautiful and supportive as though it had been consistently present in our physical experience. Families always share the lesson of communication, which is a soul lesson of great magnitude. Other soul lessons that exist within families are the lessons of truth, equality, love, unity, and personal responsibility. At this time in our soul growth, family unity and communication have expanded far beyond the level that was previously reached for the immature soul. As our consciousness expands, the closeness and love is felt more realistically than ever before as it takes on an integrated sense.

The soul always chooses the actors on its stage of life. The soul learns through the interaction with other souls that creates our physical experiences of life. As the soul is designing its next life, requests are made of other soul family members to play specific roles, which will provide an opportunity for the soul to learn through the interaction. The choices that are made by the soul create the genetic identification that science is now looking at and seeing only on a physical level.

The soul reflects the lessons through the thinking, emotions, attitude, personality, character traits, beliefs, and behavior from the chemical structure of the soul mind and emotions into the DNA structure within each and every cell of our physical matter. It is the reflection of these lessons that creates the physical experiences of our life and that creates our energy field or persona that we reflect outwardly to cloak our body. This same DNA pattern also reflects our physical being and our physical lessons of disease as soul lessons.

Each and every nuance of this tangled web is choice for our soul, and most of these experiences are subtle and totally subconscious or unconscious to our conscious intellect. We begin working on our soul lessons before we are physically born. Our lessons begin at the moment of conception and are understood by the soul and other family members even before conception takes place. The lessons will be more apparent after birth by the interaction, feelings, and emotions of the parents and the child.

Nothing is ever separate for the soul. The interactive lessons are also karmic relationship lessons that many times can only be learned with the help of the soul family member that initiated the original lesson into the soul's memory. This knowledge helps us see why each physical experience is a lesson for more than simply the individual soul that is actively learning from the lesson. Other family members are passively learning at the same time, although they may feel totally removed from the experience itself. At times the consciousness of some family members will be in denial of the lesson, and that is their role in the lesson that is shared because one of their lessons will be fear of emotions. As other family members observe the experience subconsciously as a mature soul and consciously as an intellect, they are preparing the lesson for another life time in their own physical experience.

The soul will continue living its choices whether or not we grasp the significance of the physical experiences and the support of the soul family in each soul choice. Because of our focus on soul transition, we will, as a collective consciousness of soul families, choose to create chaos to capture the attention of the emotions of love within the universe. Because our ego has the old karmic belief that death is a sin and a form of punishment that is being handed down by God, death as a soul choice always captures the attention of a group of people. The more the individual is known as a loved or admired presence, the more attention that individual's death will create and the more change we will experience in the collective consciousness.

The families themselves are aware, on a soul level, of the choice of the person to die. Death is a new beginning for the soul and gives the soul an opportunity to continue with the impact it has with other people in its new life. The choice of death is understood on an individual soul level, and when the physical family came together in its choice of the physical relationship it was understood by all as a soul memory that is subconscious. In death the role of the family members as soul support is then acted out in the physical reality. The focus of the soul family is toward changing the collective consciousness at this time in our society. Our transitioning soul is attempting to break free of its revolutionary focus and move forward into the ascending emotional soul of love. Death plays an important role because death is change for the soul and symbolizes dramatic change in the lives of the physical family left behind.

Because of death having an emotional impact on the physical family and symbolizing change in the soul family, death is now being used as the choice of some souls to expand the level of conscious awareness of our emotions. This is the purpose of many group deaths that are experienced as collective deaths in physical disasters, such as airplane crashes. Any catastrophe that causes multiple deaths acts as a greater emotional trigger for groups of souls than an average single death would. Also, younger people who are in the prime of life can create a massive collective consciousness with those who relate to them in death. Older people are expected to die in our belief system and therefore will not have an equal impact on a soul level unless the individual is widely known and publicly loved. Even public acknowledgement does not motivate the soul to the same emotional feelings as someone will who chooses death in what is considered the prime of life. Our emotional response to death is reflecting our addictive beliefs about death that we hold in our primitive soul memory. The change within each individual is important because of the emotional collective consciousness. Therefore, at this time in our history, the death rate from all manner of deaths will be higher than usual. As souls we have a determination to learn and grow. When we suppress our emotional soul evolution, we are inviting chaos to get our attention.

In the intimate family of birth and of marriage there are always chosen lessons that each person is focused upon. No one learns his/her lessons in life alone. The person that we have asked as a soul to help us with a life lesson is also working on the same lesson, although the image of the lesson may be different. We can learn our lesson and our parents may bring their lesson back into their next lifetime without a consciousness of the role they were playing for us and therefore they didn't learn the lesson. The nice thing about family relationships is we can learn from each other if we are open to the dual role of teacher and student and student and teacher. This is the perfect role because it keeps us open to knowledge without the restrictions and limitations of identity and roles to create inequality. The soul has no expectations or destinations of having learned all there is to learn. It is always our ego beliefs that limit our mind with expectations and destinations.

As we discover how our souls support each other in evolution, we can consciously appreciate every event within our life because we will see the importance of what we are learning and we will not judge or blame the person that we are interacting with in the lesson. Our soul is supported not only by our physical family on a soul level but also by the soul family on a soul level. Even when we have no conscious awareness of the soul family and its support, it is still there and it is scattered throughout the universe. Soul energy is given to us telepathically as a love energy, which is more effective than the physical support that we may be conscious of being given at the time. The physical interaction will be the primary support that we consciously acknowledge because we live our support as part of our physical life experience.

Evolving souls are always interpenetrating the dual soul consciousness to bring motivation and knowledge into the intellect. Because we are one as a spirit consciousness, we are basically one as a soul consciousness but in our soul consciousness we exist at different levels of growth, giving us our individual uniqueness. Because our soul is governed by the Universal Principles of Eternal Life and its laws, we have a wide choice of soul focuses despite the souls being in the same soul level of knowledge. The important issue for our soul becomes its level of consciousness which defines the level of knowledge and understanding that our soul is living in its physical experience. When our consciousness is expanded to include the consciousness of our dual living soul and our spirit consciousness, we have integrated our mind and emotions into a collective spirit consciousness. At this moment in time, we are attempting as souls to integrate the consciousness of our living dual soul mind and emotions. To integrate our evolving soul consciousness, we must integrate our male and female consciousness internally and externally.

If we understand the DNA and its pattern of mitosis or regeneration we can more easily understand the relationship of one soul to another. Our soul is a fractal pattern of our spirit. The DNA is the fractal pattern of our soul and our body is a fractal pattern of our DNA that gives us the precise pattern of cellular reproduction that is embedded within the soul and spirit memory. In our physical cells the soul pattern of our body is constantly reproducing itself, which shows us the soul's ability to reproduce itself at birth into more than one physical form. The soul of each of us is constantly reproducing itself into multiple lives, because we have so much to learn at this time in our evolution that the soul can send simultaneous lives into the masses to help itself with its shift into the mature soul. Our twin soul can also be creating simultaneous lives, which increases our opportunity to meet our twin soul.

Our dual soul mind and emotions evolves by the magnetic force of our chemical consciousness. We have been subconsciously and unconsciously living through aeons of time by the gravitational pull of our magnetic emotions. This is the exact method of evolution that our immature soul has experienced, and the experience of rebirth as a soul was not consciously understood because of our old karmic belief systems. Throughout our path of evolution our souls have supported each other through the crises and chaos that keeps us subconsciously in touch with our magnetic emotions even when we choose not to acknowledge them physically.

Conciliate Souls

Now that our soul is attempting to break free of its revolutionary cycle and begin to move forward again, we must consciously stimulate our emotions. Our emotional inhibitions limit our willingness to change, and therefore a soul who is well-known in the world will agree to become a conciliate soul to openly stimulate the emotions and bring people together in the unity of their mind, emotions, and feelings. Diana, Princess of Wales, stimulated the mass collective consciousness emotionally in a unique and productive way that transcends all other physical experiences of love emotions for our soul.

Many people are afraid to be emotional. Diana was not afraid of truthfully sharing her emotions and feelings. She was open and truthful about the love that she was willing to share with the homeless, downtrodden, diseased, and maimed of society.

397

Because she had lived the loss of love through the rejection and abandonment she felt when her marriage failed, she became conscious of the power of love and it was reflected into her life through the behavior of her living soul.

Our living soul is acted out in our physical life as our thinking, emotions, beliefs, attitude, personality, character traits, language, and behavior, which can be perfectly balanced or mercurial. Diana's magnetism was the reflection of the internal love of her soul and the knowledge and compassion that she felt for others who were not being loved. Her magnetism reached out to expand the emotion of love in all who related to her loss of love in her loss of life. The energy of love shone around Diana's body, face, in her language, behavior, and as the true essense of her being as she grew as a woman.

Everyone alive has felt the saddness of the loss of love, which makes us more conscious of the power of love when we personally feel love. People everywhere related to Princess Diana's rejection and abandonment in love, but many people did not become conscious of her magnetic love until they felt the loss of her love in her death. In her death Diana polarized the love emotions in billions of people, giving them the opportunity to become conscious of the power of the emotion of love within their own soul. Her loss created an expanded collective consciousness of the love that is within every person on earth. If we are a transitioning soul, we will be conscious of the love in our heart and we will very naturally react in loss and grief when we lose our physical symbol of love.

In a world that lives war, anger, judgement, and abuse through the fear of a closed mind, Diana gave the world the gift of love with her death. In death, Diana opened the soul mind and emotions in billions of people throughout the world, and even when the physical emotion is forgotten our emotions can never be as suppressed again. She expanded the consciousness of the emotions of love in humanity as no other human being has ever done. In living her love she invited the world to relate to her as an equal rather than as royalty. She shared her emotions, which increased her vulnerability to judgement. But at Diana's death many people forgot their judgement and her loss stimulated their love, which opened their hearts, perhaps for the first time, to equality, love, and truth.

Diana's family and her young sons feel their pain more intensely because of the special love and the joy and happiness of her presence in their daily lives. Our presence is our daily expression of love. They will grieve her loss and painfully miss her gentle touch, and although time will soften the pain, the loss will stay in their hearts. But Diana's death shocked the emotions of all the world and magnetically opened the minds and hearts of mankind to our equality and love emotions and the truth of our spiritual feelings. In expanding the conscious emotions and focusing the minds of billions of people into their love, she gave the world the gift of our own love. At this time in our human growth the magnetizing of love within the masses is Diana's eternal legacy of love for the collective consciousness of our soul and spirit.

Certain souls accept events that will make statements to society in relationship to the importance of the people's understanding of the experience as a soul lesson. This has happened to us from the beginning of time, and each time we have consciously grown from the experience even though we may not have had a consciousness of our growth at the time. Each time our love emotions and spiritual feelings are lived, we elevate our aware consciousness of our capabilities of loving ourself as a soul.

Throughout our immature soul, we have focused our physical nature on the physical sexual image and lived in fear as we have judged ourselves unworthy of love. To continue to evolve as souls into our mature divine nature it is necessary for all humans to open their fearful soul mind and emotions to the love of the ascending emotional soul. The fear and judgement that has humanity in its clutches is overwhelming. The collective consciousness of souls that understand love realizes that it is in the minority as an emotional force upon earth. When the world in general needs a soul lesson that can get everyone's attention, some advanced soul that is in a position of capturing the needed emotional energy force will volunteer for the assignment on a soul level. Diana's death polarized the soul love emotions of billions of people into the love within their own ascending emotional soul and created a climate of love that can be expanded to begin our ascension into the collective consciousness as an evolving soul.

Now it is the responsibility of each individual to maintain that open-minded position of emotional love. Moving from our descending emotional soul into our ascending emotional soul from our present point of inertia is essential to our evolution. As a soul we have been revolving in our superstitions and symbolic beliefs that are supported by our fear emotions for fourteen thousand years. We have essentially become stuck and unmovable in our closed mind of beliefs and descending emotional fear. Our transitional soul knows that it must begin to move into its ascending emotional soul or it will devolve back into its immature soul. Whenever an emotion of love is triggered, our soul releases some of its fear and our emotions begin to ascend.

Although Princess Diana was no longer "Her Royal Highness," she represented the many people of the world who have come from a long line of ritualistic religious beliefs and behaviors that personify the inhibition of emotion as the suppression of our female soul. She herself had moved beyond these restrictions and was seeking her personal freedom, equality, truth, and love. In death Princess Diana did what no living person could ever do before—she brought people's love emotions into balance with the mind so that we as people can truly begin our dance of life that is essential to the transition of our soul. The electricity, magnetism, and light of love touched the inner core of the spirit consciousness within the masses, and many people were surprised by the emotions and feelings they experienced.

As a soul Princess Diana accomplished the nearly impossible shift in massive numbers of souls to the love emotions within themselves. The energy of this shift is a magnetic force that will have the power to perhaps prevent what could have been dramatic changes on earth. Her death is a gift of life through her love to billions of people because she stimulated the magnetic emotional force to continue opening the closed and fearful soul minds of the masses to a higher level of collective consciousness.

With the united force of love energy, the intention and will of many souls will now change and help with the transition of the masses into the ascending emotional soul. Princess Diana has polarized the magnetic forces of our love emotions in a way that has never been done before, creating a collective consciousness that will bring the necessary changes of love into a world captured by fear and war by stimulating individual souls into a mass consciousness of love by loss and grief. The contribution of her loving soul to help mankind at this time is a gift to all of mankind as evolving souls. Her gift should be respected, honored, and lived to help the world evolve as a mature soul. We should all bless Princess Diana for choosing to live this important mission as a conciliate soul in the transition of the collective consciousness from fear to love.

Another masterful example of how souls will choose to support the masses of other souls in their evolution happened five days after Diana, Princess of Wales' death. This was the death of Mother Teresa in Calcutta, India. Many females related to Princess Diana, as did some males. The female is the love symbol of our emotional divine nature and our spirit feelings. The female emotional divine nature is now responsible for leading the human species into the ascending emotional soul. Princess Diana became the symbol of every woman and her inherent mother love as our divine nature.

Mother Teresa's death played the same role, but she reached several levels of the soul that were not affected by the death of Princess Diana. Mother Teresa magnetized many religious women and many men, but her death was designed at this time to reach many men who could not relate to the magnetic love of Princess Diana at her death because of her wealth. With Mother Teresa's death the loss of her love began the polarization of love within many men and women who are attached to their physical nature and religious beliefs. In our physical nature we live our controlling beliefs in the need for status, wealth, and material possessions as the only way to express love or to make a difference within the world. Because Mother Teresa was able to give love

from her heart without having the wealth and material possessions, she captured the love emotions of a group of men and
women who are focused into their strong physical needs and
beliefs about money, possessions, and power. The identity and
roles that are lived as expectations and destinations of money,
possessions, status, and power were challenged by Mother Teresa
and earned her the love and respect of this group.

Another group of men and women were also polarized with
love at the death of Mother Teresa, and that is a smaller group of
people who are working through the love energy within themselves and naturally relate to the selflessness and freedom from
possessions that were inherent emotions within Mother Teresa.
Mother Teresa was recognized for the tremendous differences
that she made within the lives of the poor and sick through her
love alone, without personal wealth and material possessions.
Her death will also affect everyone on earth that has been bitter-
ly and fearfully absorbed by their poverty consciousness to the
point of personally identifying with money and possessions as
love. Her example shows the world that love is valid in its own
right and does not have an umbilical attachment to money, status, power, and possessions.

Mother Teresa consciously chose poverty but she loved life
and people, showing the world that love and poverty can unite
the passionate love emotions in our physical lives. Many people
who are living within their physical nature accepted her higher
emotions of love as the inherent saintliness of her religious intention. Her religious beliefs also attracted the love emotions from
a large segment of the religious population because of their relationship to her as someone who made religion work in her life.
The people who find it a challenge to abide by the superstition
and beliefs of all religions are holding onto guilt because they
see themselves as failures in living the good within themselves.
Mother Teresa was the symbol of the "good" to millions of people who are challenged by their self-judgement and fear while
attached by their soul's umbilical cord to their religious beliefs as
a karmic lesson.

These two deaths of very different females have brought

about the polarization of love emotions to many who have never acknowledged the emotion within themselves. The enhancement of love emotions has permeated our soul consciousness as a collective mass of individual people and it can never truly go away for any person who feels the passion of love in their divine nature. With the united force of love energy, the intention and will of many souls will now change and help with the transition of the masses into the ascending emotional soul. We must honor the strength and courage of the souls of these two women for choosing to play this important role in the universal transition of the human species as a collective consciousness from fear to love. Their choice as conciliate souls has created a united force of universal love to help with the movement of the mass collective soul consciousness into love.

The soul focus of these two women was very different and therefore they each polarized the groups of souls on earth that related to their soul level of consciousness. Religion is an immature soul focus that comes from our "worship and obey" beliefs of inequality. Worship can only occur when we have fear and inequality as our lessons for this lifetime. Mother Teresa was focused on learning love through the physical experiences of worship, obedience, and poverty. These are all lessons of the immature soul of our physical nature and a large number of people are stuck as immature souls in these lessons.

Princess Diana was at a higher level of soul evolution where she found it difficult to worship anyone, including those of royal status. She was learning to love herself internally, which she acted out in her physical experiences of humility. The more she loved herself the more freedom she had in sharing her love equally and truthfully with others. Today's female is focused upon learning to love herself after countless lifetimes of being taught that women are the inferior sex of the human species and that they should not be treated otherwise. Princess Diana was learning that love doesn't come with status, possessions, power, or money but must come from loving ourself.

Both women were learning the lesson of internal love and reflecting it externally into their lives. These are different images of the same lesson, and when we look at the emotional magnetism of love that was created by their deaths, we can practically count the number of individuals that are on the same soul level that Princess Diana and Mother Teresa were on. It is these two conciliate souls that will help to bring about the transition of our immature soul. Both of these conciliate souls have allowed us to see with total clarity that love is the way of change for our dual soul of male and female consciousness.

These are only two examples of the multiple dramas in which conciliate souls can choose to play a part in affecting other souls to create the collective consciousness of change through our emotions of love. Because these two women were well-known throughout the world they had the recognition power to polarize those who were living the identical lessons that they were learning. Others, who were not choosing the identical physical experience, did share the soul level of love, which we choose to work with in our individual choice of experiences as we seek to live our divine nature. The expansiveness of these two events created one unified soul lesson for our collective consciousness.

Sexual harassment problems as well as other sexual indecencies have captured our attention for a number of years. The sexual indecencies within the different religious individuals are choices that our soul makes for the lesson of the individual but also for society. When we witness the homosexuality, prostitution, pedophilia, and the breaking of the laws of abstinence among religious men, we are seeking as a society to understand that sexuality is a biological need for procreation, sensory stimulation, and magnetism for the male and female adult soul. Sexuality is a gift of our spirit to support our soul in eternal life. Our focus on sexuality by our physical nature has created our abusive sexual activity as subjected to the religious moral law. Sexuality has been the core of our physical nature as an essential biological need. As our immature soul changes its mind, emotional, and sensory focus into the mature soul, our societal lesson is to learn the emotion of love rather than living the behavior of inappropriate sex. Examples of female inequality and sexual abuse are the Hill-Thomas case, Tailhook, teachers, priests, and other people sexually abusing children. And of course the most interesting conciliate soul sexual lesson of all is with the President of the United States.

The present sexual drama of President Clinton has been accepted by his conciliate soul as a societal lesson that will allow people to see that sexual behavior is not as important as the person's thinking, emotions, and feelings while at the same time placing our inhibited sexual behaviors in an open forum for discussion. This sexual drama becomes a multifaceted lesson for our collective dual soul consciousness in a world forum. As we live the media hype of many men and women discussing this issue, including the politicians, we are missing the major lesson of our immature soul. Our sexual activity should always be a private matter between two adults. The gossip, judgement, blame, criticism, constant manipulation, and repetition of the subject is the true societal lesson for all of humanity as we again relive the repetition of our immature soul. This conciliate soul lesson is the personification of the ego and spirit tug-of-war as it is being acted out through the anger and rage of some key players, while President Clinton shows us the love, strength, and courage of rising above the warlike behavior.

President Clinton stands alone in his actions. No other man or woman has been brave enough to openly acknowledge their own sexual behaviors, while they are vehemently judging and blaming him as though he is the first person on earth to be involved in sexual activity. Truth is a major lesson of our soul as it moves "through the eye of the needle," but who is being more untruthful, those who are "casting stones of judgement" or someone who has acted out a sexual indiscretion that has become a world issue? Moral law can never be a true societal yardstick because those who support it live their own brand of inequality, untruth, judgement, and fear, making it safer for them to judge others rather than to look within their own lives at their behavior of lying, inequality, and hypocrisy. Sexuality has been a part of our life that was created at the time of our creation and it is not going away. Any man who thinks or behaves unequally, untruthfully, or unlovingly towards his wife, daughters, or any woman is living sexual abuse. Sexual abuse, judgement, blame, inequality, lies, and fear have all been created by our male physical nature, and therefore these are the lessons for society that we are seeking to learn from sharing this sexual experience on a global basis.

The lesson of our sexuality had to be acted out by a prominent man as the symbol of our male physical nature to have impacted the world. To have taken on this societal role for the world to experience our reaction to sexuality is reason to applaud the courage, faith, and trust of Clinton's conciliate soul. Only a man that has reached the prominence, power, and recognition as the President of the United States could successfully bring this lesson to the forefront of the world's attention. No one else could have attracted the judgement, blame, criticism, and untruths that would allow all of humanity to become tired of the subject of sex. The belaboring and sensationalism of gossip as the focus of the media is also a lesson of judgemental communication that society could never have learned before. Our freedom of choice not to hear, read, or watch the terminal obsession with sex as a moral issue has helped the masses to learn freedom, independence, and self-value as our truth, equality, and love. If the media coverage was given to knowledge that would expand the consciousness of the people in the same way that media coverage is given to judgement, our society would change quickly.

The lessons of judgement, blame, and criticism are major lessons that must be learned by each and every person who wants to change and grow. When Paul began Christianity he was called the Antichrist, satan, and the devil, and ultimately he was persecuted and killed, but today he has millions of followers. Sex is not love and judgement is not love. Humility is love and respect is love. It is our ethical values that are important not the moral values that are based on inequality, lies, judgement, and fear. If we respected ourselves and our national image as a world power, we would never invalidate the world image of our Presidency and our nation by sexual judgement and blame of our world leader. The judgement and competition for the purpose of destruction of President Clinton shows us the devolution that many souls are continuing to actively live. Sexuality is a lesson of our male physical nature for the entire political, judicial, and media systems of our world.

The conciliate soul of President Clinton has accepted the role of polarizing sexuality in an open forum of world opinion to remove the subject of sex from the "forbidden fruit" beliefs of religion to the true knowledge of the essential role that sexuality has played in our soul evolution as we have believed that sex is love. The lessons that are to be learned from President Clinton's behavior are the positive ethical lessons of strength, courage, patience, perseverance, equality, respect, and love. The love and support of Hillary Clinton and their daughter Chelsea is a reflection of spiritual love and an indication of the unity that has been agreed upon at a soul level for this family. Their unity is the beauty of the unconditional love of our spirit for the soul, which they are living as they support President Clinton.

As a society we have been polarizing our sexual attitudes to become conscious of how our soul makes us aware of our sexual beliefs and behaviors that we have accepted as our expression of love. At this time the entire world is being overwhelmed with the intellectual focus on the physical sexual image, but it also includes our overwhelming reflection of self-judgement and self-punishment as it shows us how easy it is for us to lose our insight and intuition and reduce ourself to primitive behavior. It takes a very brave and evolved conciliate soul to choose a glaringly judgemental lifestyle that reaches to the very core of our physical nature to live in the public forum of the world. But being in the "eye of the media" is important to the conciliate soul in changing our thinking from our male sexual core to our female loving core. How else can everyone in the world discover what our evolving soul is beginning to realize, that its core is spiritual not sexual?

LIVING OUR PRIMITIVE SOUL MEMORY

When children begin to kill children and their parents, and parents kill children, it should become obvious to the masses that something is going on that is not understood. Old souls that return to life and are triggered by the judgement, blame, abuse, and violence in their homes, in society, and in the world will go into the memory nodes of past lives where they lived violent and abusive lives and they will act out the memory at any age. Many crimes are being committed today because society does not understand our dual soul and its transition. To transition as a dual soul the focus of our immature soul mind must cross-fertilize the mature soul mind by passing through the subconscious past life memories that are karmic and primitive in the beliefs and behaviors. Without an understanding of the dual soul minds and emotions, these primitive memory nodes will be relived at any age and will seem bizarre and out of place in our society today.

We have multiple examples of immature souls that are living past life memories without understanding what they are doing, such as Jeffrey Dahmer. Dahmer is a classic example of how we can return to primitive past life memories as we revisit our subconscious cosmic shell of primitive beliefs. Our journey as primitive beings has not always been kind or pretty, but our behavior was there to help us learn the lessons of our immature soul. When we fail to learn our soul lessons we will act them out as our lifestyle in another life until the lessons are learned. When past life memories and behaviors are not understood by the police, the medical personnel, the judicial system, and the families of criminals there is a deep guilt and shame left in our hearts, and part of this is because we all know as a soul that what is not understood will be repeated. Jeffrey Dahmer alone can be proof of the importance of each of us understanding our soul evolution and freeing ourselves of our ancient superstitions, symbols, myths, rituals, beliefs, and behaviors that are all based in ignorance and fear.

Other examples of our evolving soul speaking to us through its choices of physical experiences are all happening too frequently in today's society, such as planes crashing, ships sinking, madmen running amuck with guns, children killing children, and terrorists bombing people and places. None has yet shown the power of love that Princess Diana magnetized, but it takes a world to raise the collective consciousness of our soul lessons as human beings. We have been flirting with our intention to live our love for over two thousand years, but our addictive beliefs, superstitions, rituals, and fear have held us in our revolutionary soul journey. Judgement, war, anger, control, and fear are the revolutions of our physical nature that we have become attached to and which we must learn to release to live our love. When we look carefully at our uncivilized world, we can easily see that the outcome of our religious beliefs has been creating a world of competition, crime, rage, hate, and starvation. It is because of what we are now living that we can appreciate the love of our divine nature.

Multiple souls will choose to help open the minds and emotions of other people on an individual, family, societal, and world basis if we continue to deny and resist our internal change. It is through the feelings and emotions of loss, grief, and death that we begin to look at ourselves and expand our consciousness to the reality of our miracle of life. In creating crisis we bring ourselves face to face with emotions and feelings. In being conscious of our love and choosing to live our love, we will have less need for chaos on earth, in society, and within the family unit. As a physical nature we have lived the chaos theory, and many people have created severe addictions to chaos and crises. Chaos paralyzes our mind, emotions, and feelings as we begin our devolution.

The paralysis of thought is visible each and every day as people continue to live their dependency on other people and fail to accept personal responsibility for themselves. To live our equality, truth, and love, we must be conscious of how we are refusing to live it by our dependency on and worship of others. These are subtle lessons that we have repeated so habitually that we are totally unconscious of how we act, what we say, what we think, and how unloving we are to ourselves when we deny the love within our divine nature.

When we create inequality, untruth, and fear it is because we see ourselves as unequal. Inequality breeds the "need to be saved" within our consciousness. When we need to be saved, we see ourselves as unequal in every aspect of our life and we will reflect our inequality into our judgemental words and our critical behavior. It is through the consciousness of our emotions that we can stop being fearful and become loving. As we live in a crisis addiction, we live the role of the "savior" as a sense of power and control.

"Worship and obey" is the mantra of all cults as religious organizations. This is a major belief that is holding us back from loving ourselves. We have been taught that it is a sin to love ourselves and that we should focus our love externally to God. We are a living soul with an indwelling spirit consciousness that is abused when we worship and obey externally and deny ourselves the nurturing of our internal love. In our ascending emotional and mental soul we acknowledge our living soul and our indwelling spirit consciousness and we love ourself and life. Religions have created many false gods. Religion is the primitive foundation of crisis addictions. When we created the ultimate in false gods as we were taught to worship the "father as God," we began to live chaos in our daily life as an immature soul.

Every soul upon earth is bringing its energy together through the influence of knowledge to make a change in the focus of our thinking, emotions, and feelings. We can consciously choose to transition or we can deny the reality of change and devolve. When we accept the free choice of our mature soul, we can no longer live inequality as a female and worship our male physical nature.

In understanding the true story of our twin souls and soul mates perhaps we can overcome our terminal search for that perfect person in our life and realize that we are the perfect person that we are seeking. In understanding ourselves we never feel less than perfect or unfulfilled. As a mature soul we are seeking to integrate the male and female consciousness within us which is our living soul that is seeking internal equality as balance.

As a seed of the Creator we began as a spirit consciousness, and as a spirit consciousness we created the male and female soul consciousness as our Lord. In total unity and equality as our Lord and Spirit, we created our physical form with a chemical cellular consciousness and reflected our soul and spirit consciousness into the cells of our physical body as our living soul, which gave our consciousness the opportunity to learn from our physical experiences.

When we finished with the development of our soul consciousness of male and female and created our living soul of reflected cellular consciousness into human form, we reflected both our male and female sexual characteristics into one physical body. As we were resting after the creation of our living soul, we began to understand that we could physically live our dual natures of male and female more efficiently if we divided our body into male and female physical form. In the beginning of our human form we were hermaphrodites, or "unisexed" as a united sex. When we separated our body into male and female, we became twin souls as a male and female consciousness living in both male and female physical bodies.

When we were separated into two individual sexual bodies, we were placed into the same consciousness of our physical nature to maintain the unity and equality of the male and female consciousness. When we were both placed by our choice into the consciousness of our physical nature the female was symbolized by the emotions and the male was symbolized by the mind, creating our soul as dual in every aspect. This allowed us as immature souls to be magnetized by our emotions to the emotion of love within our female divine nature, which assured us of evolution until we could recognize our freedom of choice.

The true origin of our soul mates is the mate of our own soul that has created itself through the division of our soul. The soul has the power and the freedom of choice to focus on more than one life at a time to address different lessons or different images of a lesson. Those souls that began with the same original soul are the true soul mates of us. We frequently choose these mates in the physical world to help us learn more intensely and expansively the lessons that we have chosen. Soul mates provide us with the opportunity of expanding our dual perception. These souls are always individual souls which will integrate into one soul as we live our Cycle of Integration. We frequently choose to partner with soul mates because of our shared comfort zone and the similarity of our consciousness level. Therefore, as soul family members and frequent mates in our physical relationships, we have a long history of soul equality and unity.

Each soul maintains the integrity of itself at all levels of consciousness evolution. In thinking about ourself as a soul it is wise to think of our evolving soul as a consciousness rather than our sexual image of the physical body. Our beliefs limit our concept of ourself to our physical body, but our mind and emotions as our dual soul consciousness is never limited unless we personally limit it with our beliefs. Our living soul is our dual soul mind and emotions and the pattern of our soul as our male and female consciousness, which is reflected into our DNA or cellular memory that is present in every cell within our physical body. As a soul we are the fractal pattern of spirit which has no limitation of consciousness or cellular memory. Our limitations exist only in the addictive beliefs of our immature soul mind and suppressed emotions. Our soul chose to live with its limited consciousness during its childhood because it was necessary to gradually expand into its full power of consciousness.

Our spirit has universal memory. Our soul has evolving soul memory. Our body has cellular memory. All cellular memory is encoded within the chemicals that make up each cell and it is always at risk of mutation when the chemical cellular memory is not understood as being part of nature. Chemicals that are not a part of nature and therefore cannot be used safely within our cellular memory have the power to destroy or devolve the living soul as physical matter. Those chemicals that destroy the universal memory of spirit that is coded into physical matter will affect the brain, brain stem, spinal cord, nervous systems, endocrine system, our triplet of seven senses, and the limbic system, first causing disease and then death. Chemicals that destroy the brain will also destroy the physical cellular memory, which will affect all other parts of the body with disease, such as the kidneys, liver, and intestinal tract, which are all soul organs. Chemical excesses and deficiencies will quickly affect our heart in the same way that feeling unloved will, and our heart will clog up, wear out, or go into heart failure. Our choice to use chemicals that are harmful to our soul and our physical body are choices of our intellectual soul that is living the "I know it all" lesson. Our ignorance of who we are allows us to threaten the survival of ourselves as a human species.

As twin souls and as soul mates we all affect each other even when we are not physically connected to each other. Our effect comes from the consciousness itself, and as we live our individual level of soul consciousness we impact all souls that live on earth. Consciousness is an energy force of light that is formed from the electricity and magnetism of our soul and spirit. When our descending soul mind and emotions is veiled with beliefs, we filter only small amounts of light into our intellectual consciousness. The level of darkness that we experience within our immature soul mind and emotions is determined by the number of beliefs that we use as our multiple filters. As we have lived in the darkness of our descending soul, we have not recognized that our beliefs are creating the darkness that we are experiencing, which is acted out as war, killing, competition, suppression, discrimination, anger, rage, abuse, and judgement. All negative, judgemental behavior is being lived now as our intellect and ego choice because we are self-centered as an obsessive habit of our religious belief in inequality.

As we recognize the level that we are living as a soul, we can also recognize that we have the freedom of choice in the level of consciousness that we choose to focus within as our daily life experience. The level of our soul consciousness is no mystery because we wear it in the same manner that we wear our clothes. In observing how we live, how we act, how we speak, our attitude about life, our emotional focus, what we believe, think, and feel, and how we behave towards ourself and others, we can define the level of our soul consciousness that we are living within and we can map our level of evolution for our soul with this information. Our beliefs and behaviors clearly reflect our soul choices.

How we focus shows us very clearly who we are. If we think only in terms of our societal status, physical sexual image, the schools we graduated from, the career we identify with, the money we have, or the possessions that we own, we are firmly focused in the immature soul of our left brain. If we have religious, educational, or societal beliefs of inequality, if we feel that we are better than someone else in terms of experience, knowledge, sex, or race, if we are captured by belief limitations, fear, superiority, inferiority, inadequacy, worthlessness, and control, if we are angry, hate others, lie, cheat, steal, or take advantage of others, if we judge, blame, manipulate, seduce, and abuse ourself or others, we are in our left brain with obvious lessons that we are learning and our level of soul consciousness evolution is then weighted or pulled down by our thinking, emotions, feelings, and behaviors. During the transition of our immature soul to our mature soul we will make choices from a dual focus. Most of our life can be loving and wise, but we may have sexual behavior from our physical nature.

Our soul is no mystery to us when we look at our obsessions, habits, lifestyles, feelings, emotions, and our behavior toward other people to see where we are as a soul consciousness. If we see the world through a negative, judgemental, external, and fearful focus, we are defining our soul level to ourselves every moment that we breathe. We never hide who we are; instead we flaunt who we are in an attempt to find another person that we can attract who will have the same energy.

If we choose someone of opposite energy, we learn faster than we do when we choose someone of the same energy. If two negative souls unite together it gives them a sense of perfection in themselves and they support each other in fearing change. If two positive souls unite together it gives them the inspiration and motivation to search for truth together. If two opposite souls unite together it puts what they are afraid of facing in their daily lives so they cannot avoid living what they fear the most. A negative soul will fear change and a positive soul will not want to devolve back into fear. The action and reaction is always the choice of the soul.

By wearing our soul as our "coat of many colors," we gradually become conscious of the image of ourself and can clearly see how small changes can take place. Normally the soul moves one small step at a time. As we have been on our immature journey, we have at times moved forward two steps and slid back one step, but we still progressed in the lifetime. As our soul gets tired of its revolutions, it begins to see its intellect as the spiritual part of self. Believing that our intellect is our spirit is an ego illusion which can create devolution that will not be felt until the illusion fades and we face the truth of ourself. This is the ego's last attempt to hold on to its "coat of many colors" which it has come to love and identify with.

As our soul enters into the level of intellectual spiritualism, it is normal for the ego to believe that whatever the external focus is, it is the answer to spiritualism. Spiritualism is when we are able to live consistently from the universal memory of our spirit consciousness in the absolute truth and equality of our unconditional love. Religion lives from the superstitions of our primitive life that have been karmically stored in our ego cosmic shell of beliefs as worship and inequality since the beginning of our immature soul. Religion is based in fear, judgement, control, inequality, worship, and obedience. Spiritualism is based in unconditional love, freedom, equality, and absolute truth. It is always our freedom of choice as a soul to choose the journey that is comfortable for us.

In looking at ourself and the physical experiences that we have lived, we can clearly identify the beliefs and behaviors that no longer work for us in the transitional energy of our immature and mature soul and we will know that we have the freedom to choose what we want. It is important to look at our dual soul level and take note of those beliefs and behaviors that no longer serve us. In looking at our beliefs and behaviors we must not be afraid of change. Recognizing our freedom of choice reveals an advanced soul that is awakening.

It is normal for our ego to close our mind and emotions down and to put itself into the mode of resistance and denial. If we continue to trigger our ego it can go into a temper tantrum and distract us with multiple physical focuses that will direct our mind and physical presence away from knowledge and change. The ego functions from blind faith in itself and knowledge threatens its supremacy. Our "blind faith" ego worship has held us in tighter and tighter cycles of revolution for nearly two thousand years, and the symbol of blind faith that we are now experiencing is tornadoes, which occur as a message from our spirit consciousness. The wind is the symbol of our spirit consciousness and water is the symbol of our soul. Tornadoes become destructive when they create tight revolutions of wind spiralling to earth. Our spirit shows us how our ego mind is destroying earth.

Our ego is terrified of change because it sees change as its death and it believes that death is a sin. This shows the convoluted thinking of the ego that can't keep its facts straight. The ego believes in only one life; therefore, death is a final blow to the ego self and it sees death as a judgement from God that is killing the ego as a form of punishment for its physical sins. Supremacy, judgement, and inequality are not recognized as sins by the immature soul that has chosen these behaviors as its image of God.

Our ego wants us to blame and judge other people so that we can't recognize our soul "coat of many colors." As long as our ego can keep us looking externally instead of internally, we won't discover that we are truly seeing our own image in other people. The ego is only comfortable when it is in like energy. Therefore we choose our friends because they are like us and we can be comfortable. If we are angry, we will choose angry friends. If we are fearful, we will choose fearful friends. If we are loving, we will choose loving friends. If we are happy, we will choose happy friends. Like energy will attract like energy, which causes an expansion of the energy, and when the energy is negative it expands into societal destruction as our choice of behavior. This is the definition of our isolated societal groups, including violent gangs.

Understanding how we gravitate to the energy which makes up our soul energy will help us to recognize the level of our soul consciousness. Seeing the wisdom of our living soul as it evolves and is magnetized to the image of ourself lets us live our level of consciousness in a loving manner. We will be conscious of the energy that surrounds us being compatible or incompatible with our own energy. When we are exposed to incompatible energy, we begin to lose our mental, emotional, and physical balance and can become depressed, frantic, hyperactive or express other anxieties that will accumulate with time. If the energy that is surrounding us is compatible, we will love the comfort zone that is created and we will feel "at home."

As we have evolved through the immature journey of our soul, we have changed many things about ourselves. First of all, we have refined our body multiple times in the same way that we have changed our lifestyle and changed our beliefs to fit the times. Our core beliefs have not changed but our interpretation of those beliefs has changed to fit our evolution. Each change has occurred as a choice of our soul to grow and expand our lifestyle.

Our soul is now living in the level of knowledge. It is only in the level of knowledge that we have become consciously aware of ourselves and are attempting to understand ourselves differently. As our awareness of the importance of knowledge has become clear to us, we have begun to search externally and internally to understand our relationship to being, truth, knowledge, creation, God, love, nature, the universe, energy, and our human and Divine relationships. The changes that we have created as we have sought knowledge have all been the free choice of our soul, and they have been remarkable.

We will become truly wise when we see the relationship of ourself to all that is within the universe. As we understand the fractal pattern of geometry, we begin to understand the fractal pattern of our soul and spirit as it was created from the chemicals of the universe. As we continue to explore the DNA, we will become aware that our DNA is the fractal pattern of our soul mind and emotions as well as our organization, discipline, structure, and form of our soul and our body. As we begin to understand our dual soul, we will see how we truly are unconditional love. In understanding love we understand our relationships, and the relationship of our body to nature and earth. As we understand the relationship of our body to the universe, nature, and earth, we begin to understand our DNA, the universe, creation, and the consciousness energy that we call "God" or Spirit Consciousness. In understanding our trinity of consciousness, our understanding of eternal life becomes part of our knowledge and as a society we will begin to prove our eternal life by the pattern of our soul DNA. The more knowledge that we accumulate the more important our soul choices become, because our power of creation is expanding and, unless our choices are wisely understood, we will create devolution.

As our soul gathers its strength, courage, and love to begin its ascension, we will have access to the wisdom of our mature soul consciousness. Our mature soul mind and loving emotions is the "hard drive" of our ascending soul. In our right brain we have stored all that we have learned. The memory of our left brain can only deal with this lifetime but our right brain is now being accessed by millions of people. Because we have not been taught the truth of our soul and spirit, we see the wisdom of our right brain as a mystery that we think emits from our left brain intellect and ego. The cross-fertilization of the two lobes of our brain has been apparent for some time, but since science does not believe in the soul and spirit the medical perception of our brain is incomplete.

Religion is grounded in dependency, control, worship, and fear. Science is grounded in the intellect, ego, self-worship, and fear. Metaphysics is the science of living that studies the invisible energy of us, including the trinity of our mind and emotions as a dual soul and spirit consciousness, the matter that cannot be seen with our normal vision, the invisible cellular, soul, and spirit energy that we wear, and the unity and equality of their relationship. When we understand ourself we will understand the universe because we are a fractal pattern of the chemical universe. The interactive chemicals of the universe create all that is, as consciousness, energy, and matter. There is more energy within the universe than there is physical matter. Energy is never destroyed, it simply changes form. We are energy.

As our living soul evolves into its ascending journey as an integrated soul, we will have the love and joy of life as our everyday reality. As we live in our love and joy, we will have the power to create a "heaven on earth." In the creation of a supportive, loving environment, we have the ability to evolve in a different way, loving ourself and others as we discover how our soul uses our relationships as a learning tool for our soul and spirit evolution. It has been the perfection of our pure spiritual genius and its unconditional love to have designed us to live as we have lived. If we had been given a consciousness of our internal power before we consciously learned humility, we would have easily destroyed ourselves with a terminal devolution and we would have had to start our design again.

As we leave our paralyzed space of revolving in superstition, we must leave with a love force greater than a fear force to allow us to integrate as a male and female soul consciousness. When we are in touch with our internal source of love, we will be able to release our fear beliefs and our ego will transcend into humility. Only when we can each consistently live our humility will it be safe for us to understand the absolute truth of our power of love. When we understand love our evolving mature soul will continue as our freedom of choice, intention, and will, until we expand our spirit consciousness which is our universal purpose of life. The choice that we make as a soul must be a collective choice of all souls to bring us into a societal and universal change as we face the most important step forward that we have ever chosen as a living soul.

LIVING OUR COLLECTIVE CONSCIOUSNESS

In attempting to understand the depth of our collective consciousness, we must first understand some basic definitions that structure our thoughts, beliefs, and behaviors. Our collective consciousness is a reflection of who we are as a unified soul consciousness on earth. The largest or most massive collective consciousness on earth has the power of motion to influence our soul toward evolution or devolution. Because of the power of our thought, emotions, and feelings within our collective consciousness, we determine the physical experiences of the masses.

Our culture reflects the quality of the social and intellectual language within the human mind that is responsible for transmitting behaviors, patterns, arts, beliefs, institutions, and all other products of human endeavor and thought that characterize the community experience. The quality of our culture as a collective consciousness creates our way of living as human beings and the quality of our culture is then transmitted from one generation to another generation.

Cult is derived from the word "culture" and pertains to polarized groups within a larger culture. Cults are formed primarily as religious organizations that control the beliefs and lifestyle of their followers, especially with rituals, ceremonies, superstitions, and worship. Frequently cults offer worship as devotion and veneration to a person, ideal, or thing, and the participants adhere to the same lifestyle, beliefs, and behaviors as their leader by following an organizational doctrine or dogma. We have a human culture and religions are cults within the human culture that are varied in their beliefs, behaviors, and worship lifestyle.

Each group that forms a cult also forms a collective consciousness by living from the same beliefs and behaviors. The worship or controlled thoughts and behaviors within a cult create a collective consciousness that is equal to the members within the cult. Therefore, when religious cults have large numbers within the group worshipping the same negative, dependent, savior beliefs the collective consciousness of the group will interfere and prevent true civilization within the culture. Worship creates a collective consciousness of inequality. Civilization requires a collective consciousness of equality.

Civilizations do not at this time exist upon earth. When the foundation of a culture is based upon love, truth, equality, compassion, humility, unity, and cooperation, it is then a civilized culture. As yet, in the history of earth, true civilization has not been created. As the human culture is transitioning to the mature soul, civilization will be created by the collective consciousness of our culture because we will choose to live equality, truth, and love.

Civilization cannot occur within a culture until the equilibrium of the soul is being lived as a collective consciousness of love, truth, and equality. Cults are not based upon equality because a primary belief is the veneration and worship of a person, ideal, or thing that is seen as superior to the individuals within the cult. With this belief the devotion and veneration is given to someone or something other than ourself. Civilization occurs when we see the love, equality, and truth of ourself and understand that all of the human species is equal.

Aware consciousness is a state of awareness within our intellect and ego mind that has been reached through our knowledge of beliefs and habitual behaviors that must be changed. Aware consciousness occurs in an infinite range of awareness within multiple levels, becoming more advanced as we reach the transition of our mind and emotions into understanding. The immature soul journey has been spent in the expansion of our awareness to help us become conscious of the good within us.

Until we reach a state of aware consciousness of ourself as a whole being of matter, dual soul, and spirit consciousness, we will not be ready to transition into our mature soul. It is only when we are living from the collective consciousness of our dual soul mind and emotions that we will become conscious of the good within us. Recognizing that all humans are spirit consciousness who are learning the expansion of ourself into a collective consciousness of equality, unconditional love, and absolute truth will create a civilization for the first time on earth.

In our mature soul we have a consciousness of understanding ourself that must be lived and again expanded, allowing us to become totally conscious that we understand who we are, why we are here, and our purpose on earth as children of "God." A state of knowing within our mature soul mind and emotions will have been reached through understanding the relationship of scientific knowledge and our historical physical experience to our trinity of consciousness of being human. It is in understanding the general relativity of ourself as consciousness energy to the universe, nature, and earth that we begin to know who we are and see our purpose of creation and life. As we open our mind and emotions to understanding ourself we will see ourself as a fractal pattern of the universe and of our spirit consciousness.

Our collective consciousness is created from the thought and emotional energy that we all share. The energy streams of our collective consciousness have become commonplace as universal rivers of connected energy that are focused upon a single perception of thought and emotion, giving these rivers of energy the strength to change beliefs and behaviors within us, society, and the world.

When masses of people join together in a collective consciousness of negative and fearful thinking and emotions, destructive energy streams will occur in that level of consciousness, which will cause chaos within the culture. When masses of people join together in a collective consciousness of positive and loving energy, we will create a civilization. Smaller streams of collective consciousness are created by smaller numbers of people thinking and feeling the same way about any issue. It is the collective consciousness of the people of a nation that elects politicians and creates changes within society and our history as humans.

Original sin has become a collective consciousness within the masses of souls that live on earth. Since this belief has a long history of influence within the intellectual soul mind, it has become a karmic collective consciousness and can be present as part of the belief system even when we are not consciously aware that the belief affects our lifestyle and societal behaviors. Original sin was a belief that originated with St. Augustine in about A.D. 400 and it became part of the religious dogma. St. Augustine took the sexual superstition that had plagued man from the beginning of time and created the confusion as a Christian reality of sexual belief. St. Augustine thought that all humans are by nature depraved and sinful because of having been born from the original sexual lust of Adam which has been transmitted down through the generations to all of mankind. St. Augustine did not understand that sexuality is a biological need of all humans to assure that we live eternally as a soul. The belief in original sin became a collective consciousness with the spread of Christianity throughout the world. Our belief in original sin enhanced our judgemental thinking into a collective consciousness that has allowed fear, anger, judgement, and rage to be acted out in religious wars of violence, abuse, competition, and inequality as expected and accepted behavior.

Our belief in original sin as a collective consciousness joined with other religious beliefs about sex to create a collective consciousness of sin, guilt, and shame in relationship to all of our sexual behaviors. As a collective consciousness of souls we have been living in our depression of change for fourteen thousand years. Christianity was created during our depression with the belief that someone else would save us. Christian religion has been creating its collective consciousness since A.D. 43 and the mass consciousness energy has been growing within our soul consciousness. All souls share the collective consciousness of worship even though they may not physically support a religion.

The religious masses have always been fearful and judgemental about life after death. Without having an understanding of the invisible world, many "mysteries" were created in our thinking and emotions as primitive beings and have become multiple collective consciousnesses. Religion has preached blind faith in God and our dependency on the Messiah to save us rather than providing the available knowledge about creation. The religious belief that a single being has created the world, governs it, and controls the destinies of humanity by a specific set of laws acted out as beliefs, behaviors, rituals, and ceremonies has left many people doubting the validity of religion, and rightly so, as religion defies the power of our trinity of consciousness. Despite many who now disbelieve, the collective consciousness of religion as a cult continues.

Religion has played an important role in the expansion of awareness within the human mind and emotions of our immature soul. Once our transitional soul awareness expanded into knowledge, our soul found itself in the opposite consciousness of religious worship which has taught blind faith. An awareness of the motivation and development of religion in the human culture clearly shows how the material focus of religion was marketed to take advantage of the fear and ignorance in our soul. Religion has at all times opposed knowledge and has limited truth whenever it was possible as a means of control and dependency of the collective consciousness of mankind on religious beliefs.

Science became the collective consciousness of knowledge and deals with what is considered known fact. Science as a collective consciousness of knowledge and religion as a collective consciousness of blind faith worship began to play important and interesting roles in the collective consciousness of mankind.

The Messiah Complex is not unique only to religion but affects all of our relationships in life when we live with a worship belief as our consciousness. If we choose to see someone else as superior or inferior to us, we are living our inequality as a blind faith and our consciousness becomes a part of the collective consciousness of worship, which expands the power of inequality. Science, and particularly medical science, has set itself up as the Messiah of our physical body and mind and has jealously guarded its territory against any who appear to medicine as interlopers. Gradually through time medicine and religion have become competitors and science has become the very force that will bring about change in the collective consciousness of the masses. Insurance companies that now control the delivery of medicine to the people are raising the level of awareness that medical care is no longer being provided to serve the patient but as the monetary bottom line of control for the insurance companies. The collective consciousness that exists within the thinking and emotions of the people is the need to be saved from death and material ruin. Few people recognize that death eliminates the need to worry about the material side of life and that death is a part of life which is inevitable. The collective consciousness is again expanded by those worshipping medicine and insurance, which expands the collective consciousness of inequality.

When we have a collective consciousness of needing someone to save us, our ego is truly in competition with our spirit consciousness and the inherent design of our soul and spirit. Healing is at all times an internal transition to loving ourself and external approaches to healing are always temporary if they are not integrated with the internal transition of the dual soul from fear to love. When our collective consciousness is focused upon loving ourself, we will prevent the majority of diseases that are now considered terminal and we will change the focus of the collective consciousness.

Sexuality characterizes and distinguishes us by sexual identification and roles secondary to the accepted belief systems of the specific gender, defined by our sexual organs for procreation. Sexuality was the beginning of our soul lesson of inequality that has continued during the entire journey of our immature soul mind and emotions. For the past two thousand years we have acted out the Messiah Complex as blatant sexual inequality between the male and female which has been supported by both religion and science as they lived the inequality of the Messiah Complex. The collective consciousness of these two groups has placed women in an inferior position to the superiority of the male since their very beginning. Some slight progress is being made in both science and religion to become more equal but the collective consciousness of inequality is a challenge to unlearn and the karmic beliefs remain hidden, only to be acted out in covert tendencies of physical behavior.

It is not pleasant to look back at history and to acknowledge all of the abuse that has accompanied the lesson of inequality since the beginning of time. Looking at history in increments of one-hundred-year cycles, for the past two thousand years, will show us how we have focused as a collective consciousness on learning the lessons of inequality. The control, manipulation, seduction, and judgement of the male over the female is acted out in sexual relationships as well as every other aspect of our society. The irony for the immature soul is that we change sexes in many of our lifetimes so that we can experience our lesson of inequality through multiple images. As a soul we will always reap what we sow. When our collective consciousness expands to the level of understanding our dual soul mind and emotions, it will be important to follow the golden rule every moment of our life, rather than abusing ourself. In our mature soul we will always treat other people as we want them to treat us. When our soul mind has a karmic belief in inequality, it will be reflected into our everyday life without our conscious awareness. The collective consciousness of inequality has an impact on the individual's lesson of inequality.

The way that we choose to live our collective consciousness defines the awareness level that we have reached within our societal consciousness. Every moment that we live we think, speak, and behave from whatever level of consciousness that we have reached in our soul growth through knowledge. In the immature soul journey, it has been essential for us to become aware of ourself before we could reach the point of understanding ourself. Awareness of ourself includes our beliefs, behaviors, language, lifestyle, relationships, and consciousness from which we interact. This is the normal soul pattern of evolution that is supported by Einstein's General Theory of Relativity. We are in a state of constant movement in space and time and as a dual soul consciousness we are magnetized to the magnetic arc by the limbic system or alchemical vase of our dual soul and spirit.

General relativity is a fundamental concept of the nature of space, time, and gravitation. In the universal system this pattern is found in the expansion of space, through time and the gravitational force of energy. In us it is our expansion of consciousness, which has occurred through the relationship of space, time, and the gravitational force of the magnetic energy in the center of our brain. We do not have to believe it, be aware of it, or have a consciousness of our dual soul's constant gravitational pull for our immature soul to be moving along its journey by following the pattern of its design. Our intellect knows only that information which it has memorized in this lifetime. Our mature soul and the universal memory of our spirit consciousness have infinite knowing and continue to motivate and inspire the intellect toward greater and greater knowledge as we expand our consciousness on the mature soul journey.

If we are ignorant of ourself and life, we must expand into the knowledge of who we want to be and our limits are reflected into our ignorance or unawareness of who we are, what we believe, how we feel, and how our behavior of life is acted out. No one can give us knowledge unless we choose to search for knowledge. Exposure to knowledge will fall on deaf ears if our mind is closed. Knowledge will be absorbed like a sponge absorbs water if our mind is open. Knowledge is how we expand our consciousness. Knowledge supports our dual soul evolution into the expansion of consciousness, and gaining knowledge is our personal responsibility. It is within the dual soul level of knowledge that we transition from our immature soul journey to our mature soul journey. To deny knowledge is to deny our dual soul evolution.

We have lived from beliefs that reflect our ignorance of reality throughout the journey of our physical nature. Superstition, myths, parables, allegory, and hypnotic persuasion have fashioned our beliefs repeatedly in the shadow of our childish soul mind. These beliefs have been handed down as our karmic lessons through the generations of our soul and we have accepted them as fact through our ignorance. Our level of consciousness has changed very slowly, as our mature soul nudges us beyond our present belief system into the knowledge that we must have to bring about change. Our ego sees change as its death, and therefore resistance and denial is the nature of the ego when faced with new knowledge that is not relative to its belief systems. That is why the average intellect is motivated to read or watch dramas or crises rather than seeking new knowledge. Our intellect and ego are comfortable with repetition and will choose not to be challenged by knowledge.

We fear change because we are attached to our beliefs as our collective consciousness. Our beliefs have allowed us to repetitiously follow our perception of reality for billions of years. Our fear of change is also our ego fear of being wrong, which we perceive as our failure. These accumulated ego fears allow us to prefer ignorance over knowledge because if we maintain our ignorance as a collective consciousness, no one will see that we have been "wrong" and judge us as a failure. In our ego-focused closed mind it is better to continue our repetitious thought and beliefs rather than open our mind to new knowledge and understanding. Knowledge should be our lifetime commitment as a gift to ourself. Blind faith is our chaos of ignorance and it is the very foundation of the collective consciousness of inequality that permeates earth.

Knowledge shows us the meaning of life, our freedom, our power, our inherent wisdom, and the magnificence of the journey that we have lived as a soul that is learning to be consciously aware. Our behavior is the mirror of the level of consciousness that our mind and emotions have reached in their evolution. We can never hide our lack of knowledge or ignorance from anyone, yet we will be perceived by others through their level of knowledge. Ignorance has been created during the generations of our soul as the "sins" in the negative beliefs and behaviors of the "father," as the image of the family, which are passed on to the children. Beliefs and behaviors frequently exist as a family consciousness and a cult consciousness. This can easily be seen through our behavioral attachment of habitually going to church or as the behavior of sexual, physical, mental, and emotional abuse that is lived in multiple generations of the family and society as a collective consciousness.

Many people create the illusion of having gained knowledge and feel that they have reached their destination in life. Knowledge is our journey of life and there is no destination to knowledge because it continues to expand as we expand. Our ego will always limit our knowledge because our ego will challenge the knowledge to which we are exposed and dilute the power the knowledge has to change our beliefs. Our knowledge is in the throes of creation and expansion each and every moment that we breathe.

As mind energy we attach ourselves to like energy or we want to be like another's energy and we begin to worship that energy as the "absolute" in consciousness. This can be heard in the expression, "I want to be just like ____." Our need to copy another person's thinking and behavior holds us in the repetitious mode of a closed mind that is choosing to live through conformity. This allows us to create a hero worship for many human idols as our false gods, which we believe are superior to us. We frequently worship others because of a sexual attraction, even though we may not be conscious of the sexual component in our worship.

Since the time of St. Augustine man has conformed to the belief in original sin. This belief has become a collective consciousness of our soul which we carry with us karmically whether or not we have an aware consciousness of the belief. Therefore, sex has always led us into our collective consciousness of original sin, shame, and guilt as it has played the role of our "evil" ways. When a sexual attraction is involved in our hero worship, it can lead to violence, murder, and abuse because it will trigger our karmic belief in original sin and we will blame our depraved behavior on the one person that we are sexually lusting after. This trigger of our ancient soul belief in original sin is frequently the cause of violence in marriage and of illicit sexual liaisons. The collective consciousness of original sin supports the collective consciousness of sexual inequality between the male and female.

Sexuality was in reality created as a biological need of our individual collective consciousness of the trinity of our consciousness when we were created. As a biological need to provide procreation, sex has assured us of our return as a soul into a new physical life since the beginning of our journey as a living soul. Sex has no true connection to original sin and is not in itself sinful. Man has created his own beliefs about sin around his role of sex by allowing sex to control the physical lusting rather than allowing the ethical integrity of truth to control our passions. Sex plays three important roles in the collective consciousness of our physical body, dual soul, and spirit consciousness. Sex is designed as a means of procreation, as a magnetic energy between the male and female to keep us evolving in our magnetic arc of emotions, and for the pleasure of sensory stimulation of our spirit senses to expand our consciousness. These three dimensions of energy have kept the human consciousness focused on bringing our male and female consciousness together externally and internally.

We must be conscious of what we think, because we will create our thoughts as our physical behavior. Our integrity and our level of knowledge about sex creates the level of our consciousness reality within our mind about our sexual behavior in life. We allow our ignorance of our sexuality to control us rather than choosing to control our sexuality through knowledge. We continue to cling to and worship our basic sexual instincts rather than choosing our sexual partners wisely. Sexuality is used as a means of attraction and acts as a scale from which we then judge ourselves as unequal, inadequate, and worthless.

Our need to be loved is confused with sexuality, although sex and love are opposite and both are collective consciousnesses within our dual soul. Our intellect has never been adept at knowing the difference between sexual attraction and love. Sexual attraction also spurs us into our need to imitate those who we feel are more sexually attractive than we view ourselves. Our worship of "the sexual image" of ourself has led us into addictive behaviors that have grown into a collective consciousness within our society.

To want to imitate another individual or to worship that individual as crucial to our well-being limits our ability to grow as it creates a collective consciousness within us toward dependency on the individual who is being worshipped. There is no equality in the belief that we must think exactly like someone else and believe everything that we are told. Worshipping another person as a "physical idol" is an internal collective consciousness of our intellect and ego having reached our destination. Our worship of physical idols reaches far beyond just those to whom we feel a sexual attraction and becomes a desperate physical "need." Hero worship of sexual idols creates a collective consciousness that becomes a mass hysteria of conformity. Conformity and worship control our thinking, emotions, and feelings which keeps us a prisoner of our ego consciousness.

When large numbers of people are focused upon specific beliefs they create a collective consciousness of worship around that specific belief and see the belief as factual information. Information is always relative to the level of consciousness of the individual and can be accepted as the end of the journey for knowledge. As humans we adopt habitual beliefs and behaviors because we believe the information to be truth. Our focus on beliefs as "truth" can be handed down generation after generation and be repeated as "gospel" without being factual or having any semblance to truth.

Beliefs of antiquity are a challenge to support as fact. Because we grow consciously only when we live in the moment, we should not look back and dwell upon the past as truly representative of our present reality. When we dwell upon the past we can find our collective consciousness attaching us to beliefs and behaviors that will interfere with our immature soul evolution. The parable of Sodom and Gomorrah is an example. When Lot's wife turned to look at the cities burning she found herself dwelling upon the sins of the past and she turned into a pillar of salt. Salt is a crystal and as a crystal it was the first level of our Cycle of Development. This parable symbolizes our ability to devolve as a soul when we dwell upon the past. Both religious and Freudian concepts have managed to create a few "pillars of salt" among us.

As each of us searches for our truth, we must do so with a positive, independent, and open consciousness. We can feel truth in our heart as well as our mind and emotions. As we live the change of focus within our dual soul mind and emotions, the collective consciousness of the masses is undergoing an internal chaos. Each individual soul is challenging itself to give up its beliefs and behaviors of dependency, control, and fear as its collective consciousness. Our immature soul has lived in the collective consciousness of dependency, control, and fear as our symbol of blind faith from the beginning of its transition. Now we have the freedom of choice in where we focus our mind, emotions, and behavior. We are becoming leaders, not followers.

It is essential that we look at our beliefs, emotions, and behaviors to discover where our collective consciousness is focused. The old beliefs of inequality, control, conformity, and submissiveness are no longer valid for us as human beings, and if we attach ourselves to these negative levels of consciousness we hold ourself back from our internal growth. Old beliefs fear change. When we fear change, we contribute to our consciousness becoming stuck in the old beliefs and we react with denial to any concept of change in our level of knowledge.

Our fear is primarily based upon our fear of the unknown. "God" is the unknown. Judgement is the unknown. Death is the unknown. Punishment is the unknown. Change is the unknown. Many of our fears are based upon our fear of God, our fear of separation from God, and our fear of retribution from God. We have been taught the concept of repentance to get back into the good graces of God. The Greek word *"metanoia"* (translated as repentance) means "a spiritual transformation as a complete change of ideas and purposes." "Luther understood this fully when he wrote to Stampitz, his master and inspiration: 'Metanoia in the New Testament does not carry the ecclesiastical meaning: rather, to do penance means to transform oneself in one's inmost soul. For the Christian, therefore, doing penance is not an act that is performed at a stated time: it is a mode of conduct to be observed throughout one's whole life.'" (Marcello Craveri, *The Life of Jesus* [New York: Grove Press, 1967], 76).

Our belief that man is made in the image of God allows us to fear changing who we are because without our becoming conscious that we have made God in the image of man, we would feel we were separating ourself from God if we changed a single belief. We have a consciousness that we are not complete and lovable unless we are involved in an intimate relationship and feel loved by someone external to us. Our "need to be loved" is a collective consciousness that reflects our fear of separation from "God." In the image that we have of ourself as unworthy and inadequate, we constantly "need" that "Divine Nature of God" to save us from ourselves. We have been taught that man is the Divine Nature of God as the foundation of our collective consciousness of inequality.

We are not conscious that we see, define, and have created God in the image of our own male physical nature. We feel fearful and inadequate if we are not receiving the love that we want from another physical nature external to us. When we live with fear, we are not living with love. These are the opposite emotions of the dual soul and we focus on one or the other of these emotions, but we can't focus on both fear and love at the same time. We have created within our own mind a collective consciousness that believes we are inadequate and unworthy without someone external to us loving us in a sexual relationship, which in our collective consciousness is the image of God loving us. Our fear of not having a lover in our life is our fear of not having the love of our external "God" in our life. Since we have a belief that sex is love, our immature soul consciousness is addicted to wanting sex as love. As an intellectual collective consciousness we see sex and love as the same thing. Sex is the symbol of love in our physical nature and love is the emotion of our female divine nature. Herein lies the definition and function of the magnetic arc of our soul. Because the male and the female can be at opposite levels of consciousness, sexual communication comes from both levels of consciousness that are so far apart that understanding is impossible. Both the male and female "need to live" the perfect love story but they do not understand the dual soul; therefore, they do not have the knowledge to understand each other as love. Until we understand love as a collective consciousness internally, we will not live the perfect love story externally in our relationships. As our collective consciousness changes through our expanded knowledge, our love will create the beautiful relationships that our immature soul has dreamed about.

There is a collective consciousness of being leukwarm, or suppressing our emotions to the point of not feeling. At this time in our changing transitional soul being leukwarm means that we are stuck in fear without either thought or emotion providing us with the inspiration of life. Religious boredom and paralysis created leukwarm lives for many people. We are afraid to think, to experience emotions, or to feel. When we are leukwarm we act like a robot, simply living our beliefs by habit without thought, emotion, or feelings.

Fear is a cold emotion and it has a collective consciousness of its own. Fear is a cold emotion because it does not touch our heart. Fear functions within us from the coldness and cruelty of our fearful physical nature that lives without the emotion of love. The coldness of fear is where violence begins in our consciousness and expands into war. Anger and rage are deadly cold, but they both create the illusion of passion. Anger and rage are the iciness of ignorance, not passion.

Love is a passionate or hot emotion and exists within us as our spiritual passion for the miracle of life. Love is a hot emotion because we feel passionate about life and its issues, knowledge, change, and the love of ourself and other people. Our physical passion is a fleeting illusion. Our spiritual passion is eternal. When our consciousness comes from our loving mind and emotions and engages the entire three dimensions of our senses, we love life as our miracle and the journey that we are living becomes our passion. Passion and love can only exist when our senses are acute and our spiritual consciousness is expanded.

The collective consciousness of the masses that exists in fear must be balanced by the masses who live through their collective consciousness of love before we can overcome the fear. If we are leukwarm we have no light or whiteness in our mind and emotions; we are essentially living a colorless life captured and paralyzed in the darkness of our soul. Many souls are now living the leukwarm collective consciousness of habitual repetition, knowing not what they do to themselves or others. These are primarily souls that are captured in the collective consciousness of worship and fear and have no awareness of the repetition they are living as an immature soul.

Consciousness is the level of thought that exists within our mind and it is consistently being controlled by our belief systems. As long as we remain within our negative intellectual mind our internal level of consciousness creates our life from our unique level of conscious awareness that is limited by our interpenetrated beliefs as our ego. When our negative beliefs are predominant as our controlling mind-set of life, we hypnotize our senses, which controls the stimulation of our feelings and emotions. It is only through our emotions and feelings that we trigger our immature soul mind to release the negative beliefs. This is why we have suppressed the female or emotional part of ourselves from the beginning of our life as a living soul. Our collective consciousness of the inequality of the physical female acts as the reflection of the inequality that we feel within us towards our emotions and our internal female soul consciousness.

Each belief that we attach ourself to acts as a limitation to our divine female consciousness. When we let go of our beliefs, we are being open to explore and to understand new perceptions of consciousness by seeking knowledge. The life of every person is restricted by our belief system, which in turn restricts our consciousness. Our ego belief system does not welcome the concept of changing its rigid beliefs that we have become addicted to and accept as "fact." We use our addictive beliefs to repeat our adaptive habitual behavior and control our consciousness day after day and life after life, until we can let go of our beliefs and expand our consciousness of who we are through knowledge. Our judgemental beliefs about ourself create a collective consciousness of our fear of change. Our fear of change adds a new denial level within our immature soul consciousness.

As we adapt our habitual behavior to our addictive beliefs within a negative level of consciousness, we are personally affected. As we live our negative consciousness, we spread our particular level of denial consciousness into society and the many systems that control society. A negative consciousness level that has the energy of millions of people focused within it becomes a formidable energy force within our society. The energy of this expansive negative collective consciousness will create war, murder, chaos, and multiple external manifestations of anger and rage within people that we think are peaceful.

If a country is focused toward suppression of its people, fear and inequality is the level of the collective consciousness of the people. If a country is focused toward war, fear and inequality is the level of collective consciousness of the people. If a country believes in female suppression, fear and inequality is the level of collective consciousness of the people. If a country believes in its own supremacy, fear and inequality is the level of collective consciousness of the people. All of the multiple levels of fear and inequality as a collective consciousness are the levels that we have lived in the journey of our descending soul as a people, society, country, and nation and that are still being lived in the world society. Inequality and fear is the integrated foundation of the collective consciousness for our immature soul. Inequality and fear lead to judgement, control, dependency, and worship as the collective consciousness of our behavior in our immature soul.

Each of these collective consciousness levels has been created by an established belief system that is predominant within the people's consciousness and, therefore, each collective consciousness has controlled the way that we live as individuals. As people we become our society, race, culture, country, and nation as well as our own grandparents. We are not separate because our collective consciousness reaches out to affect everyone within the human race. As immature souls we return again and again to the same physical families to work through our beliefs as soul lessons of the collective consciousness of our individual soul agenda.

The collective consciousness within our soul and spirit, as a trinity of minds, functions from the eternal principle of equilibrium, equality, and balance that we are seeking within our dual soul mind and emotions and our spirit consciousness. The pre-

437

dominant collective consciousness of the people acts as the pre-dominant behavior within a family, group, religion, society, or country. It is through our personal level of collective conscious-ness that we create our reality with each thought, emotion, and feeling. We live our life from the level of our conscious mind, emotions, and feelings. If our consciousness is stuck in worship, foul language, negativity, abuse, violence, fear and hate, that is the focus of our behavior as a soul collective consciousness. Each individual focus of consciousness in turn creates the overall col-lective consciousness from which we behave as a group, a fami-ly, a culture, and as humanity.

As an immature soul seeking to find our equality, we must of necessity live the lesson of physical balance in every aspect of our lives. Balance is our personal responsibility, and although we may not be conscious of what we have lived as a soul, we have been choosing to consistently live the physical experiences that will guide us toward balancing our physical body, dual soul mind and emotions, and our spirit consciousness. When our intellectu-al beliefs and behaviors do not allow us to be open to our dual soul evolution, we store the real reasons for our physical experi-ences subconsciously in our ego as the cosmic shell of our beliefs that limits our thoughts and keeps us attached to fear.

At this moment in our immature soul evolution, we must become conscious of our journey as a living soul that is chang-ing and we must release all of our negative levels of conscious-ness, especially worship. In the conscious awareness of our mind and emotions, we can become aware of the hidden agenda in our intellect and ego consciousness. Our hidden agenda of denial is contributing to our collective consciousness of negative beliefs. When we are willing to examine the internal purpose of our fear behavior and feelings, we can see our change as positive and speed up our dual soul evolution. Knowing that our dual soul is our dual mind and emotions, and that it is our dual soul and spir-it that is using our physical body as a temple to experience the physical world, helps us to open our mind and emotions to new awarenesses without guilt or shame. Our fear of being wrong is a collective consciousness that allows us to judge ourself as being sinful, guilty, shameful, and worthless. Right versus wrong is a belief that has symbolized the opposite focuses of our dual soul.

When we live in fear and negativity we close down our mind and emotions, bringing ourself to the abyss of depression to get our attention. It is through experiencing depression, panic attacks, phobias, stress, anxiety, disease, drama, and chaos that we sense that we are at the bottom of our descending emotional soul and it is now time to go forward. As we become aware of our consciousness, we evolve as a soul. Our soul will challenge us over and over again to get our attention. Our challenges will happen in every facet of our life, until we feel that our life is literally falling apart and we have no concept of control left. Whenever we get too smug or too comfortable, we will create something within our lives to make us stop and look at who we are. The internal collective consciousness of our mature soul is challenging our immature soul to open our mind to change.

The collective consciousness of our mature soul is one of wisdom and love. The collective consciousness of our immature soul is one of ignorance and fear. It is our mature soul that is continually nudging us forward to look within ourself for the answers. Our mature soul mind and emotions knows the absolute truth of who we are as beautiful and magnificent humans, but our immature soul mind and emotions is afraid to look at ourself because it fears seeing its negative beliefs, judgements, and abusive behavior. Our collective consciousness of fear captures our intellect and ego in a collective consciousness of ignorance. As we have lived our immature soul journey in total ignorance of who we are, our ignorance has forced us to learn through our miracle of "life," the physical way. Our physical experiences have been our lesson of the collective consciousness in learning the art of creation as an immature soul purpose.

Our physical reality is structured from multiple levels of consciousness. Our consciousness focuses merge together to create streams of consciousness energy that exist upon earth at all times. When the rivers of consciousness are negative, earth itself begins to react to our negativity to bring the equilibrium back into balance between humanity, nature, and earth. As humans we are liv-

439

ing in the art of what we have created on earth and in nature.

As an example, a collective consciousness of disease in humans can only be balanced by restoring our physical body from the chemicals of nature and earth. Our mind and emotions can only be balanced by a collective consciousness of knowledge of ourself in relationship to nature and earth. Our spirit can only be balanced as the collective consciousness of our knowledge of the dual soul mind and emotions and our physical body in relationship to nature and earth. An individual consciousness of balance remains separate and does not have the unity of predominance as a collective consciousness to create the balance for humanity within nature and earth. Our collective consciousness of who we are, why we are here, and what our spiritual purpose is has the power to heal us, our life, nature, and earth. In our belief in separateness we have chosen to abuse earth, nature, and the heavens instead of recognizing them as our "Garden of Eden" and earth and nature as the paradise that was given to us to nurture us.

Because the consciousness of our dual soul lives within the Eternal Principle of Opposites, it has been necessary for us to experience living within separate fear consciousness before we would accept the unity of a collective healing consciousness. Our negative, fearful collective consciousness has allowed us to descend into the depths of despair and illusion before our consciousness could ascend to the peak of ecstasy. As our descending emotional soul reaches the very pit of illusion it has the power to change its consciousness and resurrect itself collectively into the positive light of love. Having the equilibrium to balance the collective consciousness into love means that each of us as people must be personally responsible for seeking change within ourselves. Without a collective consciousness of personal responsibility, we have the power to stay stuck in the collective consciousness of fear, dependency, and ignorance as we destroy everything around us.

There are many groups today that have developed a collective consciousness of fear, dependency, and ignorance. Part of the ignorance and fear of these groups is their dependency upon worshipping someone else who is also responsible for saving them. Their intense fear of what will happen to them if no one accepts the responsibility for their salvation controls their lives and keeps them from searching for knowledge. These individuals seek their saviors in idol and guru worship, religion, science, and sexuality and in each group we can define a collective consciousness of an identified savior.

Religion is a major collective consciousness of our physical nature. Religious groups are a predominant collective consciousness in the world today and their fear, dependency, and ignorance are overwhelming. Religion as a collective consciousness has begun devolution because of its intense focus on female suppression and inequality. Whether the group is a large accepted religious group or a small and unknown group, their dependency and fear controls their lives and keeps them on their path of conformity. Their fear of judgement and punishment from an external God holds them in a paralyzed mental and emotional state. Their hypnotic state of mind is an extreme form of stasis that is the final attachment of the ego to the collective consciousness of pain and suffering. Worship beliefs are acting as the elixir of hypnosis that focuses the mind into a collective consciousness of superstition, myth, and paranoid persuasion which shuts down the three dimensions of senses within the physical body.

In this last stage of pain and suffering man sees himself as conforming to the consciousness of Jesus at his death as he was ransomed by God for the sins of the faithful. This belief is a fearful interpretation of the crucifixion, resurrection, and apocalypse which has served as the basis of the religious belief system in the physical nature of the immature soul mind and emotions. All religious beliefs have their basis in the negative, fearful interpretation of the mind and emotions of our male physical nature which is not a true interpretation of Creation, God, or Jesus. Man has proclaimed his image as God, and through his art of creation of religion he has created the illusion as fact in the collective consciousness of the masses.

All religious groups are cults that control the beliefs and lifestyles of their followers while teaching them that without this

441

control they will not be saved. When we focus on Jesus saving us we live through the fear of blind faith and we are dependent and controlled by our fear of punishment from God if we change our focus from our blind faith to knowledge. Blind faith is a collective consciousness of immense proportions at this time for humanity and as "blind faith" it depends upon ignorance, which is the opposite of knowledge.

Science is another major collective consciousness of our physical nature. Science is also a predominant collective consciousness in our society, and it is dependent upon a lack of emotion and consciousness of the invisible energy within us, which limits its consciousness to relative truth which is ignorance. Scientists are also prone to fear because death in a one-life philosophy is the unknown. It is for this precise reason that medical science has waged a war of competition between life and death from the beginning of its existence. Our fear is expanded into a collective consciousness of "blind faith" in medicine to save us from the unknown, and death remains the unknown when the dual soul and spirit is not understood.

Science teaches mankind fear in its perception of medicine as our only path of healing. Our dependency upon science as another savior is another consciousness of blind faith and ignorance because all of science is relative to the limited consciousness of the scientists themselves. The focus of science on external cause reflects the limited consciousness of the perception of humanity, nature, and earth. The need of medical science to have all of humanity conform to its way of thinking shows the power of the ego's fear and dependency. The blind faith that man has in medicine's power to save the body is also a collective consciousness of immense proportions. At this time there is a collective consciousness that is shared between religion, science, and sexuality that holds the human species in the bondage of inequality and this allows our fear of change to pivot on the sexual issue because of the male control of science, religion, and our world cultures.

The first major collective consciousness that is attached to our physical nature is our belief in the inequality between the male and female. The male and female inequality issue has allowed sexuality to constantly perpetuate the belief that the male is supreme over the female. The male belief in inequality has created fear, dependency, and control over the female from the beginning of our immature soul. Male sexuality as a collective consciousness has exercised tremendous power as a fearful method of control within humanity that has increased with the increased descent of our emotional soul. Sexuality has been misinterpreted by our physical nature as the physical act of love and as humans we have judged ourself in relationship to our sexual image. The sexual image controls our society and all of its multiples of collective consciousness. This collective consciousness is so intense that it controls our economic foundation as corporations, government, politics, judicial system, health care, education, and the entire media complex, and it has become the "life-force" of our society. The male physical nature on earth has a collective consciousness of itself as superior to the female that lives as a karmic belief within the cosmic shell and is acted out in the sexual behavior.

Both the male and female live in their physical nature throughout the immature journey of the soul. The male is focused upon the mind and the female is focused upon the emotions to enhance our awareness of the duality of our soul. The collective consciousness of the mind and emotions within the physical nature of both the male and female has played the game of life as a scripted drama of sexual interaction. Our limited collective consciousness of the roles that are played by both the male and female has allowed us to live our dramas of sexuality as the mature soul lesson of equality while being acted out in our physical nature as inequality, control, abuse, and dependency.

At this point in our transition both the male and female have an intellectual and ego attachment to their physical nature that is being acted out as a resistance and denial of change. The resistance and denial, which we live in learning to let go of our focus on our physical nature, is our collective consciousness of sexual need. Sexual needs spawn sexual abuse, pedophilia, pornography, explicit sexual behavior, violence as sexual crimes, promiscuity, adultery, and teenage sexuality, which our addictive beliefs live as conformity in our fear of change.

Our belief in an external God is a collective consciousness that exists karmically within our immature soul whether or not we have a conscious belief in God during this lifetime. We had to believe in a judgemental, fearful, and angry God during our past lives for us to reach the opposite belief in a loving God during this lifetime. Our soul mind and emotions function from the Eternal Principle of Opposites, so first we must have a consciousness of our beliefs before we can become conscious of the importance of releasing the belief and living from the opposite perception of life. Our God consciousness has kept us aware of our indwelling spirit consciousness and has acted as the bridge for our dual soul to learn to acknowledge itself. As we have created each of our beliefs as our external world, we have surrounded ourselves with our fears and our rage. It is our fear and our rage as a collective consciousness of worship that has denied our indwelling spirit consciousness.

Our belief in Jesus is a collective consciousness that has overwhelmed society within the past nearly two thousand years as a dependency on being saved. This belief has escalated during the period since Jesus fulfilled his mission on earth in A.D. 30, although the belief in the Messiah occurred many years before Jesus' birth. Many other "gods" have played the role of the needed "Messiah" for our physical nature as a way of guidance and teaching. We have a collective consciousness that expects Jesus as the Messiah or Christ to save us, which allows us to avoid the personal responsibility that each of us has to save ourself and it reflects our need to create our sexual image as our savior. Only superstitious fear of "evil spirits" is the basis of our belief that we need to be saved.

In 2030, two thousand years will have passed since Jesus refused to accept the role of the Messiah and left his mission on earth. In leaving Jesus gave man the opportunity to save himself by seeking the truth of his personal responsibility to transition into his mature soul. The need to be a savior or to be saved is another image of the immature soul lesson we are living as

444

inequality. We have no recognition of our personal power of creation. To set ourself up as a savior or want to be saved reflects how we live our collective consciousness of fear and inequality because we must see ourself as better than or less than to play either role in life.

Historically our beliefs in Jesus are patterned from the earlier beliefs in Hermes and various other "gods" that were worshipped in various periods of our ancient cultures. Both Hermes and Jesus were known as "The Good Shepherd" and "The Lamb of God." The image of Jesus on the cross has developed a collective consciousness of Jesus being crucified that has become "fact" for many people. Because people believe in the pain and suffering that God "allowed" Jesus to suffer in death, the collective consciousness of death as pain and suffering has been created since the image of Jesus is seen as superior to the image of ourself.

The Christ Consciousness is a collective consciousness of our indwelling spirit consciousness that is expanding within the divine nature of our soul. It is the internal divine nature and spirit consciousness that is the collective consciousness of our mature soul that is designed to be the internal journey of saving ourselves as we evolve as an integrated soul. Our belief in Jesus saving us has acted as a bridge to the consciousness realization of how we are to live as Jesus lived to save ourselves. Many of the interpretations of Jesus and his life are relative truth and should not be worshipped as "fact." By experiencing the collective consciousness of dependency on being saved, we can now understand the independence that we must live to save ourself and experience our internal Christ Consciousness.

As we have descended as an immature soul we have lost touch with the memory of our creation as part of earth. Our earth consciousness is returning as the bridge to create the collective consciousness of understanding our chemical relationship to earth within ourselves. We are a trinity of consciousness energy that lives in harmony as humanity, nature, and earth. During the billions of years of living in the darkness of our immature soul journey, we have had little and many times no respect for nature or earth. We have lived as a collective consciousness with the illusion that we can destroy nature and earth and continue to live as humanity. With the power of our scientific belief "that all food is good food" we have seen ourself as separate from nature and earth. We have created this illusion of separateness from nature and earth as a collective consciousness. It is this misguided scientific belief that has created the widespread diseases of our present society, which also includes the separateness approach to healing as treating our various body parts with the use of toxic chemicals.

Our collective consciousness has existed from ignorance, greed, and materialism and has led us into disease without our having the knowledge to see the destruction that our unaware consciousness has brought unto itself. Despite our ignorance the earth consciousness has been here to support us and will continue to be here as our support unless we destroy it. Nature and the weather events of earth have joined together to raise our level of consciousness and bridge the separateness belief that we have lived. When we love and nurture both nature and earth, they will nurture humanity.

The inherent earth consciousness of humanity is the consciousness of being matter as part of earth. It is our earth consciousness that has allowed us to live at a different vibrational energy in matter and to experience our dual soul lessons through our physical experience. The earth consciousness provides a strong collective consciousness energy for all of humanity that protects, nourishes, and teaches the mental, emotional, and physical being of all humans. As we experience the balance of our descending soul emotions and our ascending soul mind we can consciously hear the diva spirits of nature talking to us to help us understand the collective consciousness of earth.

Our universal consciousness is inherent within our unconscious universal memory. It is through our spirit consciousness that we begin to fully understand our relationship to the universe. The multiple universal collective consciousness streams are always supporting us and giving us the time that we need as human beings to grow into an understanding of ourself. The universal consciousness is the guardian consciousness of our dual soul and spirit consciousness and provides for us the consciousness streams that bridge the physical world as we know it with the soul and spirit world that we remain unconscious of in our immature soul mind and emotions.

The universal consciousness acts as a storage of consciousness energy. All energy that has been is today. Energy that is stored in the universal collective consciousness has the light of spirit within it and it is used to protect the universe, earth, all planets, and all species that live on those planets. The universal consciousness moves with total harmony and rhythm, creating synchronicity, fluidity, and balance within the universal collective consciousness when the collective consciousness is positive. When the consciousness streams are negative, the universe, earth, and nature will experience chaos.

Collective consciousness streams that are negative cannot be stored in the universal consciousness but exist as part of the earth collective consciousness within the souls that are captured by the immature soul mind and emotions. The universal consciousness is a collective consciousness of love, truth, and equality combined with faith, trust, and understanding. This is the collective consciousness of the Spirit Realm of the Universal Consciousness. The immature soul consciousness can be and is negative as an earth consciousness.

The consciousness that we have been living is the intellect and ego mind consciousness of our immature soul and it is affecting earth and humanity as a collective consciousness. We have lived with a collective consciousness in this focus for billions of years. Throughout these years we have developed multiple collective consciousnesses from the belief systems that we have attached ourself to by our intellect and ego mind consciousness with each belief that we accept as fact. This is the negative collective consciousness that affects people on earth today as chaos, which is inviting all slumbering immature souls to awaken to change.

We have lived this collective consciousness as our beliefs and behavior since the beginning of our living soul. Our collective consciousness of placing blame on an external focus, judging others by our own belief systems, competition, war, fear with its accompanying judgement, control, dependency, anger, conformity, rage, worship, and rebellion have all been the focus of our immature soul mind and emotions. Our religious, scientific, and sexuality beliefs have all become collective consciousnesses of our intellect and ego mind and they are the primary source today of our collective consciousness of worship. All three of these major collective consciousnesses are interpenetrated and act as one negative stream of consciousness for humanity.

Our blind faith has been external to us and we have become dependent upon someone else saving us, which means that our collective consciousness continues to be external as an earth consciousness rather than an internal consciousness of personal responsibility and power. The collective consciousness of inequality is an example of the interpenetration of our collective consciousness. Faith in our immature intellect and ego is lived as a dependency and denies the knowledge of our dual soul and spirit that gives us independence. Our collective inequality consciousness between the male and female has been conformed to as "the word of God," and some women today have the belief that "submission is an honor." Others have found the control and dependency, the inequality, and the mythical religious beliefs totally unacceptable. This collective consciousness must gain in strength to become the greater collective force to bring about change.

Our intellect and ego mind has created multiple cultures with various religious cults with different beliefs that have formed into the collective consciousness of controlling and dependent cults. A cult is: "any religious organization that controls the beliefs and lifestyle of its followers especially with rituals, ceremonies, etc." (*The New Shorter Oxford Dictionary,* 1993, s.v. "cult."). The collective consciousness of humanity has been controlled by various cults from the beginning of time, and long before we began the level of knowledge as a soul. Religious rituals and beliefs have held us in a collective consciousness of judgement, shame, guilt, sin, and powerlessness as we have been taught to be controlled and dependent on the beliefs of the "leaders" of these religious cults to save us. The collective consciousness that we "need" to be saved by an external God has shut out the image of our divine nature and spirit consciousness within our intellectual mind. By creating a collective consciousness that we are a "child of God," we will be capable of changing our image from being saved to an image of saving ourself when we accept with an open mind new concepts of God as our indwelling spirit consciousness. Having a collective consciousness of ourselves as a trinity of consciousness lets us create our world with the power of love.

Our collective consciousness that the Old Testament is the undeniable "word of God," which is believed to have been recorded around 1650 B.C., allows us to think that no one else has the power to hear the "word of God." As we enter into our mature soul we will realize that each of us, as a child of our spirit consciousness, can hear the voice of "God" speaking to us within our trinity of consciousness. There is no logic to the belief that only a few rather old Jewish men that were alive about four thousand years ago could at one time hear the "word of God" but no one else has that same ability. As humans we all have equal capabilities but we focus on only a certain number of lessons in a lifetime.

The Torah was spoken by "God" to Moses and is used as the first five books of the Old Testament known as the Pentateuch. The Zohar was spoken by "God" to Moses de Leon (1255-1305) and uses many passages that were given earlier to the older Moses with a different interpretation that was essential because of the difference in the time. The Zohar is said to consist of approximately 2,500 pages. In the mid-1500s A.D. another Moses, Moses Cordovero, and Isaac Luria produced additional Hebrew manuscripts. As far back as Moses of Egypt there was speculation that Moses was plagiarizing the teachings of Hermes. History shows that our beliefs go a lot further back than 1650 B.C. The parables have been passed down for many thousands of years as mythology and have been repeated for aeons of time. The collective consciousness of our religious beliefs is stored only in our subconscious ego mind and can be repatterned into our intellect in each lifetime until the beliefs are learned as soul lessons. Our beliefs that have evolved from our myths, superstitions, symbols, and rituals all have expansive collective consciousnesses in our immature soul today. Truth is stored in our mature soul of the divine nature and our universal mind of spirit consciousness.

When Moses de Leon was communicating with "God" he was well aware that revealing the information as it was spoken to him through his own mind as he sat silently at his table would leave it unmarketable to the average man. Once again Moses de Leon, as the Moses before him, concealed the secrets of the information and wrote in a vernacular of the times that would sell itself to the masses. The concealed information is cloaked in symbolism and allegory that was popular at the time, and that made it easier for the people of the day to believe in their mythical gods, superstition, and ritual. When Jesus came he, as those before him, spoke in parables, conveying his messages allegorically, wrapped in the garments of the time that could be recognized. "The word of God" is always given for the times, as it is being given today. The collective consciousness of these ancient beliefs remains with us today as karmic beliefs. Now we have grown into the level of revelation and rebirth for our immature soul and we have the ability to hear the truth and recognize it from our heart of spirit memory.

Spiritual information always allows man to see why it is important to live by the spiritual values that are inherent within us. Our spirit consciousness has kept humanity on the immature soul journey of searching to understand ourself through love. In each instance all spiritual information is around for awhile before it hits the best seller list. True spiritual information has always had its dissenters because of our collective consciousness of worship and dependency. But once "God" as an external presence became the belief of the collective consciousness, this ancient information, more than any other information, has remained the foundation of our collective consciousness beliefs on a karmic basis because truth is concealed within the words.

As humanity reaches the time of change from the immature soul mind of knowledge to the mature soul mind of understanding, we must examine the collective consciousness that we have been living and accept that our fear and inequality do not serve us anymore. Karmic beliefs have occurred as the beliefs of our immature and unaware consciousness, and as the focus of our soul changes we must be willing to let go of the collective consciousness that was formed from within our superstitious mind and fearful emotions as external fear and inequality.

All of my books are given to me as "the word of my indwelling spirit consciousness." Reading them over and over will help you move yourself through the infinite levels of your mind consciousness until you reach the level of understanding knowledge. Each one of us possesses the same capability as the sages of old. The difference now is that we are all moving into that precise understanding and emotions of love in greater and greater numbers. Information is now being given as truth and not relative truth that wears the garments of the day as a cloak to create an illusion.

We live as vital members of humanity and we must work with a loving collective consciousness of our truth. Some people are ready to transition into their mature soul and others are not. Those who are ready for understanding will be empowered through the truth of knowledge and become the leaders of our society as we flirt with our first level of civilization. Those who are not ready for the current force of our mature and loving soul will be dissenters living in denial of self in the same way that people have before them.

Our dual soul lives within the Eternal Principle of Opposites with the only difference being our conscious internal knowledge of our freedom of choice, intention, and will. Searching for knowledge with a true understanding of how all knowledge relates to us is our personal responsibility. Our mature soul is now seeking knowledge with the intention to understand all available knowledge in relationship to ourself, nature, and earth. When we live the collective consciousness of our equality, absolute truth, and unconditional love, we will be firmly into our integrated soul consciousness and fully in touch with our spirit consciousness. The power of our conscious knowledge when it is understood in relationship to our human body will give us answers as quickly as we can ask questions.

It is with the advanced souls who are ready to transition that living the collective consciousness of change is of great importance. Our dual soul is organized by the Eternal Principle of Equality. The collective consciousness of understanding ourself must be able to have dominion over and balance the fearful and unequal collective consciousness of humanity on earth before we can begin the journey of our mature soul. The collective consciousness of the physical world and the fear and inequality experiences that we live in our physical nature will not change until the masses begin the ascension of the emotional soul. When this soul rebirth happens we will have a new world that is changing because we are changing our collective consciousness as humans and we will perceive life as good and loving.

There are many collective consciousnesses that exist within our unique society that can act as a deterrent to evolution. Two of the most intense ego collective consciousnesses of the mind focus upon blind faith and worship. We are living in the soul level of knowledge and being stuck in blind faith and inequality is the exact opposite of knowledge. Blind faith and inequality both severely limit our knowledge and our awareness of reality, because to have blind faith and to worship we must be stuck in the ignorance of inequality and live the expectation that someone external to us will save us.

The consciousness of blind faith has been taught throughout the world by religions and dictates that we follow the dogma of different religions without asking questions such as, "why?" Accepting dogma without knowing why the rules have been made, the value of the rule to you, what is the purpose of the rule, does it serve everyone equally, leaves us in the ignorance of blind faith. Accepting scriptural interpretations that are not understood, where the interpretation is not equal, where the history of the religion itself is not known, is placing blind faith in the religious beliefs.

Blind faith in anything creates a dependency on the information being truth. Blind faith removes our curiosity, motivation, and inspiration to expand our mind and emotions. Blind faith also creates a dependency on someone else saving us, taking care of us, feeding us information, finding us a job, providing us with money, entertaining us, and generally taking our creativity away from us because we do not understand the value of self-motivation and personal responsibility. Blind faith allows us to live our inequality. Blind faith is a collective consciousness that comes from the primitive soul mind and suppresses our female emotions.

When large groups within a society live in blind faith and inequality they live with a closed mind and the creativity within that society is limited, making others responsible for that part of the society that is dependent. Collective consciousness streams affect daily life and belief patterns in all of society. Buying into beliefs that are established through blind faith and inequality creates adaptive habitual behaviors that are destructive and reflect the repetitious mentality of a follower. We have lived the collective consciousness of our immature soul by blindly acting out our adaptive habitual behaviors as our perception of reality. Now our beliefs and behaviors are not creating harmony in our world and both our beliefs and behaviors must change for us to evolve as a loving and mature soul.

Our present collective consciousness of drugs being a quick-fix for all of our ills is a good example of beliefs and dependency. When we have a collective consciousness of drugs curing all of our ills we will not differentiate between prescription drugs, over-the-counter drugs, and street drugs. Each collective consciousness that we have creates a "mind-set" of fact within us that allows us to follow the herd. Our herd mentality is a collective consciousness of blind faith that keeps us from asking questions. The collective consciousness of dependent beliefs and behaviors that was created from the dependency on prescription drugs by the parents and society is now repeated in the child as a dependency on street drugs. The "sins" of the parent can always be found in the next generation of the soul as it is repatterned in the child by the family and society. Our "mind-set" that drugs can heal us has gone out of control and become our nemesis. A transitioning soul will attempt to break the repetitious pattern of the collective consciousness of the parents and not accept drugs on blind faith.

Other children will be followers of the collective consciousness, which slows down the growth of society by stopping the creativity of individual thought. Whenever a society adopts the "herd" mentality, as it has with religion, inequality, and drugs, it creates a victim and poverty consciousness that is overwhelmed with fear. Fear allows the collective consciousness to continue with habitual behavior and beliefs until the individual can absorb the knowledge to balance out the collective consciousness mentalities that have the power to lift the mind out of the fear belief system. Our consciousness is always limited by our awareness of "ourself" in relationship to our internal consciousness. When the focus is upon the external realities and is a consciousness of blind faith, dependency and addictions are the normal result because personal responsibility is not accepted as part of our behavior.

When parts of society focus on the collective consciousness of materialism they do so at the expense of the follower and the marketing intention is to connect to the collective consciousness of the dependent mind that accepts what it hears on blind faith. Each and every person has free choice, free intention, and free will. As we come into the period of transition of our dual soul, we are being challenged to use our mind freely and independently as we make our choices wisely. The materialism and greed in our society has become self-centered and unequal and people create fear within their lives as they become victims of their need for materialism.

Each individual consciousness creates a belief that is seen as truth for that specific mind focus and is relative to its specific level of awareness. This allows those souls that have blind faith and dependency to act them out in the behavior that is appropriate to their level of awareness. The more ignorant a mind is of the internal self and the responsibility that we have to use our freedom of choice, intention, and will, the more dependent we will be on blind faith. As we live in the follower mentality and create a poverty and victim consciousness as our collective consciousness with fear, inequality, and dependency, we will also fear change.

Group cultures come closer to having a like mind than others in society. Groups are made up of families, friends, co-workers, interest groups, career groups, politicians, races, ethnic groups, religions, scientific, sexual, and military focuses, schools, and any other group that has similar beliefs. When any one of these groups tries to control the "flock" with a specific organized set of rules, rituals, ceremonies, beliefs, and lifestyle behaviors they create a collective consciousness among the group. These groups then become a "cult" because of the blind faith and dependency upon the collective consciousness of the group. Today our society is formed of multiple cults that compete for power and control. All cults worship a "leader" who focuses upon control, dependency, and blind faith to survive.

There has been an ongoing hostility between the "cult" mentality of blind faith and gnosticism or knowledge since the beginning of the level of knowledge for our soul. Knowledge has the power to change the collective consciousness and open the mind to our creative powers. Blind faith and knowledge are opposites within the dual soul mind and emotions. Blind faith is the "I believe" approach that is opposite to the "I know" approach of science. "I believe" suppresses our mind and emotions and "I know" limits our mind and emotions. Knowing occurs only when information can be directly related to understanding ourself. Knowledge can result in true knowing only when we have an understanding of the relationship of the knowledge to our internal self.

Our ego fears its own emotions, which are judgement, anger, and rage, that are acted out in our behavior at multiple levels of intensity. The personal responsibility that we must accept to learn all that we can learn and make our own free choice about life is not a popular concept because we have been taught blind faith which supports our fear of the unknown. Knowledge sets us free. Knowledge changes the unknown to the known. It is important to create a collective consciousness of knowledge as the truth and understanding of ourself.

Our male and female role and identity is another widespread collective consciousness that has had a dramatic impact on our evolution as a dual soul. The collective consciousness of our role and identity as either a male or female has been defined by religion and we have accepted the religious collective consciousness as our belief and lifestyle. Our acceptance of the religious role and identity of the sexes has controlled our belief and made dependency and control part of the blind faith of the relationship since the beginning of the level of knowledge for our immature soul.

We still worship the sexual role and identity in many respects, especially if we are religious. This worship has led to the soul lesson of inequality that we have lived as human beings. Very few females challenged the submissive, unequal role that was cast as the life of the female until this century. Until recently no one successfully challenged the belief of male possession of the female and children as male chattel. When we accept in blind faith that the female is owned by the male, then abuse is permitted at the discretion of the male. Our belief in inequality has supported the abuse of women, children, and non-aggressive men from the beginning of our immature soul. This blind faith approach to the male and female roles and identities has held our soul evolution in the abyss of ignorance for billions of years.

The collective consciousness of homosexuality has been increasing over the past few decades. Homosexuality as a consciousness has always been present within the immature soul journey. Its role as a collective consciousness has come into being in the past thirty years. Homosexuality is playing an important role in the life of humanity today because it is allowing us to learn to love our own self-image. Society has accomplished wonders in causing us to worship our sexual image, not only in our sexual roles and identities but also in our physical sexual self-image. To use the love of the same gender as a way to love being male or to love being female shows us that as a soul we are both male and female and this helps us learn the internal soul lesson of equality and love.

In the dual gender focus of our dual soul, we can behave as either a male or female regardless of our physical gender. In homosexuality the individuals are matching the focus of the soul persona image of gender rather than attracting the physical opposite of the body. As a soul mind and emotions homosexuals will continue to attract the opposite. As a soul lesson homosexuality is also bringing equality into our collective consciousness with an intensity that we have experienced before in the struggle for equal rights for women, ethnic cleansing during World War II, and the race riots in our society. These lessons of discrimination are soul lessons of equality that have all been designed into this last one-hundred-year cycle of our immature soul. Each has been a valuable lesson at this time for our dual soul because we are learning to balance our mind and emotions as well as the male physical nature with the female divine nature of our soul to see that all humans are equal in every aspect of our being.

The other major collective consciousness that is affecting all of our society today and many other nations on earth is the material collective consciousness. This collective consciousness motivates many collective behaviors among the masses that are seen in our daily living. Our attachment to materialism allows us to live a collective consciousness of poverty, victimization, greed, untruthfulness, meanness, and paranoia and at the same time feel that we are superior to others. The material collective consciousness is our immature soul acting out our fear of survival. Money and possessions have become the way of self-judgement of our fear of survival.

Money and possessions only have value within our mature soul when they are used to help others, but our belief in hoarding comes from the superstition and myths that we need our money and possessions to go with us to be accepted by God. The old myths that we are ransomed by God before we can enter heaven are no longer acted out in our burial practices but that does not mean that we are free of the karmic belief that makes us obsessively and compulsively feel the need to accumulate great wealth. Our fear of survival is connected to our fear of death and fear of God as a massive collective consciousness that allows us to hoard more money and possessions than we can ever use or enjoy. These fears create a collective consciousness within the mass consciousness that allows fear to control our living and self-judgement to be rampant.

Whatever belief that we have is undoubtedly shared by millions of other people as a collective consciousness. It is the sharing of beliefs that creates a collective consciousness as an energy stream within our universal soul. It is these precise energy streams that we are intimately dealing with as we face the change from our immature soul to our mature soul. In understanding how the force of these energy streams creates resistance to change, we can acknowledge our need to change and let go of our beliefs that create each collective consciousness of resistance and denial for our dual soul.

These are only a few of the collective consciousnesses that we are actively living today that are beneficial and loving to our soul. The numbers of collective consciousnesses are infinite in our minds and emotions, and, therefore, within the universal system of earth. When two or more bind together on earth, they bind together in the universal energy of thought. So as we share our thoughts with others we always create a collective consciousness of those who think as we do. In sharing our lessons of soul evolution we touch the heart and emotions of those seeking knowledge. Understanding ourselves as a spirit consciousness that is learning to be human is the collective consciousness of our divine nature.

THE MATURE SOUL AND
OUR POWER OF CREATION

As we have lived in our immature soul, we have been learning the art of creation by creating our thoughts, emotions, and beliefs externally as our physical reality. Because we are living in our physical nature, creating our thoughts, emotions, and feelings as our physical reality has been perfect to help us become comfortable with our external art of creation.

As our consciousness expands and we become aware of how we create externally from our negativity and fear, we will see the wisdom of choosing to create from our internal, positive thoughts and emotions of love. The more we change our focus of thinking, emotions, and feelings into our loving self the more positive and loving we become and our society becomes. As we have created externally, we have not been consciously aware that we create our own reality moment by moment as we live. One reason that we suppress our consciousness of our art of creation is because we do not look at our own thoughts, language, and behavior but we look externally at the thoughts, language, and behavior of others and copy or conform to our external observations.

Each time that we have had a perception of reality, we have "struggled" to make it real as a part of our physical reality. As we heard prophecy we turned the words into our perception of reality as a belief, created the physical belief into "fact" as a superstition, and supported it with an external, physical place, object, ritual, or symbol that fit our vision of the words. When we were given the information on the Ark of the Covenant we created a physical box, covered it with veils, and created beliefs about the box, which we worshipped as sacred. We made our "God Consciousness" into the image of man and then we worshipped man. We made our perception of heaven and hell into real physical places that we imagined to exist and we put gatekeepers in place to manage these physical places. Our image of "God" was given the gates of heaven to manage and our image of hell was handed over to the "devil." This has all been the physical part of learning the art of creation for our immature soul.

What we have proven to ourself is our ability to create from our thinking, emotions, and feelings. We have not proven that everything that we have created along the path of our immature soul has been truth, but we have proven that we can take our thoughts, emotions, and feelings and make them real as our external physical creation. Because of our need to worship someone or something as superior to us, we have not lived truth as part of our creation. Worship is our focus on inequality. Inequality is not our truth because we were created equally as a male and female consciousness. If we worship man as superior to woman, we create inequality for the woman. If we worship our dependency and the control of religion as superior to our independence and freedom, we create inequality within our physical lives by discrimination, especially between the male and female, but it also spills over and is created as our mental and emotional beliefs in every facet of our external physical lives. As we have been learning the skill and knowledge of the art of creation, we have been learning to respect our own ability to create.

If we worship science we limit our knowledge because of our perception that science has all of the intellectual answers, but science holds our emotions as unequal to our mind. Because science has separated itself into individual disciplines the communication of scientific discoveries within the separate disciplines has been held concealed within the individual sciences for many centuries. Revealing the discoveries of science was seen as an emotional exposure for many centuries, and scientists were fearful of judgement from their colleagues and religion. The competition and the fear that exists within the mind and emotions has always served to conceal truth in our external society as we have lived our immature soul journey.

In the dance of life within our descending soul, we must balance our emotions with our mind or we limit our perception of reality. Worshipping our intellect as superior to our emotions is the behavior of inequality within our own soul mind and emotions of our left brain consciousness. We create our reality within our level of consciousness when we see ourself as superior or inferior in any way to another person. The inequality and emotional suppression that we have lived is teaching us to respect and value our power of creation.

Our beliefs in inequality have allowed us to create the physical behavior of discrimination of the sexes, races, education, handicapped, aged, money, possessions, and status. As we have made our thoughts, emotions, and feelings into the physical reality of our beliefs and behaviors, we have created the world that we know. Our fear has created our need for competition instead of cooperation. Some societies have created more sophistication and others have created more war and abuse. What we create depends upon the knowledge that we have learned, which changes our consciousness of our art of creation to our power of creation. Knowledge that is learned only as "fact" has no emotions that help us relate our knowledge to the reality of us as human beings. It is only when we balance our ascending mind and our descending emotions that we can create the equal dance of life that will transition us into our power of creation.

We have lived in the physical nature of our immature soul as both males and females. Our soul is our mind and emotions. As the soul of our physical nature has descended it has moved further away from the memory of our dual soul and spirit consciousness and has created itself as the superior intellect of our physical reality. Our belief that our intellect is superior shows us the magnitude of our emotional soul descent. The more intensely we have focused on the intellect the more intensely we have

461

suppressed our emotions. We have created our suppression as real in the physical world by suppressing the female as the symbol of our emotions.

Our emotional soul descent is accomplished by the suppression of our loving emotions as we descend into our fear emotions. When we think of the descending emotional soul, we must understand that our soul is our invisible dual mind and emotions, not an external physical substance. Therefore our emotional soul descent has occurred within as we have been suppressed during female lives. As we return as males living in our physical nature we suppress our emotions because we relate our emotions as "female" and unworthy of a strong and secure male. Our intellect has continued to ascend in knowledge and descend in emotions in both men and women, which has created our state of mental and emotional imbalance and physical disease.

It is the imbalance of our expanded knowledge to our suppressed love, truth, and equality that keeps us from being balanced and open to the revelation of our loving soul. If our emotions had been part of the consciousness of our expanding intellect, we would be more balanced as human beings. Our depression with all of its myriad of fear emotions is the result of making our fear beliefs our physical creation of society, which continues to conceal the expansion that our emotions seek.

Our emotions want to ascend in the same way that our intellect ascends, and until the ascension of our emotions occurs, we will continue to be stuck in our revolutions of fear beliefs as our daily art of creation. The female is the physical external symbol of our internal emotions. The male is the physical external symbol of our internal intellect and ego mind. We act out or create female suppression as a physical reality to show us what is happening to us internally as a soul. We have used our immature soul mind and emotions in our physical nature as a perfect way to experience our art of creation as a state of mental and emotional imbalance for our immature soul. We have made our imbalance physical by creating a state of imbalance between the physical male and female as inequality of our thinking, emotions, and feelings, which we again create physically as our beliefs and behaviors. And the cycle of our art of creation has been set in place by our revolutions of experience.

Our worship of the male as the image of "God" has been a gradual creation of our intellect that we have come to worship in the past two thousand years of our religious beliefs. During the past two thousand years the multiple religious focuses have been directed toward female suppression. Because of the focus of religion the female has become more suppressed than ever before in history as we have consciously suppressed our emotion of love and created our suppression as a physical reality by suppressing the female. In the male intellect sex has been believed to be love, but love is an emotion not a physical act or behavior. Making the act of sex into the illusion of love has added to the internal suppression of the emotions, while keeping the inequality of the male and female as our daily creation of reality. Creating an imperfect illusion of a perfect image has kept our immature soul confused about the perfection of who we are.

Our mature soul is clever, humorous, fun-loving, humble, and totally loving of its physical children. Our mature soul gives us all of the space that we need to learn our power of creation. So far we are the prototype or primitive version of the true product of our mature soul because we live unequally and without a consciousness of the unconditional love of our spirit.

Imagine Michelangelo as he began the sculpture of David. Michelangelo knew that the perfect image of David already existed in his block of marble and it was his personal responsibility to uncover the beauty of the hidden image. As Michelangelo chipped away at his block of marble, it was hard for other people to see the image of David. Many imperfections seemed to become real under his chisel but Michelangelo always knew that he had to chip away until the perfection of David was revealed. He didn't become discouraged as he created a new prototype by his daily labors because he knew that under a few more levels of marble was the beauty of the David that was clear in his mind and heart. His labors were subjected to intense judgement as he toiled away, but others could not see the perfect image of David that Michelangelo knew was hidden within the marble. In his labor of love the days seemed to speed by and by evening his strength was depleted by the external judgement that he heard. But before the sun could rise once again in the sky Michelangelo returned to his beloved David and continued with the perfection of his art of creation.

Think of your immature soul as a work of art in progress as the sculpture of David was, and think of your mature soul as Michelangelo, the tireless artist that is determined to bring out the perfection within you. Everything that we create in our physical world is created by this same universal pattern, and each of our lives is filled with an identical symbolism. Our mature soul always sees the image of who we are in our dual male and female consciousness and it will continue guiding us through our physical experience until the perfection and beauty of our mature soul is revealed.

Because we are focused on inequality, untruth, and fear as our art of creation we have not yet reached the consciousness level of civilization. Civilized people do not treat others in an unequal manner, fight, kill, maim, judge and they do not live in fear. Civilized people live their love and create peace, equality, and truth. When we use our power of creation as civilized people, we always treat others as we want others to treat us with equality, truth, and love. In our perfection of love we live our truth and equality through compassion, cooperation, communication, and the sharing of our love as the way that we create our lives and our society. When we are not afraid to reveal the beliefs that hold us in bondage and grow beyond them, we can become civilized as our power of creation.

As our immature soul has descended as a physical emotional nature, we have created our ego from our fearful thinking, our fear emotions, and our primitive superstitious beliefs, and we have created our beliefs as the "fact" of our physical reality. It is our ego that limits our ascending intellect and suppresses our emotions, which has caused them to descend into our pit of depression and desperation. It is our descending soul emotions that keep us from evolving from our physical nature to our divine nature. Our ego/spirit tug-of-war is responsible for our depression as we move back and forth between the physical nature and divine nature of our dual soul. As we create our depression, we will judge ourselves in relationship to our beliefs and accept the scientific belief that we are mentally ill.

In accepting the scientific theory that we are mentally ill, we use our art of creation to support our beliefs and we create a "mind-set" of mental illness. Our attempt to find a scientific cure for the normal change that is occurring within our dual soul is misguided by our external beliefs, and doomed to failure because we use our art of creation to fulfill our belief that we are mentally ill. With each physical step that we take in a forward intellectual motion to support disease, we enhance the strength of the belief in disease as our art of creation. At the same time we increase the disparity between our intellect and our emotional balance and reflect our imbalance by our perception of healing.

We are constantly reinforcing our intellectual and ego beliefs as the art of creation of our physical reality. As we increase our abusive approach to disease, we are triggering anger as the emotional response of the masses to being abused. Experiencing anger is good. If we simply conform to the habitual behaviors of abuse, we will not learn. Once we feel anger we are willing to seek knowledge and change the reality that we create. Once we have the knowledge to understand our consciousness and how it is evolving, we will heal ourselves by changing the way that we think, the emotions that we live, and our feelings that limit our sensory response to life, which will open our mind to the knowledge that helps us to understand ourself and our power of creation.

Multiple government and private organizations have been formed in our society as a result of anger and as a form of physical security. Many of these organizations are focused on money, health care, insurance, inequality, disease treatment, physical violence, family abuse, spousal abuse, crime, drunk driving, alcoholism, all types of addictions, and essentially our society and in many respects, our economy is supporting the masses by primitive forms of punishment and dependency. We have created our government and society as our art of creation from our fear and inequality.

When we reach the level of consciousness of civilization, we will no longer focus on our security needs because they will no longer be needed. We will focus on the expansion of our consciousness by the seeking of knowledge. Creative education will be available for all students, as memorization is not possible for the mature soul mind of knowing. Our society will change the focus of businesses and will provide multiple services for nurturing ourselves, eating the foods of nature, drinking pure water, breathing pure air, keeping our earth in harmony, and clear communication. Religion will no longer be the focus of our mature soul that does not worship, but socialization as the beginning of what we now call religion will return through the community influence. The media will become a primary source of knowledge and will no longer focus on judgement, analysis, crises, and sensationalism. The self-centered approach to commercial ventures will disappear and the community approach will prevail as we begin to use our power of creation.

Our ability to create our physical reality will expand and we will create our heaven on earth instead of living the hell that we have created. Within every culture we can see the level of consciousness that is being created. We have learned our art of creation by not truly knowing what we wanted; therefore, we have created to the best of our ability what we thought that we wanted. In many instances what we think we want is not always what we really want. Many relationships have status, education, sexuality, physical image, money, possessions, family, or happenstance as their foundation. None of these criteria makes a loving or lasting relationship. It is our belief that these external requirements will give us happiness in our life relationships and they have become the foundation of our art of creation.

The value or lack of value of our physical criteria is never more obvious than when we create relationships and find ourselves unhappy. We created the relationship because we thought it was what we wanted. After the unknown became the familiar, we could then define our disillusionment by seeing that the relationship was not what we thought we had created. Recognizing that our relationship was not what we wanted does not teach us to change and create what we do want. Instead of looking internally to examine the beliefs and fears of our soul, we look externally and blame our partner in the relationship, which allows us to repeat the relationship over and over again without learning why we have such "bad luck" in finding someone to love us. Our art of creation has never been perfect as an immature soul, but the perfection of us is concealed within us and will be revealed as we integrate with our female divine nature and begin to use love as our power of creation.

Our immature soul is totally self-centered as an intellect and ego. It is because we are self-centered that we look externally. As an ego and intellect, we create the illusion that we are superior because we believe that we are made in the image of God. All males and all females who are focused upon their intellect and ego, rather than their emotions, subconsciously live as self-centered people. Living the illusion of superiority or inequality creates a multitude of fear emotions within us that we use to habitually create every aspect of our life. It is the art of creation of our self-centered intellect and ego illusion that has controlled us during the journey of our immature soul.

Our intense beliefs of fear, guilt, sin, pain, and suffering have given us the skill and knowledge to create our "victimization" of disease as our physical reality. The more negative our thinking, emotions, and feelings become, the more disease we create as the reflection of our soul into our art of creation. As we use our art of creation to create disease as our physical reality, we are attempting to show ourselves how we image our thoughts, emotions, and feelings as our physical creation into our physical body and mind. Once we have the knowledge that it is our thoughts, emotions, and feelings that are toxic to the cellular structure of our body and mind, we can accept the wisdom of change as we use our power of creation of our thoughts, emotions, and feelings to restore our health.

As we create all of our negative beliefs and emotions as toxins within our cellular structure, we will abuse ourselves at the same time by not eating, drinking, and breathing the chemicals that will support our body. When we take on this self-abusive behavior, we will frequently start smoking, which is one way of externally suppressing our spirit senses by an excessive contamination of the air that enters our lungs as our lifeforce energy. We will deny personal responsibility for our art of creation when we find our body full of disease.

It is the purity of the air that we breathe that enhances the neurons and increases the feelings or senses throughout our body. Our senses are the indwelling spirit that enhances our consciousness. Our consciousness is the sensory response within our body to our thoughts, emotions, and feelings. Therefore, when we smoke, inhale, or breathe any type of cigarette, drug, weed, chemical, pesticide, or fumes, we suppress our sensory response and suppress our mind, emotions, and feelings, which paralyzes our consciousness. We become a "victim" in our mind and deny that we are always responsible for our art of creation.

When we live in fear we suppress our emotions and therefore we suppress our sensory response, which paralyzes our consciousness, and we will frequently not relate the physical experience to our art of creation. Our feelings trigger our emotions that spirals into our thinking and creates a sensory response that expands our consciousness. Our consciousness expansion is our soul evolution which we create through the physical experiences that we live each and every day. We create our physical experiences as our behavior from our beliefs which, in turn, creates the opportunity for our feelings to stimulate our emotions which stimulates our thinking, and the energy spiral evolves into an expansion of our aware consciousness as a sensory response. We live this spiral of action and reaction countless times each day, which acts as a stimulant to our senses, although our immature soul can remain unaware of our art of creation as the cause and effect of every nuance of our life.

The evolution of our soul into its ascending path requires that we balance our mind and emotions before we can do the dance of life that will carry us through the abyss of our ego. Our ego will become angry, rageful, controlling, manipulative, seductive, and totally out of control in its intention of winning the dance of life that allows our ego to bask in its superiority. Our ego will focus on money, status, possessions, education, relationships, science, religion, and it will become involved in various ways of feeling sorry for itself before it will be open to change. Once the ego truly believes that the mature soul is becoming strong enough to use its power to create change, the ego will go into temper tantrums of revenge, punishment, pain, suffering, victimization, poverty, and abuse to prevent change from happening. External, negative, and fearful temper tantrums are used by our ego to deny our emotions, feelings, and thinking from an awareness of our expanding consciousness. The fear that our ego creates essentially shuts down our thinking, emotions, and feelings and sends a message to our intellect that it is in control.

Education and knowledge are not the same physical experience for our ego. Education is based upon the memorization of information that is considered "fact" by the intellect. True knowledge requires us to look at all information and relate each piece of knowledge to ourself and to all other pieces of information. True knowledge gives us a complete picture of who we are and why we are here. Education is linear and focuses upon the tunnel vision of one discipline of thought. Education was designed to provide knowledge but in the past one hundred years it has become more linear and separate than a unity of mass thought as knowledge.

In our physical nature we think, suppress our emotions, and become addicted to our beliefs as a substitute for our emotions and feelings because we fear change. Our ego beliefs act as our limitation of thought, emotion, and feelings, which creates expectations of destinations that paralyzes our immature soul evolution. We only descend and ascend emotionally and intellectually in our immature soul. Once we ascend emotionally to balance with our ascended intellectual mind we become balanced as a mature soul and we become balanced as a male and female consciousness. Balance brings about love, truth, and equality for our male and female consciousness, which gives our integrated soul the power of creation.

The immature soul of our male physical nature has always been focused on its sexual core. The mature soul of our female divine nature has always been focused on its love. Our immature soul has evolved itself through our physical experience without memory of our art of creation or a consciousness of our mature soul and spirit. Both our male and female physical being have been living in our male physical nature, with the male being focused upon the intellect and ego and the female being focused upon the emotions. Our obsessive compulsive addiction to this unequal structure has finally brought us to our knees as a form of subconscious ignorance. In our ignorance our ego distracts our intellect with any subterfuge that it can find to shock our senses and keep us from our knowing and feeling love. This has created the suppression of the female as the symbol of our divine nature which we are also suppressing as a soul as we have externalized our judgement and blame and denied our responsibility for our art of creating our physical experiences.

Our immature soul is our left brain and our mature soul is our right brain. Because we have lived the past fourteen thousand years in our transitional state we have emotionally descended through seven primary levels of depression. During the past three thousand years our revolutions in depression have been lived as an accumulation of suppressed emotions that are continually descending. During the past one hundred years the accumulation of our ascending intellectual knowledge has expanded greatly and created an astounding diversity between our emotional, feeling, and sensory response of consciousness and our intellect. It is the relative distance between our thoughts and our emotions and feelings that creates our sensory response of depression.

Our transitional phase is the period of our lives when we are changing the focus of our thought, emotions, and feelings from the left immature brain to the right mature brain. For fourteen thousand years we have been cross-fertilizing our left and right brain as our immature and mature soul. Our right brain is the hard drive of our mind in which we have been consistently storing everything that we have learned when we die. As we get close to our transitional phase, we have been able to access some of our stored knowledge while we are storing some of our learned intellectual knowledge through cross-fertilization. Therefore, as we exchange our knowledge back and forth from our left and right brain, while at the same time suppressing our loving emotions and feelings, we have expanded our depression and increased the relative difference between our mind and our emotions. We know that things are happening in some minds that are not consciously happening in other minds so we label these people as depressed or mentally ill.

Everyone alive as a human being today is living some level of emotional depression simply because we are living in a left brain world of fear, anger, judgement, and control. As we cross-fertilize our mind, we become aware of knowing things we have not learned in this lifetime. We also hear voices, the music of the spheres, see visions, become conscious of our past lives, and develop an understanding of the energy that creates us as human beings. Science has created our cross-fertilization as a physical reality in the laboratory by genetic engineering. As humans we have created cross-fertilization of the human species by marrying outside of our culture, race, or ethnic group. In agriculture we cross-breed animals, plants, flowers, and herbs to produce new and stronger species.

As a dual soul we are striving to create cross-fertilization in our physical experience to help expand our consciousness of what is happening within our mind and emotions. Genetic engineering can be a method of devolution for our soul if we fail to become conscious of the purpose in learning this art of creation. As we are integrating our male and female consciousness as a soul, our physical bodies, our intellect, our emotions, and our feelings are showing us our level of evolution on a daily basis as we physically create what is happening internally with our dual soul minds.

Enormous numbers of people are being born today who do not feel the identity and role that religion attaches to their physical lives. The degree of difference that is felt is so totally overwhelming that it enhances the fear emotions and increases the rebellion of the soul to belong to some group where they will be understood. Many of these souls will use alcohol and drugs as a

471

method of blocking out their feelings. Each generation brings individuals who are more balanced as males and females into a new life. As our thinking, emotions, and feelings are lived from our equality, truth, and love, we will also find our physical bodies becoming more balanced. The advancement of these changing souls far surpasses the souls that are addicted to religious beliefs of fear and rage. The religious belief in one life blocks out the understanding of the eternal life of each soul and the evolution that we are living. To use our power of creation our mature soul must be comfortable and free in its thinking, emotions, and senses.

Homosexuality is frequently used as a soul lesson as we create the balance of the male and female soul by learning the lesson of loving ourself. Our world is full of male and female homosexuals that are being seen as sinful and guilty. What is missed in this relationship is the persona of the soul's energy. Homosexuals always attract from the soul persona and not the physical gender or sexual core that our physical nature identifies with itself. The religious roles and identities that have structured the "moral values" of our society are based on fear and inequality and they do not teach us love and equality of ourself or anyone who is different from our religious beliefs.

When a soul chooses a homosexual relationship they are seeking the soul lesson of loving self instead of seeing themselves as sinful. The emotions may not become balanced in one lifetime of living as a homosexual because the opposing energy from society does not allow the lesson of love, truth, and equality to be learned in harmony. The inequality and judgement that is lived toward homosexual relationships is another way that we create and live inequality in our physical lives. As a soul we will use our art of creation to provide the physical experience that we must live to learn our soul lessons and allow ourselves to expand as a soul into our power of creation. Our dual soul has no limitations in its power of creation.

Inequality, untruth, and fear are lessons of the immature soul. Love, truth, and equality are the lessons of the mature soul. As humans we can look at these emotions alone and see where we are focused in our art of creation. Life is our miracle and we create it by living our unique level of consciousness as our creation moment by moment in our daily lives. It is only in our mature soul that we will be able to live our love, truth, and equality with the wisdom of our power of creation.

Our immature soul always creates as an art of creation as we seek the skill and knowledge to become aware of "how" we create. Our mature soul always creates from its power of creation as we seek an understanding of "why" we create. As a transitional soul we can create from both levels of consciousness as we balance our thinking, emotions, and feelings on our journey home.

HEALING AS THE INTEGRATION
OF OUR DUAL SOUL

Healing has held a position of magic and mystery within our intellect from the beginning of time and it will continue to trigger the entire spectrum of our thinking and emotions until we gain the knowledge to change our beliefs from external healing to internal healing. A healing consciousness is the opposite of our disease consciousness and both can be the attitude that we create from our dual soul consciousness.

There is an intense focus within a segment of the medical community to find a "new paradigm" of healing. Healing would not be necessary if we understood who we are. When we understand the internal cause and effect of inequality, we discover the key to imbalance. Healing as a physical process to treat disease can be used as an example of how the intellect searches for external answers. Our physical body is a fractal pattern of our soul and spirit, our internal soul pattern is a fractal pattern of our spirit, and our soul and spirit are a fractal pattern of the chemical universe. We are a perfect pattern of biochemistry. The "paradigm" of healing cannot be changed by our ego as a new drug, a new physical process of detection and treatment, or any other external protocol. We are seeking to understand the relationship of us to the chemicals of nature.

The organization and discipline of our soul and its healing abilities are inherent within our cellular structure as part of the fractal pattern of our spirit and soul design. The ignorance of our design does not change the inherent pattern of healing, it simply changes the longevity of the physical body and our immature soul mind and emotions through death.

Healing can never be a new paradigm. It is the Universal Law of Cause and Effect, which is restoring balance within our body and soul. The healing pattern that is inherent within us is as old as our soul. Healing ourself through the lessons of disease is exactly what we are doing as we evolve as a soul in each physical life. Our healing cannot be separate as an external process because we have been healing ourself as a soul and physical body since we became a living soul experiencing the miracle of life.

When people speak of "New Paradigms" of healing they are essentially trying to come up with a new physical process, including new drugs, for external healing. Our external perception of healing is a perfect example of how our immature soul mind and emotions have created everything that we think as a physical fact on our immature soul journey as we have descended deeper into the "pit" of our physical nature. Our immature soul has focused upon detection, as a physical process of becoming conscious of disease, and followed through with an external physical treatment as a process of healing the disease, which is the current medical paradigm. Our immature soul is evolving into the divine nature of our mature soul that is enlightened by our spirit essense because this is the spiritual path of our dual soul journey. We are evolving as a dual soul into healing ourselves. We must recognize what our soul is and learn to live as spiritual beings before we can understand healing as an internal gift of our dual soul and spirit consciousness.

Our physical design is also the design of our soul and spirit that is integrated into each and every cell within our body. Until we destroyed the perfection of our design we had perfect cellular balance, dual soul equality, and spiritual freedom of equilibrium. Medicine has externally applied "Band-Aids" to heal cancer and other terminal diseases that can only be healed by an understanding of our integrated, internal cellular structure. As souls it is time for us to change our linear, tunnel vision to cyclic thinking that allows us to see the whole picture of who we are rather than focusing upon a singular part of our body or mind with an external perception. When we understand ourselves, healing will occur spontaneously. Spontaneous healing happens to some degree all of the time. Some people are living with the power to create spontaneous healing.

Medicine's external search for a new paradigm simply shows us that we do not understand the trinity of consciousness that motivates and inspires us because we are still captured by the addictive beliefs of our immature soul. Life is the miracle for our soul and we have done everything within our power to limit our mind and emotions, to kill our physical body, and to paralyze our spirit senses. As our ego has become dominant over our intellect, disease has become the "mind-set" of our immature soul consciousness. It is important for us to unlearn our abusive and addictive beliefs and behaviors and we will heal ourselves.

In the Bible we can read of the longevity of the human species over aeons of time, which is telling us that the length of our physical lives has a hidden meaning for our paralyzed immature soul. We can also become mentally hypnotized by the repetitious "begats" that are recorded and want to ignore them because we do not understand that we are being exposed to the knowledge of the Law of Continuation for our incarnating soul. Primitive interpretations of life have kept us from understanding ourselves.

Realistically there could not have been a mind focus upon disease if an individual could live for more than 900 years and "begat" numerous children. These primitive souls were obviously smarter than we are now about the focus of the mind because they were more concerned with living and reproducing than they were with disease and death. We don't see anywhere in biblical literature that Methuselah lived to be 969 years and died of cancer. Instead we read that at 187 years he had his first son. Is this information sending us a message that how we think is everything to our body? In our society fifty-year-old men are taking drugs for impotency.

In biblical times the attitude of people was focused on staying alive instead of being obsessed with dying as we have been during our period of revolution. Now we take life for granted as we live out our unhappiness and boredom, but we obsess over our "fear of death" because we have never been taught the truth about our soul and spirit. Our religious beliefs have instilled the fear of death into our ego as a belief that "death is a sin" and death puts us at "the mercy of God's wrath and judgement." Our fear of death is essentially the foundation of our fear of change that is holding us captive within our immature soul. Medicine expands our religious fears by competing with death and denying our soul and spirit.

In the days of Adam and Eve mankind was only just beginning its descent into the shadow side of the immature soul to experience its physical nature. In the beginning of our creation, we understood our purpose of being human as a male and female better than we understand it today. As we descended into the very pit of the immature male soul of our physical nature, our memory was lost. As we have reincarnated into each lifetime, we have returned without the memory of our past lives. Our thought focus as an immature soul has been on the "blank slate" of our intellect and ego mind and fear emotions.

With the love and wisdom of our mature soul as the female divine nature influencing the balance of our physical body and the equality of our soul mind and emotions, disease will gradually cease to be an issue. As we have descended further into the shadow side of our soul in our physical nature, we have lived shorter and shorter life spans, because we have created inequality between the divine nature of the mature soul and spirit consciousness and the physical nature of our immature soul of intellect and ego.

At this time we are midpoint in our soul journey and many souls are beginning their ascent into the light side of their mature soul. As we can sense the pattern of our life spans lengthening again, we are becoming conscious of the love in our divine nature beginning to restore our mental, emotional, and sensory cellular balance.

Understanding the soul pattern that we have been living will help us to understand that looking for a new external paradigm of detection and treatment has the ability to once again attach us to the scientific focus of "needing to be saved" from death by the physical, external world. If we simply change our belief about the cause and effect of external therapy, we will create harmony again for our immature soul that is seeking the knowledge to understand itself. The pattern of life was clearly established when we became eternal spirits. As medicine searches for a new paradigm, it is searching for a new external approach to healing, which will not change the cause and effect of a new dependency on the new paradigm. Our external path of searching is an ego distraction that keeps our mind and emotions limited to one perception, which keeps us in ignorance of the internal reality of our soul and spirit. We reflect our unique level of soul growth by the way that we think, speak, and behave; therefore, when we are fearful of opening our mind and emotions to expand our knowledge, we are defining the personal level of aware consciousness for our immature soul consciousness. Without the knowledge of real-life philosophy, we will continue to focus on our disease "mind-set."

We must look within ourself to find the pattern of creation, and when we understand the pattern of creation, we will understand the pattern of our own eternal survival in the physical world. We will discover ourself to be a timeless fractal pattern of creation that is now healing ourself as a dual soul. We created ourselves and we will continue to recreate ourselves until we understand the wisdom, love, and creativity of who we are. We are responsible for seeking and discovering our own power because we are at all times our own creator. As we open our immature soul to the knowing of our mature soul, we will realize that we have within our trinity of consciousness the knowledge and understanding of who we are. Our intellectual linear mind is afraid for us to discover our potential of healing ourself through the internal balancing of the electromagnetic energy of our consciousness. Our trinity of consciousness is our supraconsciousness that we use as a cyclic and integrated mind and emotional consciousness that far exceeds the capabilities of our linear intellectual and ego mind, which separates all of life by the use of its tunnel vision within the cosmic shell of beliefs.

To acquaint us with our own potential of healing by using our trinity of consciousness would create equality within the human species. Many minds cannot yet grasp the true perception of equality. We must begin to accept that we are a masterpiece of creative design that our intellect can never truthfully unravel by itself. We are only now capable of understanding the truth about who we are when we are willing to integrate all of the knowledge that is available to us. Our intellect separates knowledge into separate "disciplines" and does not organize and relate all information as a unit of knowledge. The logic of the design of the fractal pattern of the human species is a level of understanding that has been beyond the imagination within our intellect. But we have constantly been given pieces of the design which we have lived. When we look at the computer and its evolution of capability, we can sense the journey of evolution for our immature soul mind. When we look at fractal geometry, mathematics, chemistry, biology, physics, history, astronomy, and environmental science, we can see the truth of our own creation. All of the knowledge that is important to understanding ourselves is available in different disciplines. When we change our perception of the knowledge it will be understood.

Healing is first of all an internal balance because disease is an internal imbalance. We cannot truly heal disease through external influences, but only through the internal influences that change our addictive beliefs that are limiting us. Knowing that our physical nature creates disease as a lesson that our immature soul is seeking to learn helps us to understand why traditional medicine has not succeeded in healing disease. External processes interfere with our internal landscape and allow our diseases to become multi-complex and multi-virulent as we destroy the hierarchy of organisms that are essential to the validity of our elemental physical matter. As chemical beings we are creating a dramatic imbalance within our chemical self in multiple ways. Our excessive use of chemicals destroys the internal chemical balance that is the very foundation of our cellular body, dual soul, and spirit.

If the truth of healing were understood by medical science, we would not have disease. The perception and the reality of disease itself proves the limited understanding of the intellect and the futility of repetitiously continuing with an approach to health that has proven its inadequacy by its outcome. Our beliefs about disease have innocently led us to where we are in our own self-destruction. To evolve from where we are, we must be willing to dramatically change the way that we think, the emotions that we live, our feeling response, and our physical lifestyle.

The only true healer is found within our soul and spirit which is the very essense of us. Without our soul and spirit being present within our physical body we are dust. We have no lifeforce. We are an eternal spirit consciousness and we are using the physical matter of our bodies as a tool to learn how to be human. Disease captures our attention and makes us look internally at ourself. Without the emotional crises of life, such as disease and death, the immature soul would not use its emotions and feelings to grow and change, which it must do with or without our conscious awareness and understanding. As immature souls we are learning the art of creation and our immature soul creates in the negative. Learning the art of creation is learning the skills and knowledge of creation. In our immature soul we have been focused on learning the skills and knowledge as part of our evolution into our mature soul. Our mature soul will live the power of creation. When we understand ourself as a soul, we will transition into our mature soul and learn the power of creation in the positive, and we will heal ourselves.

We have been patterned to believe that our emotions and feelings are inferior to our mind. For our immature soul to evolve and integrate with our mature soul we must first learn how to balance our thinking, emotions, and feelings within the immature soul. Our intellectual mind cannot move as a linear mind into an integration with our divine nature. Balancing our mind and emotions gives us the dance of life that is essential to our soul evolution. Our multiple addictions, high risk adventure, crises, disease, and fear are all there to show us how to use our emotions and our senses to trigger our feelings. We focus on physical activities to produce the internal hormones that will give us an emotional high. We jump out of airplanes, climb mountains, bungee jump, and take multiple risks to stimulate our internal hormones. We watch horror shows that scare us half to death because they make us feel our emotions and they provide sensory stimulation for our senses. Sometimes we are literally killing ourselves in our attempt to awaken our immature soul mind, emotions, and feelings to balance and heal ourselves. Our four biological needs are also playing extreme roles in our soul transition. Our inherent need for pure air, water, and nature's foods and our inherent need for sexual procreation are all at risk during this transitional period.

The goal of our spirit consciousness is to merge the divine nature with our physical nature to create an integrated dual soul consciousness, which gives us the power to create consciously as physical beings rather than subconsciously from soul, or unconsciously from spirit. Each time that we live an emotional experience that emphasizes our finite nature as physical beings, we expand our level of conscious awareness of our eternal Divine Nature. Bringing our male and female consciousness together as a soul is an art of creation that we have been practicing in our physical experience since the beginning of our immature soul. The reflections of our internal male and female consciousness learning balance have been acted out as the inequality drama of our physical lives. The closer we come to our divine nature the more dramatic we have become as individuals and as society in our attempt to heal ourselves by awakening to our equality. We have reflected our art of creation into creating diseases of our body and mind as a way of learning our power of creation.

We have become hypnotized by the physical world and we have therefore learned to equate and judge ourself relative to our beliefs. We have also learned to seek healing through the externalized beliefs and physical processes that have been handed down within our immature soul memory as social and family customs, as well as our religious, political, scientific, and educational beliefs. The lives that we have lived have been perfect to teach us how to balance the physical, mental, emotional, and feeling energies of our consciousness. We are also learning the balance of our physical body, the equality of our dual soul, and the equilibrium of our spirit. If we have an open mind, we can absorb the skills and knowledge to understand ourselves without getting stuck in our fear and self-judgement.

Because we live consistently within our three dimensions of electromagnetic energy, we must learn to know and accept our internal power as greater than our external beliefs. At present our conscious awareness only relates to our physical body and intellect, as it denies the integration of our soul and spirit. We are matter but we are also three dimensions of electromagnetic energy that we wear daily as our cloak of consciousness that has its source in the chemicals from which we support our physical body, mind, and emotions.

Knowing who we are removes the necessity of disease as we evolve into our mature soul. Disease today is an internal lesson for our immature soul and it is a very important lesson of our evolution and our awakening to our eternal life. Countless lessons are being learned through our experience of disease, and the lesson of healing ourselves is a major gift to ourselves. Physical healing is only an issue of the physical body that is captured by the intellectual and ego mentality. Disease is a means through which we seek conscious mind-shifting during our physical life or physical transformation into another physical life by death. Either choice provides change for our dual soul and its evolution. There is a soul advantage to our conscious mind-shifting during each life, because it allows us to remember the lessons that we have learned and to consciously change and grow from those lessons within each lifetime. Knowledge removes us from the cave of our intellectual mind that we have been hiding in for years. We learn best by living the experience of our physical life which we can then relate to our intellectual knowledge. If we refuse to participate in life and we refuse to seek knowledge, we are acknowledging to our soul that we are paralyzed or stuck in our fear of change. Disease will give our soul an opportunity to awaken or choose death as a new beginning. Disease is also the primary lesson of shifting our mind internally rather than remaining in an external focus.

Physical disease reflects the misdirection of our subconscious and unconscious energy through our conscious fear. Therefore disease is our own creation, although the memory of the creation is not conscious within our intellectual mind since we create from our denial and resistance and not from our conscious intention. Because we have not understood that we are a chemical human, we have used chemicals in all aspects of our lives without realizing the effect they have upon our cellular structure.

In all aspects of our lives, chemicals have been creating a perpetual state of internal and external imbalance. The physical cause of all diseases is a chemical imbalance. It is normal for our left brain thinking to make us victims of external organisms. If our internal chemicals were not out of balance, we would remain the highest living organism on earth and not feel threatened by other organisms. The reality of our physical life is so overwhelmed with chemical contaminants that we cannot escape from unwanted chemical exposure. The air that we breathe, the foods that we eat, and the water that we drink are all polluted with unhealthy chemicals to create an imbalance within our body. We have created disease because of our external, negative, fearful thinking. Because we have not understood our creation, we have innocently sabotaged who we are and our art of creation with chemicals that destroy our balance. Now we can change if we can unlearn our addictive beliefs.

Our scientific attachment to external cause, detection, and treatment continues to focus our intellect, money, and time on various issues such as blame, judgement, and fear which expands disease dramatically. Disease occurs because our veil or cosmic shell acts as a shield around our intellect, which resists our soul and spirit consciousness and misdirects our thinking. Attempting to cure diseases by adding another toxic chemical to our body is distorted thinking. More chemicals create more imbalance and our body collapses into pools of decaying matter internally as disease or externally as expressions of anger and violence that expand the diseases of our society.

Both the internal and external expressions of disease play a role in capturing our attention and directing our thoughts to our thinking, responsibility, attitudes, lifestyle, and behavior. Our mature soul is determined to get our attention and it is very clever at bringing us back to our emotional self through events of our family, community, society, nation, and the world. Our mature soul allows us to experience what we don't want, to prove to us that we can change and grow. When we become totally disgusted with the outcomes that show us that healing is not happening, we begin to realize that we must change our approach, which can only be done by changing our thinking, emotions, and feelings.

Our healing is dependent upon the beliefs, behaviors, and emotions that create healing of our diseases. Our society, as a whole, focuses upon the fear of disease which escalates the creation of disease. As individuals and as a society we have developed a disease consciousness instead of a health consciousness. We believe we are destined to be sick, not healthy. Our disease consciousness creates fear, dependency, and worship of doctors, medicine, and testing. At this time we have lost our freedom of life and we have become a slave to our fears as the only emotional stimulus that we allow ourselves to experience.

An understanding of ourselves and the power that is contained within us must be reached before people will be willing to change their definition of disease, its cause, and its cure. Healing occurs when the negative energy from fear and the pollution of chemicals are removed from our body and we seek the balance of our emotional and chemical restoration. In our chemical society we are challenged to find a place where we can detoxify our body and mind to restore the electromagnetic energy to its true level of balance. Even our food is genetically engineered with viruses, bacteria, and pesticides without our knowledge. With our present level of chemical contamination, we are innocently creating chaos in our cellular structure and energy form.

Healers who are consciously using their soul and spirit energy can teach others to balance their body and mind. Our personal belief in the healer allows a temporary healing to occur;

485

whether it is a physician, spiritual healer, a place, or a thing, the belief that we are healed initiates the healing. Because the power within us is contained within our mind and emotions that are controlled by our beliefs, we must all learn to heal ourselves by looking internally to discover the beliefs that are no longer serving us. As we heal we create a collective consciousness of healing that will be effective throughout the world. In healing ourselves we will think positively, live our loving emotions, and allow our internal emotions of love to be the primary sensory stimulus that expands our consciousness. In changing who we are we can prevent disease and live long and happy lives.

Any external healing is only temporary unless we willingly open our soul mind and emotions and live our cyclic consciousness that keeps our mind, emotions, and feelings open. We must also restore the validity of our cellular chemicals. Healing can be documented by the many thousands of people that have experienced temporary healings at Lourdes and the sixty-five that have been documented as truly healed. Temporary healing, which is a misnomer in itself, can also be documented in traditional medicine as the patient continues to create other diseases after being pronounced "cured." It is no accident that we continue to create one disease after the other. Disease is an internal lesson that helps us stay focused internally. With the external magnetic force of negative beliefs to overcome, disease will help an advanced soul to resist the negative influence of primitive beliefs, except where medicine is accepted as blind faith.

Many individuals live with the presence of annoying symptoms because of their resistive beliefs that misdirect their thinking and emotions into a dependency on drugs, surgery, and other physical therapies. Pain and suffering always challenges us to change internally, but we misdirect our perception of change and believe that someone else can help us by an external therapy. Many harmless symptoms can expand into multiple diseases, allowing the person involved to become confused and angry because no one truly "healed" them. We have an expectation that a doctor can "heal" us from our lifetime of self-abuse because we have given medicine the power of "God" in our mind. Many diseases are the result of our chemical excesses and deficiencies that make it impossible for us to heal ourselves until we change our lifestyle behavior and our attitude.

On a spirit level the purpose for the entire human species is identical for all of us. It is our spirit intention to merge our physical nature with our divine nature. On an individual basis each person is living the lesson of soul evolution at a personal level. Internal healing is the correction of our intellectual error of thinking negative, external, and fearful thoughts. We have lived in ignorance of the relationship of our trinity of consciousness, physical body, nature, earth, and the universe. We have been missing some vital keys of knowledge as we have lived our immature soul journey. The most important key is the understanding of who we are as a soul and spirit. Without the knowledge to understand our soul and spirit nothing else makes sense to us. Our addictive religious beliefs defy the logic of our mature soul mind and act karmically as our resistance and denial of change.

Our different levels of evolution of consciousness become glaringly evident in our beliefs, communication, language, behavior, attitude, emotions, and in our perceptions of life. The difference in our levels of consciousness is becoming more pronounced as some souls are evolving and changing the veil of their addictive beliefs, others are revolving in their ancient beliefs, and others are devolving into their ancient ego memories. Experiencing the ego tug-of-war is a constant challenge as we change our beliefs and behavior. Each level of consciousness reveals the difference between an open mind that is willing to change and a closed mind that denies all change. All change occurs one step at a time. We literally meet our challenges with each step that we take. When we reach the level where our perception of life is moving back and forth between our left and right brain, we can experience the chaos of anxiety, fear, phobias, stress, and depression, despite the reality that everything in our physical life is going beautifully.

Our family, friends, contemporaries, and lovers are all in our lives as either positive or negative support of our soul lessons.

Those individuals that we feel a closeness to, especially our family, friends, and lovers, are usually members of our soul family and are in our life by choice. We chose these souls to be actors upon our stage because of our eternal soul and spirit relationship. We never journey through life alone. We also never come back into a life alone. As we choose our parents and physical family members, we are revisiting with our soul family.

We have full and individual responsibility for ourself. Our life is about us and our soul journey into our Divine Nature is an individual journey of personal responsibility. No one else can do it for us. It is our personal responsibility to learn the power of creation. We are using ourself as our example of creation. If anyone tries to save us, it destroys us. It is our negative beliefs of karmic origin, which reach from the very beginning of our soul journey to our present survival fears, that create our ego cosmic shell to conceal and veil us from our mature soul and spirit. Our soul and spirit have been seen as a mystery to our intellect because our intellect is limited by our ego and cannot see the remainder of our trinity of consciousness with clarity.

It was at the time of the completion of our cosmic shell that we began to see our power as external to us. This shift from internal to external perception occurred during our immature soul journey. This was the beginning of what we know as religious thought. We had already begun our focus on science as we examined what we thought was the reality of life. It was science that prepared us as an immature soul for our addictive religious beliefs. As we tried to find some logic in our sexuality and the universe that we could observe, we didn't have enough pieces of the puzzle to put the entire picture together in our mind and we began to symbolize. In our ignorance we began to believe the symbols as fact and the conclusions that we came to early in our evolution became the religion that we worshipped; now we are challenged to change our earliest conclusions.

Our negative, external, and fearful beliefs separated our soul mind and emotions and allowed us to see "God," healing, and our physical power only as an external and negative force that threatened our survival. Our fears and beliefs were then reflect-

488

ed into our everyday lives through our thoughts, our words, and our physical behavior to create disease, abuse, crime, war, and life crises. As we have descended as an immature soul, we have expanded on the negative, external, and fearful focus of our immature soul and we have sincerely believed that what we are living is all there is in life. This belief has created the expansiveness of our physical, mental, and emotional diseases.

Healing will occur within each individual when we no longer live in fear. Fear is at all times a fear of change because we fear for our survival. Survival is not an issue for us as eternal spirits. Survival is only an issue when our belief in ourself is defined in relationship to our belief in one life and the power of the external forces to control and destroy our finite existence here and in the hereafter. Our focus on our physical body, which is finite, has kept us in ignorance of our eternal life as an evolving consciousness with a purpose of learning the power of creation.

Change must occur in our beliefs and in the way that we support and expand each dimension of our consciousness energy as physical beings. When we can change our beliefs and our behaviors, healing will become a reality for us. When we begin to support the integrity and viability of the physical dimension of our consciousness energy, which consists of the physical body, intellectual mind, fear emotions, and the ego, and respect our consciousness, we will be on the path to healing ourselves.

The viability and integrity of our intellect has its foundation in truth, love, and equality. For our intellect to evolve it must merge with our mind of wisdom, and our ego must change to humility to survive to enfinity as an integral part of our dual soul. Our ego is the cosmic shell of our intellect which is subconscious to our intellect. Our ego controls our intellect as a buried electromagnetic energy of old karmic beliefs that is concealed from our intellect. All of the thinking and emotions in our left brain are subjected to the limitations of our ego and its electromagnetic shield of beliefs. Our physical body is a dramatically slowed down electromagnetic energy that must be restored through the chemicals of nature to be viable and useful to us for long periods of time.

We must change our beliefs to understand that when we are through being physical and choose death, that part of our electromagnetic energy that slows down to become physical will once again speed up to become spirit. This is the explanation of what happens to our soul and spirit at the death of our physical body. Our soul and spirit changes from the liquid and solid state that they exist in within our body to a gaseous chemical state. In this ethereal or gaseous state the soul and spirit leaves our old physical body as our last breath of life, but our soul and spirit will return within three days as a new conception within another physical body and we begin our power of creation as a new life.

Our physical body seeks pure air, water, and nature's nutrients from pure foods to restore and rejuvenate the viability and integrity of its lifeforce energy. These natural elements support our cellular structure and maintain the integrity, viability, and credibility of our internal hierarchy of cells. Nutrition, including air and water as well as nature's foods, is the very foundation of vibrant health for our physical body and the chemical excitement for our mind and emotions.

If pure organic nutrition was used as the first step in disease prevention by traditional medicine, disease would be less prevalent today. Hippocrates' simple but profound words, "We are what we eat" impart wisdom beyond our present imagination. The value of nutrition has been consistently denied by medical science for the past fifty years, and this has allowed the vain attempts to restore our body through chemicals to fail. Improper nutrition allows the credibility of the body to break down and the body to be invaded by internal and external organisms which create disease. Our body and mind function from love, symbolized by the nurturing of ourself with the proper chemical nutrition, which is the action of loving ourself. Truth symbolizes the supporting of our body and mind with the knowledge of its integrity. Equality symbolizes the absolute balance within our cellular structure that enhances the evolution of our dual soul and the balance of our physical body and our spirit. We have been learning our spiritual values by living what we don't want in our physical experience.

When we create disease we are creating cells within our body that are not capable of reproducing themselves in the original pattern of their design. This is all of the evidence that we need to understand that we are creating a chemical and cellular imbalance, which promotes decay within our body. It is time to ask ourselves, "Why are we decaying?" Science has not accepted the value of these natural elements as necessary to prevent disease, although massive amounts of research has been done over the past forty-plus years that has emphasized inadequate nutrition, polluted air, and polluted water as causes of disease. Our internal fear for our physical survival is directly related to our physical body's need for pure air, water, and nutrients as food for our cellular memory. We feel threatened internally on a cellular level. The value of air, water, and foods in their pure form can easily be researched within existing literature and will be found as the most accessible prevention for all diseases. We continue on our path of physical self-destruction because of our greed and the influence that our way of life has in supporting the economic greed of our society. Our intellect and ego believes that money is our path of survival. As we create self-destruction internally, we will live self-destruction externally as a society as we become unbalanced on all levels.

The intellectual mind is the next physical level of ourself that we must heal through change. When the mind is living in fear from the negative beliefs that we are attached to, it is living in a box and repeatedly externalizes blame, judgement, resistance, and denial. We close our mind to expanded thought, and we live in ignorance that allows us to keep our left brain intellect and ego separate from the rest of our brain, which is our mature soul and spirit consciousness. When we are focused on judgement we are sick, and we have the power to destroy ourselves, society, and the world.

Our intellectual mind completely enslaves itself to the negative beliefs that we live within our primitive social culture and creates the shell of the ego as our personal defense system of unlearned karmic lessons in the form of addictive religious beliefs that are seen as moral law. Moral law is a creation of man and changes with man. Our intellect prides itself on memorization and regurgitation within its closed system of beliefs. Our intellect does not have the insight to understand our soul and spirit mind from its closed position of control and judgement. As our intellect is limited by our beliefs, we always look externally to blame and judge everything that happens to us on someone or something else, and by doing so we begin the disease process on all three dimensions of our physical reality. Our intellect must unlearn its belief system and be open to new philosophies before healing can become a reality. Our key to unlearning is the knowledge of ourself that relates us to all that we know about nature, earth, and the universe. Our knowledge base has expanded greatly in the past one hundred years and we have the opportunity to look back at history to observe how uncivilized we have been in our perception of life and equality. Our society and the societies of the world are as diseased as our body as we struggle to understand our divine nature and change our beliefs so that we may become civilized.

Our ego worships our intellect as supreme and denies, resists, and separates itself from the influence of any thought that does not meet the standard scientific and religious criteria of examination that has been devised by our intellect. Our ego is terrified of change because of the beliefs that have created the ego as our bastion of self-defense. Our ego is arrogant, judgemental, fearful, unfeeling, and an insatiable know-it-all. Best of all, our ego is an Emmy-award-winning performer that can out perform the greatest actor or actress alive. Our ego is a magician that creates illusion in every performance. The ego pulls lies out of the sleeve of the intellectual consciousness as quickly as a magician pulls rabbits out of his hat.

When we can sense our ego and intellect as a child that is obstructing our soul and spirit, we can take back our power from the spoiled and hypocritical child of our mind by choosing to accept our soul wisdom, love, creativity, and ingenuity. The unconditional love, truth, and equality of our spirit will then be available for us to use within our physical lives. As we have used our intellect and ego, we have forgotten that our spiritual ethical values are waiting to be used in our physical lives. It is our ego that is attached to the "moral values" of religious law. Moral values are based upon the judgement between right and wrong, good and bad, white and black, male and female, and the judgement continues ad nauseam, as the symbol of living our lesson of inequality.

We have been taught as part of our religious beliefs and social customs to give away our power. Our entire societal system fosters dependency in all facets of our life. Giving our power to an external God, the church, medicine, education, politics, money, physical possessions, love relationships, or anyone that we feel controls us, removes our internal power by ignoring and denying our equality. As we have lived our multiple lives with the religious belief system as the foundation of our society, we have become depressed, diseased, violent, greedy, self-abusive, and bored with the repetition of our lives. In seeing the outcome that we have created in our society by living our religious foundation of addictive, fearful, and unequal beliefs, we can see the wisdom of change.

When our internal power is removed, we instill fear for our survival into our intellect and ego by the very act of separation and our body and mind react with disease to alert us that we are losing our balance. This is the way in which we have chosen to live and experience the ultimate lesson in inequality that allows us to see the need for balance and equality within both the internal and external focus of our physical reality. Living our physical balance, soul equality as a male and female consciousness, and the equilibrium of our spirit values is an absolute healing for us as humans.

We have approached our lesson of inequality through every facet of our physical world, and it began with our lesson of sexuality as we sought to understand the equality that exists between the male and female externally and to balance our male and female energy internally within us. Medicine is our soul lesson of inequality that denies a partnership between the physician and the patient. Inequality is the lesson that bridges our physical nature with our divine nature. Equality is the lesson that we are now seeking to learn by integrating our male and female soul consciousness as an external and internal healing. Our mature soul wants us to live the exact opposite to what we have lived as an immature soul.

Physicians teaching us that we have the internal power to heal ourselves, rather than creating self-fulfilling prophecies by telling us that we are going to die, would help to change our mind-set in relationship to disease. The ego of the physicians and scientists will find the metaphysical approach a hard pill to swallow. Because of the external healing beliefs and mind-set of the medical community, we must all accept personal responsibility for our own health and stop our blind-faith believing in the medical perception as the only perception available to initiate healing.

Acknowledging and accepting personal responsibility for our individual freedom of choice in our healing and health becomes a motivational energy that inspires our thinking, speaking, and behaving to change in a healthy and positive way. Accepting our power of choice is inspirational and motivational as it integrates our soul and spirit with our intellect and it puts us on the path to healing ourself.

Disease is not an unhealthy condition for the soul. When the mature soul does not have the conscious cooperation of the intellect to learn a lesson, it chooses disease as a method of living the internal lesson. Our mature soul lessons of personal power, patience, strength, courage, humility, faith, trust, and giving and receiving love are frequently learned through our experiences of disease. If we choose to stay healthy we must live with an open mind, heart, and hand. We must live simply, patiently, and compassionately as a part of the whole of humanity. Judgement, isolation, and separation are lessons of our intellect and ego, but the communication, cooperation, and compassion are the behaviors that we live as a mature soul.

Our ego controls our attitude toward our lifestyle and our longevity. When our ego accepts untrue beliefs, we live by those beliefs and practice our art of creation. Beliefs that are not valid in Universal Law create an imbalance in our body and mind. Only the pure foods of nature support our body in Universal

Law, because that is what we used in the creation of our physical body. Massive amounts of dietary information and the health effect upon the body are inaccurate and are creating disease in our society. Our mind has been switched from pure foods to processed foods as an economic and convenience factor because of our addiction to money and instant gratification.

If we believe that all food is good food, we will not be concerned about what we eat. If we believe that the "doctor" alone has the power to heal us, we won't be willing to accept any personal responsibility in the healing process. If we believe that we will only be accepted by our friends if we drink, smoke, and indulge in promiscuous sex, that will be the behavior that we live. If we believe that judgement is right, we will "wrong" others to redeem ourselves. If we believe that we are going to have disease or die because of hereditary factors, we will create the disease and we will die. If we are told we are going to die, we will die because it will become part of our belief system.

It is only when we have the power to say "No, I am not going to die" that we have the chance to live and heal ourself. If we fear going beyond what we are told to think, we are choosing to ignore our internal power to change. Our attitude towards disease reflects our self-image into our daily behavior and defines the lessons of inequality and externalization for our immature soul consciousness. Our attachment to disease and its symptoms consumes our life and controls our daily activities, words, and thoughts. Our denial of change is a reflection of our addictive "disease" mentality.

Our disease obsession creates an attitude that becomes an ego defense against opening to our soul and spirit healing. Our life reflects our attitude into society as an expanded resistance and denial of our internal power. Society becomes obsessed with disease behavior on all levels as the reflection of the collective consciousness that is coming from millions of people who are living in fear of disease. We are now in the throes of this expansive and magnificent lesson of inequality as individuals and as a society that continues to live lives that are mentally and emotionally dependent on "being saved." The "being saved" mind-set allows us to destroy ourselves, society, and the world with judgement, as a mental disease, which becomes a physical disease.

Scientists have examined our thinking and our attitude for many years but they have examined it from the intellect and ego perception of the external cause and effect of the family, the fear within our own minds, and not from the spirit energy of our supraconscious mind. Each of us can only perceive life from our individual level of consciousness and scientists are no different; therefore, all research has been biased by our limited intellect and ego beliefs. When a scientist has an open mind and no fear of truth, the results will be valuable. The fear that is supported by our religious beliefs has allowed science to research disease and not health. It is in the miracles of healing where the answers are waiting to be found. Our soul consciousness directs the perception of the mind. We can consciously deny religious beliefs and still find that our scientific thinking is limited by the hidden karmic beliefs that we have not unlearned. It is our addicted beliefs that create our fear. If we honored spontaneous healing and studied the thoughts, emotions, feelings, and lifestyle changes of those individuals, we could define the patterns of physical healing. Spontaneous healing is not truly spontaneous healing, but healing occurs over a relatively short period of time as the cellular structure detoxifies itself.

Prejudice is rampant among scientists and medical disciplines. At the mere mention of soul and spirit or "spontaneous" healing the intellect begins to convulse and the denial shields strengthen. Prejudice is contradictory to the true meaning of science, but that has not stopped the reaction of the intellect and ego of many scientists that are attached to their karmic beliefs and fear. Our intellect has become so frightfully restricted by our ego that the mere thought of an unknown mind power existing outside of the intellect is intolerable. Our resistance and our denial beliefs and behaviors serve as a good example of the ego and its need to control. The linear or tunnel vision of our ego and intellect can never compare to the cyclic thinking that we experience in our trinity of consciousness. Today's science is the Model T of the mature soul.

In reality the intellect is simply a grain of sand in an ocean of our mind consciousness. Yet any and all concepts of change threaten the physical nature of our intellect and ego, allowing prejudice, judgement, and denial to rear its fearful head. Inequality, discrimination, and prejudice are rampaging through the intellectual minds and religious communities that feel threatened by different perceptions of reality that challenge our common beliefs. The fear of being wrong is the fear of failure, and both will act as shock waves in our society when exposed to real-life philosophy. There is no right or wrong because what we live is perfect for our soul growth. Effective changes occur through attrition, which is why death expands our evolution through compulsory change and growth. Death is a choice for our soul because it is a new beginning and a soul healing. For the soul, death is a time of celebration. When we focus on living life in a healthy and beautiful way, we learn more as a soul. When we choose death and begin again in a new life, we must repeat any and all unlearned lessons, which is repetition for the soul. All knowledge and all emotional and feeling lessons are the only part of our life that we store forever within our mature soul as growth.

Choosing death will allow soul change more rapidly than physical vegetation, and therefore competition between life and death should be governed by the quality of life and not the quantity. Death can be a healing for the soul when the body and mind can no longer function at will. When we live our beliefs we also live the cause and effect of our beliefs in the outcomes of both life and death. When change is not possible in life for the intellect and the ego but the soul is ready to change, death brings about a transformation, a healing, and a new beginning for the dual soul. In terms of activity it is the evolution of our immature soul into our mature soul that is important, not the image or the activity of the physical body. Some individual souls will choose to limit the physical body to change their mind and emotional focus from the sexual, physical image of self to the soul mind and emotional image of self. Expansive growth can occur when the soul makes this dramatic choice.

The intellect and ego functions as a rigid, cold, linear energy that refracts and reflects illusions endlessly upon itself as a sexual, physical image with a superior intellect. This is our ego illusion created by the restriction of harmony and fluidity within the imposing energy fields of our addictive beliefs. The soul and spirit is warm, soft, and pliable and functions through an eternal cycle of expanding consciousness energy that moves faster than the speed of light. As we know from nature, those plants which stand rigid and brittle before the changing seasons are broken and lost in a storm, but those that are soft and pliable continue living through the chaos until a new season arrives and they spring back into vibrant physical beauty and life. Our soul is ready and eager for a new season.

We can only recognize our soul and spirit when our perception changes to the internal focus and we know what to look for in our search. Our spirit consciousness is the core of our lifeforce energy and reflects into the physical world as varying degrees of light, sound, vibrations, color, smell, thinking, emotions, and feeling. Our immature soul energy essense has individual degrees of reflection and refraction in its cosmic shell and therefore is not clearly represented as our spirit consciousness. The intellect and ego separates the trinity of consciousness into separate realities and denies the mature soul and spirit consciousness as it accepts the religious image of beliefs as its ego denial. In universal reality the spirit energy exists in all things at all times. Whether we are conscious of our spirit or not depends upon our level of consciousness evolution. Our spirit energy exists within our trinity of consciousness but our intellect denies our spirit and mature soul because our ego is blocking it out. In biblical terms ego refraction is called concealment.

The most dramatic view of our soul consciousness is always found in the thoughts, words, and behavior of the human being as the integrated reflection of the spectrum of energy that we accept within ourselves and our life. Our internal persona of unconditional love is concealed from our awareness when we are living in our immature soul. We must understand our physical nature before we can understand our divine nature and live our unconditional love. Our physical nature is an identical but opposite pattern of our divine nature, and both our physical and divine nature are a fractal pattern of our spirit consciousness as an androgynous energy of male and female consciousness. Each level of our consciousness energy moves at different vibrational speeds which produces different physical effects that are dependent upon the level of consciousness evolution of our soul. The difference in vibrational speed accounts for all consciousness differences within the human species and within all levels of life that is not in human form. The consciousness of a rock or an animal is vibrating at a different level than we do as human beings.

Acknowledging that we have an integrated soul mind as a superconscious mind and an eternal trinity of minds as a supraconscious mind will allow us to go beyond the intellect and use our cyclic mind in all walks of life. We can examine our superconscious mind by exploring the consistency of how we live our equality and love, which creates truth through the unconditional love and equality of our language and behavior. We can look within ourself to see if we are living with a consciousness that is consumed with fear, judgement, disease, and death, or are we living with a consciousness of being happy, healthy, and creative in our life?

We cannot separate the effect of our dual soul and spirit from our physical life. The influence of our internal power is clearly defined in the health, happiness, joy, peace, and humility that we live in our daily life. We can only become conscious of our soul and spirit from the power of our thoughts, our words, and our resulting behavior. If we think that we have no fear but we continue to judge ourself and others, and have frequent doctors' appointments for annoying symptoms of disease as we live in fear, we do not know our own mind. If we believe that we are dependent upon Jesus or Allah to save us, then we do not know our own mind.

To discover our controlling beliefs we must look at what we manifest in our body, our mind, and our life as the physical behavior and lifestyle that we live. To discover the health of our body and mind, we must look at our beliefs, our attitude toward personal responsibility and power, and our lifestyle as our behavior toward ourself and others.

Our challenge in looking at health is not to replace one external, physical process with another external, physical process but to look at our integrated body living an integrated life through our thinking, speaking, feeling, emotions, and behavioral experience. The separatist approach of the medical community toward patients, science, and research will never be successful in healing, because we are not separate pieces as a mind, emotions, feelings, and body parts. Looking at us as only physical beings is another level of the separatist approach that interferes with healing. Acknowledging that we are a spirit, dual soul, and physical body that is totally integrated is our first step to healing.

Once our attitude toward ourself and our life changes, balancing the physical effects of nutrition, emotions, personality, character, attitude, beliefs, lifestyle, and behavior will create all of us as a balanced person, society, and the world. As our change occurs we will begin to reflect our harmony, love, and balance into society and the world. As a mature soul we can create a "heaven on earth" as we live the ethical values of our spiritual divine nature instead of the moral values of our physical nature. As we move into the level of understanding as a mature soul, we will no longer create disease except by free and conscious choice for a specific experience of healing for the soul.

We always live within our personal creation of the physical world as we perceive it in our mind. We have only to observe the difficulties of our personal relationships, family, society, and the world to see that multiple changes are at this time essential to our growth if we want our immature soul to evolve. Change must be initiated by us as we release our beliefs and behaviors. Beliefs and behaviors that worked for us as an immature soul will not work for us as a mature soul. As a spirit and dual soul consciousness, we are invisible as an electromagnetic energy, but it is the same electromagnetic energy that creates new life as a body and mind and that is integrated with our invisible lifeforce energy of our invisible soul and spirit. We are never separate.

The pattern of our soul and spirit consciousness is found in our DNA. It will be the biochemistry of our cells that scientifically shows us the pattern of life and how that pattern created our life from our trinity of consciousness by using our dual male and female DNA as our consciousness and our soul pattern of life. The proof of our ability to heal and regenerate our cellular structure is simply waiting to be discovered. As scientists become comfortable and humble with their internal discoveries, we will solve our problems of earth and create a civilization of unconditional love with a passion for understanding ourselves. Science now has the capability to prove reincarnation, soul families, to design programs to heal the mind and body, and to prevent crime. If our scientific abilities were put into positive use, we could quickly see our society and earth as a unified world begin to heal. The days of war are gone from the core of many people and change is occurring as communication and sharing becomes universal. Unfortunately there are many souls who are continuing with their immature beliefs and behaviors and the immature soul consciousness is a threat to our soul evolution.

Science also has the ability to become greedy and destroy the beauty of our perfect pattern of life that has supported us through billions of years of evolution. If we focus on the external commerce of money and ignore our soul and spirit, we will devolve. As all of the scientific knowledge is looked at in relationship to us, we will not be dependent on the religious beliefs that are esqued to fit the consciousness of the times for the immature, judgemental soul.

We are a Higher Universal Mana, or the highest living organism on earth. We are HUMAN and we are a miracle of life as a physical being. We are a male and female soul consciousness evolving into an expanding spirit consciousness by fulfilling our mature soul purpose of learning the power of creation of ourselves as a trinity of consciousness.

THE MIRACLE OF LIFE

Aeons of time, thought, and action goes into the making of one reflective human being traveling through the space of enfinite lives. The miracle of our being is our evolution of consciousness as our dual soul mind and emotions. We have become creatures of habit and our adaptive habitual thoughts, fears, and behaviors sap the strength and courage from the miracle of our lives. It is the uncommon person who has the strength and courage to be reflective beyond the ordinary and accepted beliefs and behaviors of the cultural system in which each life begins.

We began as male thought and female emotion and in that state of being we have continued throughout our immature soul journey. At last we are completing our journey home to our mature soul consciousness where we will integrate our physical nature and divine nature as one.

Inspired thought comes from our spirit. Intellectual thought comes from the filter of our ego beliefs, which distorts our spirit inspiration. The wisdom of thought comes from our mature soul that has expanded with knowledge as we have lived our art of creation as our physical experience. As dual thought and emotion we create that which is us, our body, our mind and emotions, our feelings of spirit consciousness, and the reality of our physical lifestyle. It is a miracle when we suddenly realize and accept that we create the cause and effect of our being. We are the miracle of life. Life is our miracle of being. We are our own creation as the miracle of life as a chemical spirit consciousness. We are a living dual soul as a male and female consciousness. We have thought of life as a mystery or as magic, but it is truly our miracle of creation.

When Jesus was born the Magi of old recognized that his birth was creating a new beginning of intense revolutions. These ancient magicians came bearing gifts to the magic of his life and what it was to mean to the dual soul within us. They understood the magic of life better than many and chose to celebrate the coming to earth of an integrated consciousness who would consciously remember the learning within his own soul and spirit. Jesus came to show us the example of what a reflective and advanced human can be on earth and he lived his power of creation.

In our perception of self and earth, we reach distorted perceptions of our reality. The fear and unconsciousness of our inner reflection into the external world of other people, places, and things allows us to be led without needing to think, experience emotions, and feel. We unconsciously reflect our internal fear externally to those around us, while simultaneously blaming and judging the other people in relationship to our own fear, unconscious reflection of thought, and emotional reaction. Our attachment to judgement begins as self-judgement, which we then reflect externally to other people. The crucifixion is the symbol of our self-judgement as we constantly persecute ourselves with the pain and suffering of self-abuse and ignorance.

Our human ranks bulge with the ignorant whose minds harbor only useless external facts surrounded with the emotions of fear. There are those who we ask to think for us as we lamely follow behind, part of the controlled herd, unable to think beyond someone else's thoughts and example. The multitudes do not think, or feel, or allow their emotions to support them because this would require internal reflection and the magic and power of life would be too much for the faint of heart. The habits and beliefs that we have attached ourselves to are seen as fact and we fear any concept of change.

Internal reflection causes a searching thinker to differ from habitual beliefs and behavior as we carve a journey of love for our internal trinity of consciousness that has lost its comfort zone in our external fear and anger. If we want to be whole of dual soul mind, spirit, and body we must learn to listen. Let he who hath an ear, hear.

THE MUSIC OF THE SPHERES

Logic is the absolute of being.

I am that I am.

Today, I am. Now is.

Tomorrow is illusion of the mind

The time and space of another universe

In rhythm with being,

Being is the miracle of life.

The unconscious force

Of forward motion

Consciousness expanded

As we open to the wisdom

Of understanding self.

Being is the Magic of life

The light of truth

The inspiration of thought

The joy of celebration

The passion of understanding

The eternal equality of being.

I am that I am
The harmony of love
Whole in every way.
A trinity of consciousness,
Male, female, and spirit
A symphony of unconditional love.

A miracle of human life
Consciousness on earth,
A magic child
Of the Universal Creator,
In harmony and rhythm
With the eternal
Music of the Spheres.

GLOSSARY

Absolute Truth - Knowledge that is understood by the mature soul and that is consistent with Universal Law.

Abuse - A soul lesson of learning to love ourself in which we accept abuse or inflict abuse upon ourself physically, emotionally, or sexually as part of our life design. When we learn the lesson of loving ourself, we no longer tolerate abuse.

Advanced soul - The immature soul that has reached a higher level of aware knowledge and is in the vibrational path of transition while releasing the cosmic shell of ego beliefs.

Aeons - Enfinite time that cannot be measured by human systems.

Apocalypse - A prophetic disclosure or revelation.

Arbor Vitae - Tree of Knowledge which defines the dual soul journey of our male and female consciousness as it evolves within our Trinity of Consciousness.

Attitude - The mental and emotional response to our perception of ourself and life.

Aura - The auric energy that surrounds the physical body as our first dimension of invisible energy that is detectable as color by our eyes. Auric energy shows the color reflected from our personality and character that forms the initial layer of "invisible" energy around our physical body.

Callosum commissura - The neurological bridge between the left and right hemispheres of the brain, which acts as the seat of our dual soul.

Causative energy - The third dimension of our invisible energy which is our spirit consciousness.

Chemical consciousness - We are made as a consciousness from the chemicals of the universe. Carbon, oxygen, nitrogen, and most of the minerals have created our consciousness and our physical body as a fractal pattern of the universe. Earth and nature are also a fractal pattern of the universe and support our chemical restoration, rejuvenation, and procreation with air, water, and food.

Civilization - When the foundation of a culture is based upon love, truth, equality, compassion, humility, unity, and cooperation, we will be civilized. As yet in history upon Earth, true civilization has not been reached.

Closed mind - A mind firmly encased behind a cosmic shell of ego beliefs that can see nothing beyond its own mirror image of fear.

Collective consciousness - A mental and emotional response that has become commonplace as connected energy streams within groups of people, giving it the strength to change beliefs within our society and our world.

Common sense - The knowing of our mature soul memory.

Competition - A superiority intention of the ego that is based upon fear and judgement and is the beginning of all conflict which expands into crime, abuse, and war.

Conciliate soul - A very advanced transitioning soul that agrees to polarize a macrocosmic soul lesson to create understanding of the lesson within the collective consciousness of the masses. The conciliate soul is seeking to bring unity to the masses. The conciliate soul will not be conscious of the role it is playing.

Consciousness - Is our awareness of and understanding of the interaction that occurs as our thinking, emotions, and sensory responses are stimulated by our physical experiences of life.

Conscious mind - The level of awareness from which we live under the control of the intellect and ego while we are learning as an immature soul.

Cosmic energy - The enfinite energy of thought, emotions, and senses as consciousness that is our gift from the Spirit Creator or "God."

Cosmic shell - The ego shell of beliefs that surrounds our intellect and mirrors our own image back to us as our perception of reality.

Creativity - The resulting action of the inspiration of the spirit and the motivation of the soul being put into physical action by the intellect and physical body.

Criminal mind - The self-centered ego mind that is created by reflecting our primitive beliefs of survival and security into fear, greed, and violent behavior.

Cross-fertilization - A transition of our dual soul mind and emotions from the left brain to the right brain. As learned knowledge passes from the left brain to cross-fertilize the right brain, the light of understanding passes from the right brain to cross-fertilize the left brain, which brings the balance of loving thoughts and emotions to equal proportions within the dual hemispheres of our brain.

Cults - Used as a metaphor in the present society. "Cults" denotes worshipping cultures within a society that ascribe to differing beliefs under the leadership of someone or some group of people that establishes laws, ideology, and practices for the people to live by. The more excessive the control of worship behavior, lifestyle, money, and thinking, the more cultist proportions they are displaying. Religions are cults as defined by their controlling beliefs and behaviors, although they do not recognize their own mirror image. Cults control sexual activities, religious beliefs and worship, and lifestyle behaviors by fear and reward, which are patterned from the judgement and wrath of the leader of the cult.

Culture - A group of people brought together by common beliefs, rituals, and behavior.

Cultural prejudice - The judgement directed against a group based upon differences in beliefs, rituals, behavior, sex, color, or ethnic origin.

Cycle of Awareness - The physical nature purpose of living as the immature soul during the first half of our soul evolution. It is the intention of the soul to become aware of our physical nature and our need for physical experience as growth during this cycle.

Cycle of Development - The spirit thought purpose of developing the human form and structure as physical, using an exact fractal of the cosmic pattern.

Cycle of Expression - Three levels of soul energy that move us from the beginning to the end, such as our thoughts, words, and actions from which we create our birth, life, and death.

Cycle of Integration - The spirit purpose of living as the integrated energy of our physical and divine natures during the last cycle of our spirit expansion.

Cycle of Understanding - The dual soul purpose of merging the male and female consciousness to search for the absolute truth of creation and the purpose of being human during the last half of the soul journey of evolution.

Day - As interpreted biblically, "day" means aeons as spirit time rather than a "day" of physical time.

Demon - A word of Greek origin (daemon) meaning "divine being" that was later interpreted as "evil spirit."

Dimension - We live with three dimensions of constantly interacting electromagnetic energy as a physical cellular body, dual soul mind and emotions, and spirit consciousness. Each dimension of our energies consists of an enfinite number of consciousness levels.

Disease - The degeneration of physical matter and energy due to an obstructed or static energy flow resulting from the excesses and deficiencies of life, which create an imbalance.

divine nature - The female soul and spirit in human form.

Divine Nature - The integrated energy of our physical nature, divine nature, and spirit consciousness that is consciously aware and in full understanding of self, creation, and our purpose of expanding the fractal pattern of our Creator energy.

Doctrine of Two - Our soul is organized as opposites, creating the Doctrine of Two, which allows us to live and learn from two diametrically opposite perceptions of reality. The soul is dual in every aspect.

Dream - Messages that are sent to the intellect from the soul and spirit during sleep periods. Dreams are a method for the soul and spirit to capture the attention of the intellect by transforming the message into physical symbols that can be understood by the intellectual mind. Each symbol is unique to the life activities relating to the individual soul and spirit and the symbols will always be true to Universal Law, not our physical beliefs.

Dual soul mind and emotions - Our dual soul consists of a double helix of mental and emotional energy that exists in dual polarities of external negative descending energy and internal positive ascending energy. As an invisible electromagnetic energy our dual soul mind and emotions are seated within the left and right brain and the invisible chemical consciousness vibration becomes the chemical cellular fractal pattern of the DNA as a double helix.

Earth consciousness - A fractal pattern of the Cosmic energy that was created as a school for the creation and growth of humanity. We are a fractal chemical energy pattern of the Earth, which is the primary support energy for the physical matter of soul and body. The responsibility is clearly understood by the Earth. Because of the Earth consciousness, Earth will continue to replenish its life to sustain our life if we do not interfere.

Ego - The interwoven fiber of our physical, fear beliefs that creates a veil as a cosmic shell to encase and inhabit our intellectual mind. Our ego beliefs are subconscious to our intellect. Once the veil is dissolved the ego changes into humility, and unity replaces separateness for our dual soul.

Elan vital - Lifeforce energy, breath.

Energy - We are electromagnetic energy as electricity and magnetism that exists in three different force fields of physical energy, soul energy, and spirit energy. Energy by its very nature must move and change, and therefore as human energy we must move and change or decay will result. Energy never dies but it can change its form.

Enfinite - The immeasurable energy of eternal life. Time as it relates to our spirit consciousness.

Enlightenment - The coming together of our immature and mature soul minds. Enlightenment describes the releasing of our old primitive beliefs that have held our intellect in bondage and the creation of equal integration of our male and female consciousness.

Ensphere - To be enclosed within an impenetrable sphere of ego beliefs as our cosmic shell.

Enspirit - To be enlightened with the power of creation by the unconditional love of our spirit shining through the perforations of our cosmic shell.

Equality - The balance that we seek in the energy of our male and female self as we begin to understand that all of humanity is equal as consciousness. Our internal equality as a dual soul can only be learned from the physical experience of living equality as males and females in our physical nature on earth.

Equilibrium - Our third dimension of equality that we reach when we are equally balanced in the physical as males and females, are living equality as a male and female soul, and living equilibrium as a spirit in our Trinity of Consciousness.

Essense - Energy of our eternal spirit senses.

Eternal life - An energy of spirit consciousness existing as a seed of the Creator. Our life is eternal as Spirit and as we grow and expand we will become One with the Creator existing into enfinity as Spirit Consciousness.

Ethereal energy - The second dimension of our invisible energy that surrounds our physical body. This ethereal field contains the soul pattern of our past lives that exist as soul prints of consciousness.

Ethereal self - Soul energy consciousness that exists as an ether or chemical gas that we are not conscious of in our physical nature except through the acuity of our soul and spirit senses.

Ethical values - Values that are lived from the love, truth, and equality of our heart as inherent values of our spirit consciousness.

Evil - The worship of ignorance as the illusion of truth.

Evil spirits - A contradiction in terms. Spirits are not evil. Humans are evil only by definition of our ignorance which we live as destructive beliefs, behavior, and inequality. Since we are of spirit origin as humans, the concept applies only to the inhumane behavior of man. (See "demon".)

Evolution - The change and growth of our dual soul as we learn and spiral into the next level of consciousness.

Fact - That which has been learned by the intellect and defined in relationship to theory, observation, or experimentation relative to beliefs.

Fractal Pattern - An exact smaller or larger pattern of something else. A human baby is a fractal pattern of an adult human.

Genetic karma - The soul lessons that we work through in each physical life that have their genesis in our primitive soul growth and are reflected into the cellular consciousness of our DNA.

Genetics - The chemical fractal pattern (DNA) of our eternal soul and spirit.

Good- The truth of us that is found within our mature soul and spirit consciousness which we live as equality and love. The "God" in us.

Heal - To make whole. Healing is the unity of our physical body and our Trinity of Consciousness reaching the perfect state of balance, equality, and equilibrium. Our first level of healing is the integration of our male and female consciousness as a dual soul, which heals our physical body.

Health - From the root word "heal," a condition of physical, mental, and emotional balance which we learn as we evolve our dual soul into a whole soul.

Higher Universal Mana - The spirit consciousness found in the physical matter of a human being.

Homologous thought - The integration of our dual soul with our spirit consciousness to form an equal relationship of cyclic thought.

Human - The highest energy form of physical life upon Earth.

HUMAN - The first anagram denoting the Higher Universal Mana of Spirit Consciousness in human form.

Ignorance - An uninformed state of mind that is produced by ignoring change through physical resistance, rejection, and denial of knowledge.

Immature soul - The embryonic infantile soul mind and emotions that began the descending path of our male physical nature billions of years ago and that we continue to live as we face our transition into our ascending mature soul. The immature soul is focused externally with a negative polarization of thought and fear emotions.

Infinite - Immeasurable in physical time and space. Time as it relates to the dual soul.

Inspiration - The energy of the spirit as it transcends to the intellectual mind. Inspiration can be recognized as an idea or as imagination, and it will always be felt with enthusiasm and excitement as it is unconsciously accepted by the intellect. The ego distortion then determines if the inspiration progresses to creativity as a physical reality.

Instinct - The wisdom and ingenuity of our mature soul that is given to us as a soul sense of knowing which can be directly communicated to the intellect. The intellect has the ability to receive or deny this communication.

Integrated mind - The merging together of our dual soul mind and spirit mind into one mind that functions in an unbroken cycle of energy with total harmony and rhythm. An integrated mind is a supraconscious mind using all levels of consciousness as a unified energy of one mind.

Intellectual creation - The physical energy of the mind that lives and creates in fear, separateness, and greed within the external world, protected by the ego cosmic shell from the influence of the soul instincts and spirit intuition.

Intellectual soul mind - The immature soul mind that has entered the level of knowledge in our soul growth. Our intellectual soul mind continues to have karmic strings attaching it to our primitive soul memory that challenges the ego to release old beliefs.

Intellectual spiritualism - A sense of being spiritual that is conveyed by the ego to the intellect. Once there is an opening within the fiber of the veil that allows images beyond the veil to be discovered by the intellect, the ego convinces the intellect that it has become spirit and there is no further need to search for change and growth.

Intuition - The truth of our spirit consciousness that is consistently given to us as a spirit sense of understanding and inspiration.

Karmic beliefs - Beliefs that have their origin within past lives but have been continued into the present life as a lesson that is not yet learned. Karmic beliefs create the subconscious cosmic shell of our ego and are captured in fear.

Karmic energy - Relationships that exist between people that are continuing a lesson from a past lifetime. Karmic energy is never punishment but it is a lesson that will be approached from different images to allow it to be seen with clarity. Karmic energy includes lessons for everyone that is involved and it is never exclusive to only one person. Disasters of all types are frequently the result of shared karmic energy for everyone involved.

Karmic memory - Misunderstood in present society as memory originating in this lifetime rather than karmic memory from past lifetimes. As the soul is evolving, our conscious intellectual mind is being bombarded with electrical current from the soul and spirit which opens the intellect to karmic lessons of soul memory that are not yet learned. Karmic memory will be a frequent occurrence in the decades to come as we rend the veil of the ego and develop a conscious awareness of soul memory. This phenomenon will expand the judgement in many egos as it searches for someone physical to blame. Until karmic memory can be accepted, the intellect will remain under the fear and judgement influence of the ego.

Law of Continuation - The discipline of our soul that provides us eternal life through procreation, magnetism, and sensory response.

Law of Sevens - Universal levels of physical growth that reflect our pattern of soul growth as seven primary levels relative to seven times seven to infinity.

Life design - Each physical lifetime is designed by our soul and spirit to include our lessons of choice. Our life experiences symbolize images of the lessons that we are learning. Many alternatives are designed into each life regarding specific experiences, but the soul and spirit has the freedom to change the life experience if the lesson is learned or the need for intensity within the lesson changes. We have total freedom of choice with each soul experience. There is never absolute predestination or predetermination in a soul life design. Our life design is an integrated mind choice that is open to change.

Lifestyle - A specific level of beliefs and behaviors that we create and live as a reflection of our unique thoughts, emotions, and feelings.

Love - The predominant energy of our mature soul consciousness that is searched for in the physical discovery of self in relationships. We are unconditional love as spirit consciousness and all searching within the physical world is symbolic of the internal search for the love of our divine soul and eternal spirit.

Macrocosm - The electromagnetic energy field of the world.

Mana - Spirit consciousness.

Mature soul mind - The ascending path of our dual soul mind and emotions that is seated in the right brain. Our mature soul has been formed from billions of life experiences and the information is stored as soul memory within our female consciousness as our divine nature. The mature soul is focused internally with a positive energy polarization and it lives the emotions of love. All mature soul memory is recognized as an instinctual knowledge.

Mesocosm - The electromagnetic energy field of society.

Metaphysics - The study of the visible and invisible energy of our body, dual soul, and spirit.

Microcosm - Our individual electromagnetic energy field.

Mirror image - A reflection of our own energy of fear emotions, beliefs, and behaviors that are mirrored back to us by the ego veil that surrounds our intellectual mind and that we reflect outward from ourself to other people as judgement and blame.

Moral values - Religious laws that are lived from the judgement of right and wrong in the immature soul and have their source in religious beliefs.

Motivation - The energy of our mature soul as it transcends into our physical consciousness, subconsciously accepted by our intellect as an inherent knowing.

Nature consciousness - An awareness of nature that allows us to see, feel, taste, smell and touch Earth as our life-giving connection.

New soul mind - A soul that resists and denies knowledge as it lives ignorance.

Occult - Hidden, concealed.

Open mind - A mind that is open to changing habits, beliefs, and behaviors. This intellect is no longer imprisoned behind a solid shell of ego beliefs as it searches out and welcomes change and creativity.

Paradigm - A pattern of thought, belief, and behavior.

Pattern - Making a consistent impression through identical repetitions of thoughts, beliefs, and behaviors.

Perception - The intellect and ego conscious mind response to reality, which defines our impression of our self-image, sex, life, and our physical world by our pattern of thoughts, beliefs, behaviors, and habits.

Perfection - Living through a balanced, equal, and cooperative behavior of love and truth toward all of humanity, nature, and Earth.

Personal civilization - When an individual lives from love, truth, and equality as the way of physical life, and our positive perception is consistent in all thoughts, words, and behaviors.

Personal responsibility - Using our power of creation as our conscious freedom of choice, will, and intention.

Perview - The internal personal review of our beliefs, emotions, and behaviors as our perception of physical reality.

Physical energy - The male, external focus of beliefs and behaviors that is based upon fear, judgement, competition, separateness, greed, inequality, and supremacy.

Physical nature - Our personality and character traits that reflect the beliefs and behaviors of our male consciousness and that we direct with an external focus into the world around us. Our physical nature is our embryonic soul that is developing awareness as an immature soul through our sexual focus.

Power Naps - When the ego is dissolved into humility, we will use power pauses or naps rather than sleep to go deeper into our soul and spirit consciousness to restore our balance.

Prayers - Repetitious thoughts of our immature intellectual soul mind.

Primitive soul mind - The immature soul mind that we used to begin our evolution that was self-centered and focused only on survival and security through fear, deceit, war, and greed. Today our primitive mind is strongly connected to money as our present belief in our survival and security. The same self-centered thinking and emotions of fear, deceit, and war continue to exist in the pursuit of money and ignorance with no communication, cooperation, and compassion being lived.

Primitive times - Aeons of time that were spent by humanity living and growing in the early levels of the immature soul. The most primitive level is the first level of soul growth when we left our focus as spirit consciousness to enter the physical nature as a "living soul."

Prophecy - Information given to humans as divine predictions in the spiritual attempt to save us from ourselves. As humans we receive visions, insight, knowing, and intuition which comes to us through the acuity of our spiritual senses. There are an infinite number of levels from which prophetic realities come, which depends upon the mind focus of the prophet, but they occur in three primary fields of sensory energy - seeing, hearing, and feeling - although any of our senses can be used.

1. **Psychic prophecy** - Information given from the intellect (immature soul) and its ego cosmic shell. This prophecy is generally identified as a very physical informant such as a warrior or a human of negative character and personality using the physical senses of the prophet. Normally the informant will have physical identities and roles to which

the ego is attached which will be emphasized verbally and acted out physically usually in male form. This is frequently considered as a form of external possession by the physical prophet, but it is the intellect assessing a past life that is captured in the ego and being lived as an identical lesson in the present lifetime.

2. **Soul prophecy** - Information that comes as insight and knowing from the infinite mature memory nodes found in the right brain. This is a more ethereal vision if seen and the information is always positive and focuses on the lessons of the dual soul. At times identities are used to help the informant understand the material. True mature soul information normally comes from the dual source of the male and female consciousness with roles and identities. This is frequently received as a form of external communication from energy that is believed to be angels or Saints in the spiritual world. These are past life memories in the mature soul.

3. **Spirit prophecy** - Information received as inspiration from the spirit consciousness intuitively speaking words from universal memory and mature soul memory. Intuition and inspiration appear as an energetic causative force without material substance. Information is universal to help all of mankind and reveals the reasons why the information is given at a particular time. Spirit prophecy will be positive and interpreted positively because of the level that we have reached as a soul. Spirit prophecy (biblical) of the past has also been positive but has been interpreted from the dark side of our immature soul. Spirit prophecy is heard as the internal voice of "God" through the spirit consciousness within us and has no physical role or identity. Spirit is purely electric and magnetic in nature and can create an animation for life. Electricity and magnetism create light, which allows the information to reveal knowledge of enlightenment.

Prototype - Primitive and constantly changing design.

Relative truth - All fact that is determined as knowledge during our immature soul evolution. Information is relative to belief and will change as life circumstances change to become true knowledge. Relative truth is based on our perception of life relative to our ego beliefs and behaviors.

Religion - An organized culture that worships with devotion and zeal a deity that is considered superior to self.

Revelation - To reveal "occult" or hidden knowledge that releases our immature soul from the bondage of our beliefs.

Ritual - A belief and behavior that is acted out repetitiously in our life, society, or the world, which we endow with sacred meaning.

Sabbath - To set in place to stay with a time of rest.

Self-centeredness - The singular focus upon our external physical needs as the behavior of our physical nature.

Self-love - Loving ourself as a whole person of equal value.

Senses - The partial design of our Spirit Consciousness that is embedded into the physical body and dual soul. Our senses exist on three dimensions and in our physical body the cerebellum, brain stem, spinal cord, and all nervous systems are responsible for life as our spirit senses.

Sensing - Consciously using our physical senses as well as our soul and spirit senses to increase our soul and spirit connection to self and others as a method of expanding our consciousness.

Sexuality - The core energy of our physical nature which pertains to our sexual organs, desires, and reproductive capabilities, which we have used to label and define our identities and roles in life.

Sexual promiscuity - Indiscriminate sexual activity that has no love, commitment, or responsibility of mind intention but is indulged in with the intention of physical pleasure and release. A dramatic soul lesson of self-abuse that becomes the external search for the internal peak experience that symbolizes the loving self.

Simultaneous lives - Multiple lives of our soul that are spent in physical reality at the same time.

Sin - Misunderstanding of choice, intention, and will.

Sleep - Our way of giving equal time to our subconscious soul and unconscious spirit by focusing away from the conscious mind of the intellect and into the soul and spirit consciousness.

Soul devolution - Sliding backwards into primitive physical beliefs and behaviors that imprison the soul in a downward spiral.

Soul evolution - Consistent change and growth of our soul in forward movement.

Soul family - Our spirit consciousness has followed the fractal pattern of our Creator and focused all souls into seven soul families with seven specific purposes that will allow our integration to occur as a collective consciousness of homologous thought when we enter the Cycle of Integration.

Soul revolution - Repetitious physical behavior that captures the soul and holds it in the same pattern of life experience, preventing forward growth and in time creating devolution.

Spirit consciousness - The seed of "God" that was given to us as the purity of thought at our moment of creation and that is eternally connected to our dual soul, with both our mature soul and spirit being symbolized as the female energy of our divine nature.

Spiritualism - Living our unconditional love, truth, and equality in every aspect of our life.

Stagnant energy - Our physical body and immature soul mind and emotions in a state of stasis, obstructing the flow of our energy pattern, allowing inertia and decay to create disease in our mind and body. This can be found in people who refuse to change their habits, beliefs, and behaviors to allow growth.

Static energy - Our physical intellect, ego, and body that is in a state of imbalance, allowing fragmentation and confusion to interrupt and divert the flow of our soul and spirit energy. This energy creates hyperactivity, frenetic activity, anxiety, depression, and disorientation.

Subconscious mind - The mature soul mind that is always available and motivating to our intellect but remains separated and unacknowledged by the ego. The ego is the subconscious mind of our immature soul.

Superconscious mind - The integration of our dual soul as a male and female consciousness.

Supraconscious mind - The wholeness of our Spirit Consciousness as an expanded superconscious mind.

Survival - The constant forward movement and change of our dual soul energy.

Thoughtform - Our original form of human creation as our spirit consciousness that created our male and female consciousness and subsequently designed our physical creation.

Trinity of Consciousness - The dual soul of male and female consciousness in unity with our spirit consciousness.

Twin soul - The original external separation of our physical body into the male and female sexual gender symbolizing the dual nature of our internal soul as male and female consciousness.

Unconscious mind - Our spirit mind that consistently inspires our intellect but is dramatically resisted by our ego, allowing only an unconscious influence to occur within our intellect.

Universe - Another fractal pattern of the Cosmic energy that is populated by other planets and beings.

Universal consciousness - Massive streams of energy that collectively merge to strengthen humanity and create changes within the world of Earth, as well as other planets.

Veil - The interwoven energy of the beliefs of our ego that acts as an unbroken cosmic shell around the intellectual mind.

Victimization - The acceptance of inequality as what we deserve as a way of life.

Void - The emptiness that our dual soul feels as it reaches the transitional level of our dual soul mind and emotions after releasing all of its cosmic shell of beliefs. Void is another word for freedom which we must adjust to.

Walk-in - A choice of the soul to spend one or more lives in a different soul family with a different purpose. To "walk-in" the soul must experience physical death and choose to design the next life and birth as a member of a different soul family.

KATHY ODDENINO
A Philosopher for our Time

Kathy has been intimately involved in understanding the "science of living" ever since she was born in Salem, Illinois in 1930. As the second of five children, she came into life sick to present her parents with an additional challenge during the Depression years. At six months old she had the whooping cough, which went into double pneumonia, and gave her parents the shock of their lives by dying. The family physician declared Kathy dead and the blankets were pulled over her face. While the physician sat at the dining room table signing the death certificate, she began to cry under her shroud.

Kathy's mother told her this story after Kathy was an adult, a mother, and very sick with another disease. Kathy always thought her mother told her about dying because her mother was still trying very hard to understand why her daughter was still living and why she had spent her life with a passion and a mission to overcome any disease that had the audacity to challenge her. To Kathy, this experience is a normal part of her life as an evolving consciousness. Her passion and mission of personal healing are the same passion and mission she feels to teach the simple truth of who we are as spirits learning to be human.

Kathy is a "real-life" philosopher for our time because in sharing her own wisdom, in the Metaphysical tradition of Pythagoras, Socrates, Hippocrates, Hypatia, and other great philosophers of old, she defines our dual soul and spirit consciousness in relationship to the miracle of our body. To Kathy, every question about the nature of our human life is important. If you feel stimulated by the knowledge of what it means to be human and the power of our creation in everyday life, then you are a Seeker of Knowledge in the same tradition which drew great crowds of thinking people in ancient times. We are all equal as teachers and students, yet at this time in our world philosophers in the Metaphysical tradition of practical wisdom are few.

Annapolis has been Kathy's home for nearly twenty years. Kathy's great-grandfather was married in St. Anne's Church in 1728, so choosing to live in Annapolis is for her a "journey home"—just as Metaphysical Philosophy teaches, the generations of life fulfill their cycles. Since 1984 Kathy Oddenino has been teaching classes, seminars, and retreats in Annapolis and around the country with a focus on understanding our human consciousness. She has written six books published by Joy Publications entitled, *The Joy of Health: A Spiritual Concept of Integration and the Practicalities of Living; Bridges of Consciousness; Sharing: Self-Discovery in Relationships; Love, Truth & Perception; Healing Ourself: Growing Beyond the True Cause of Disease;* and *Depression: Our Normal Transitional Emotions. The Journey Home: Our Evolving Consciousness* is her seventh book. Joy Publications has also audiotaped for distribution over 150 of Kathy's self-actualization seminars. Kathy is a noted speaker on a diverse range of humanistic topics and has been a frequent guest on radio and TV talk shows.

Kathy's forty years of experience as a registered nurse include twelve years of medical research in transplant and immunology, sixteen years of health care administration and management, and twelve years of emergency health care. She speaks with an honesty and depth of understanding seldom found in the medical arena. Since we have not been taught about the power of our internal spirit, the belief system of our culture has focused upon an external God and an external physician as being responsible for saving our soul and our body. Kathy's life experiences taught her that our belief systems must change for us to become healthy as individuals and as a society. Her interaction with personnel, families, patients, and with individual clients as a Metaphysical consultant has created an expansive understanding of the personal power of healing within each of us and she is a living example of the truth of her Metaphysical philosophy.

For Seekers of Knowledge

Knowledge is the key to continuing our evolution as human beings. True knowledge stimulates an open mind to expand the consciousness of who we are and our purpose of life. We have been searching for the truth of who we are since the beginning of our creation. The journey of our living soul and spirit embedded in physical matter is within our memory and can be understood by studying our history if we understand how to relate the knowledge to who we are internally. Metaphysical Philosophy teaches us to relate the knowledge of how we live to who we are. As a philosopher for our time, Kathy Oddenino offers the comfort, excitement, and purity of truth for anyone who feels they have a "mission" in life. We are all philosophers at heart and therefore we all have a "mission" to understand the truth we feel within our heart and the purpose of our experiences to us as an evolving soul. By taking us into the invisible energy of Being, God, Truth, Knowledge, Energy, Creation, and Human and Divine Relationships, Kathy Oddenino's evolving body of work expands the core teachings of the ancient philosophers whose passionate purpose was to create a truly civilized society.

Kathy's books are written in a spiral of energy which gently expands the consciousness of any reader who is searching for the truth within himself or herself. As spirits learning to be human, we have the gift of freedom of choice, will, and intention. As Kathy has written, "Evolution is a personal choice." Choosing to read Kathy's books is a gift to yourself you will never forget.

OTHER BOOKS BY KATHY ODDENINO

The Joy of Health: A Spiritual Concept of Integration and the Practicalities of Living
ISBN #0-923081-00-3, QP, $14.95, 300p.

Bridges of Consciousness: Self-Discovery in the New Age
ISBN #0-923081-01-1, QP, $14.95, 298p.

Sharing: Self Discovery in Relationships
ISBN #0-923081-02-x, QP, $14.95, 354p.

Love, Truth & Perception: Spiritual and Philosophic View of Human Destiny
ISBN #0-923081-03-8, SP, $14.95, 288p.

Healing Ourself: Growing Beyond the True Cause of Disease
ISBN #0-923081-04-6, QP, $24.95, 600p.

Depression: Our Normal Transitional Emotions
ISBN #0-923081-05-4, QP, $24.95, 348p.

Kathy gives seminars and retreats, as well as teaching courses in Internal Spiritual Healing Therapies. For information on these events and any of her titles, please call 1-800-542-1400 or visit http://members.aol.com/joypub. Joy Publications books are sold nationally by Borders Books, as well as many local stores, and are carried by several national distributors.